MW00718708

Retina and Vitreous

Section 12

2007–2008

(Last major revision 2004–2005)

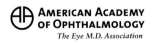

**AMERICAN ACADEMY
OF OPHTHALMOLOGY**
The Eye M.D. Association

LEO

LIFELONG
EDUCATION FOR THE
OPHTHALMOLOGIST®

The Basic and Clinical Science Course is one component of the Lifelong Education for the Ophthalmologist (LEO) framework, which assists members in planning their continuing medical education. LEO includes an array of clinical education products that members may select to form individualized, self-directed learning plans for updating their clinical knowledge. Active members or fellows who use LEO components may accumulate sufficient CME credits to earn the LEO Award. Contact the Academy's Clinical Education Division for further information on LEO.

The American Academy of Ophthalmology is accredited by the Accreditation Council for Continuing Medical Education to provide continuing medical education for physicians.

The American Academy of Ophthalmology designates this educational activity for a maximum of 40 *AMA PRA Category 1 Credits*™. Physicians should only claim credit commensurate with the extent of their participation in the activity.

The Academy provides this material for educational purposes only. It is not intended to represent the only or best method or procedure in every case, nor to replace a physician's own judgment or give specific advice for case management. Including all indications, contraindications, side effects, and alternative agents for each drug or treatment is beyond the scope of this material. All information and recommendations should be verified, prior to use, with current information included in the manufacturers' package inserts or other independent sources, and considered in light of the patient's condition and history. Reference to certain drugs, instruments, and other products in this publication is made for illustrative purposes only and is not intended to constitute an endorsement of such. Some material may include information on applications that are not considered community standard, that reflect indications not included in approved FDA labeling, or that are approved for use only in restricted research settings. The FDA has stated that it is the responsibility of the physician to determine the FDA status of each drug or device he or she wishes to use, and to use them with appropriate patient consent in compliance with applicable law. The Academy specifically disclaims any and all liability for injury or other damages of any kind, from negligence or otherwise, for any and all claims that may arise from the use of any recommendations or other information contained herein.

Basic and Clinical Science Course

Thomas J. Liesegang, MD, Jacksonville, Florida, *Senior Secretary for Clinical Education*

Gregory L. Skuta, MD, Oklahoma City, Oklahoma, *Secretary for Ophthalmic Knowledge*

Louis B. Cantor, MD, Indianapolis, Indiana, *BCSC Course Chair*

Section 12

Faculty Responsible for This Edition

Carl Regillo, MD, *Chair*, Philadelphia, Pennsylvania

Tom S. Chang, MD, Los Angeles, California

Mark W. Johnson, MD, Ann Arbor, Michigan

Peter K. Kaiser, MD, Cleveland, Ohio

Ingrid U. Scott, MD, MPH, Miami, Florida

Richard Spaide, MD, New York, New York

Paul Bennett Griggs, MD, Seattle, Washington
    Practicing Ophthalmologists Advisory Committee for Education

The authors state the following financial relationships:

Dr. Kaiser: research funding from Alcon, Bausch & Lomb, Eyetech, Genentech, Novartis, and QLT

Dr. Regillo: research funding from Alcon, Eyetech, Genentech, and Novartis

The other authors state that they have no significant financial interest or other relationship with the manufacturer of any commercial product discussed in the chapters that they contributed to this publication or with the manufacturer of any competing commercial product.

Recent Past Faculty

Gary W. Abrams, MD

William E. Benson, MD

Neil M. Bressler, MD

Susan B. Bressler, MD

Gary C. Brown, MD

Ronald E. Carr, MD

John C. Cavender, MD

Elaine L. Chuang, MD

Harry W. Flynn, Jr, MD

M. Gilbert Grand, MD

W. Richard Green, MD

Steven J. Guzak, Jr, MD

John R. Heckenlively, MD

Leonard Joffe, MD

Michael F. Marmor, MD

Travis Meredith, MD

Robert P. Murphy, MD

Robert C. Ramsay, MD

W.A.J. van Heuven, MD

In addition, the Academy gratefully acknowledges the contributions of numerous past faculty and advisory committee members who have played an important role in the development of previous editions of the Basic and Clinical Science Course.

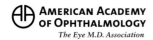

Contents

PART II Disorders of the Retina and Vitreous 49

General Introduction

The Basic and Clinical Science Course (BCSC) is designed to meet the needs of residents and practitioners for a comprehensive yet concise curriculum of the field of ophthalmology. The BCSC has developed from its original brief outline format, which relied heavily on outside readings, to a more convenient and educationally useful self-contained text. The Academy updates and revises the course annually, with the goals of integrating the basic science and clinical practice of ophthalmology and of keeping ophthalmologists current with new developments in the various subspecialties.

The BCSC incorporates the effort and expertise of more than 80 ophthalmologists, organized into 13 section faculties, working with Academy editorial staff. In addition, the course continues to benefit from many lasting contributions made by the faculties of previous editions. Members of the Academy's Practicing Ophthalmologists Advisory Committee for Education serve on each faculty and, as a group, review every volume before and after major revisions.

Organization of the Course

The Basic and Clinical Science Course comprises 13 volumes, incorporating fundamental ophthalmic knowledge, subspecialty areas, and special topics:

1. Update on General Medicine
2. Fundamentals and Principles of Ophthalmology
3. Clinical Optics
4. Ophthalmic Pathology and Intraocular Tumors
5. Neuro-Ophthalmology
6. Pediatric Ophthalmology and Strabismus
7. Orbit, Eyelids, and Lacrimal System
8. External Disease and Cornea
9. Intraocular Inflammation and Uveitis
10. Glaucoma
11. Lens and Cataract
12. Retina and Vitreous
13. Refractive Surgery

In addition, a comprehensive Master Index allows the reader to easily locate subjects throughout the entire series.

References

Readers who wish to explore specific topics in greater detail may consult the journal references cited within each chapter and the Basic Texts listed at the back of the book.

These references are intended to be selective rather than exhaustive, chosen by the BCSC faculty as being important, current, and readily available to residents and practitioners.

Related Academy educational materials are also listed in the appropriate sections. They include books, audiovisual materials, self-assessment programs, clinical modules, and interactive programs.

Study Questions and CME Credit

Each volume of the BCSC is designed as an independent study activity for ophthalmology residents and practitioners. The learning objectives for this volume are given on page 1. The text, illustrations, and references provide the information necessary to achieve the objectives; the study questions allow readers to test their understanding of the material and their mastery of the objectives. Physicians who wish to claim CME credit for this educational activity may do so by mail, by fax, or online. The necessary forms and instructions are given at the end of the book.

Conclusion

The Basic and Clinical Science Course has expanded greatly over the years, with the addition of much new text and numerous illustrations. Recent editions have sought to place a greater emphasis on clinical applicability, while maintaining a solid foundation in basic science. As with any educational program, it reflects the experience of its authors. As its faculties change and as medicine progresses, new viewpoints are always emerging on controversial subjects and techniques. Not all alternate approaches can be included in this series; as with any educational endeavor, the learner should seek additional sources, including such carefully balanced opinions as the Academy's Preferred Practice Patterns.

The BCSC faculty and staff are continuously striving to improve the educational usefulness of the course; you, the reader, can contribute to this ongoing process. If you have any suggestions or questions about the series, please do not hesitate to contact the faculty or the editors.

The authors, editors, and reviewers hope that your study of the BCSC will be of lasting value and that each section will serve as a practical resource for quality patient care.

Objectives

Upon completion of BCSC Section 12, *Retina and Vitreous*, the reader should be able to:

- Describe the basic structure and function of the retina and its relationship to the vitreous and choroid

- Recognize specific pathologic processes that affect the retina or vitreous

- Choose appropriate methods of examination and ancillary studies for the diagnosis of vitreoretinal disorders

- Incorporate data from major prospective clinical trials in the management of selected vitreoretinal disorders

- Explain the principles of medical and surgical treatment of vitreoretinal disorders

Introduction

The retina is a delicate membranous structure that lines the posterior aspect of the eye, adhering firmly at the optic nerve head posteriorly and at the ora serrata anteriorly. Divided into central and peripheral zones, this photosensitive layer makes possible the various kinds of visual function:

- detail discrimination
- color perception
- vision in dim illumination
- peripheral vision

In general, retinal disorders do not cause ocular pain. Chapter 1 of this volume covers retinal anatomy in greater detail.

The normally transparent ocular media allow clinical examination of the retina. Routine diagnostic techniques include direct and indirect ophthalmoscopy as well as slit-lamp biomicroscopy. Ancillary tests, such as fluorescein angiography, indocyanine green angiography, echography, optical coherence tomography (OCT), scanning laser ophthalmoscopy (SLO), diagnostic x-ray, and electrophysiology, may provide additional diagnostic information in eyes with transparent media or in selected eyes with media opacities. Documenting clinical findings, either descriptively or by illustration, is an essential element of a complete posterior segment examination. Understanding of the vitreous/retina/choroid relationships is emphasized in Section 12.

Examination of the posterior segment is facilitated by maximal pupillary dilation, which usually allows evaluation of the retina from the posterior pole to its anterior margin at the ora serrata. Scleral indentation, combined with indirect ophthalmoscopy, is a valuable technique for observing the peripheral retina and examining it in profile. Slit-lamp biomicroscopy in conjunction with precorneal contact lenses or non–contact lenses are useful in examining both the posterior pole of the retina and the retinal periphery. Biomicroscopy is also critical in the diagnosis of macular thickening, as well as in the diagnosis of various vitreoretinal and choroidal diseases. Fluorescein angiography is a commonly employed ancillary test, and indocyanine green angiography is another technique that adds to our understanding of the pathophysiology of chorioretinal vascular diseases, especially age-related macular degeneration. Many of these techniques are discussed in Chapter 2.

Electrophysiologic tests and their significance in diagnosis are reviewed in Chapter 3. OCT shows anatomic relationships of the retina, vitreous, and choroid, which may provide further understanding of pathologic changes in various posterior segment diseases.

Ultrasonography, or echography, employing both A- and B-scan techniques, is useful in patients with clear or opaque media. Echography is particularly important in determining axial length, but it may also help to diagnose choroidal lesions. Furthermore, it is a quantitative measurement that can be used for follow-up evaluation over time. However, as with ophthalmoscopic evaluation of the posterior segment, the physician must use consistent, methodical techniques of examination and documentation to allow meaningful comparisons.

X-ray techniques are useful to determine the presence of intraocular calcification or bone formation. Plain-film x-ray and computed tomography (CT) are useful in determining the presence, number, and location of radiopaque intraocular foreign bodies. Magnetic resonance imaging (MRI) can be helpful in cases of orbital disease processes that affect the posterior segment, such as thyroid eye disease, or in inflammatory diseases of the posterior segment itself, such as posterior scleritis. However, MRI is *contraindicated* if there is a possibility that the patient has an intraocular, orbital, or intracranial metallic foreign body.

Depending on their location, developmental or acquired alterations in the posterior segment may or may not be symptomatic. Some diseases, such as diabetic retinopathy, may be asymptomatic until advanced stages are reached. When present, symptoms caused by posterior segment abnormalities may include the following:

- transient or persistent reduction in visual acuity
- alterations in color perception
- metamorphopsia
- floaters
- photopsia
- scotomata
- loss of visual field

Part II, Disorders of the Retina and Vitreous, discusses diseases of and trauma to the posterior segment in Chapters 4 through 14. Diagnostic techniques are included throughout these discussions. Management and therapy of the retinal disorders covered in Part II are informed by the many clinical trials being conducted or interpreted in these areas. Several of these trials and studies have been set off from the text for easy reference.

Part III, Selected Therapeutic Topics, offers more detailed information on three important posterior segment treatment options: photocoagulation, photodynamic therapy, and treoretinal surgery. Treatment strategies, complications, and outcomes are covered in detail. Clinical illustrations help provide better understanding of these vital tools of the retinal surgeon.

Throughout this volume primary reference sources are supplemented by appropriate and up-to-date text references. See also the Basic Texts and Related Academy Materials that appear at the end of the book.

PART I

Fundamentals and Diagnostic Approaches

CHAPTER 1

Basic Anatomy

The Vitreous

Occupying 80% of the volume of the eye, the vitreous is a clear matrix composed of collagen, hyaluronic acid, and water. It is bounded anteriorly by the posterior lens capsule and posteriorly by the internal limiting membrane of the retina. The vitreous body is composed of two main portions: the central, or core, vitreous and the cortical vitreous. The central vitreous has collagen fibers that insert in the vitreous base, a region where the vitreous fibers adhere firmly to the retina and pars plana. These fibers arch posteriorly. In between the collagen fibers are hyaluronate molecules, which bind water molecules. These hyaluronate molecules, with their associated water molecules, act as fillers and separators between the adjacent collagen fibers. The collagen fibers in the second part of the vitreous body, the cortical vitreous, are much more densely packed and course in a direction roughly parallel to the inner surface of the retina. The vitreous is most firmly attached to the vitreous base, but it is also firmly attached to retinal vessels, the optic nerve, and the macula. The attachment of the vitreous to the macula is arranged in 3 circumferential zones centered on the foveola. Focal traction on the retina may produce retinal tears or holes. The vitreous may also place traction over a somewhat larger area. Because of the larger area, the resultant tensile force on the retina may be below that required to cause tears. This force may distort the retina or cause tractional elevation of the retina. One example of this process is the vitreomacular traction syndrome, a condition where the patient develops blurring and distortion of the central vision because of tractional elevation of the macula by the vitreous.

Neurosensory Retina

The area defined by anatomists as the *macula lutea,* or yellow spot (Fig 1-1), is that portion of the posterior retina containing xanthophyll (yellow) pigment. The conventional boundary of the macula, as defined histologically, is that area with 2 or more layers of ganglion cells that is 5–6 mm in diameter and is centered vertically between the temporal vascular arcades. Oxygenated carotenoids, in particular lutein and zeaxanthine, accumulate within the central macula and cause the yellow color. These carotenoids have antioxidant capabilities and also function to filter bluer wavelengths of light, possibly preventing photic damage. The yellow pigmentation in the macula contributes to

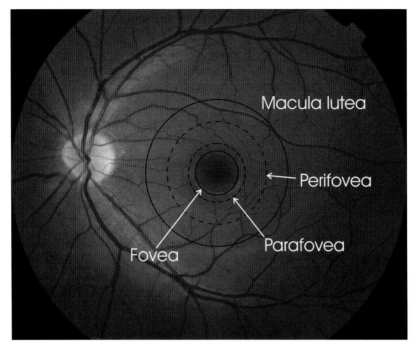

Figure 1-1 Anatomic macula, also called *area centralis* or *posterior pole*. The anatomic fovea and foveola are contained within the center of the anatomic macula. *(Photograph courtesy of Richard F. Spaide, MD.)*

hypofluorescence in fluorescein angiography, and it may become more apparent in certain pathologic conditions such as cystoid macular edema or early stages of macular holes.

The central 1.5 mm within the macula is occupied by the *fovea* (or *fovea centralis*), which, by its anatomy and photoreceptor composition, is specialized for high spatial acuity and for color vision. Within the fovea is a region devoid of retinal vessels known as the *foveal avascular zone (FAZ)*. The geometric center of the FAZ is often taken to be the center of the macula and thus the point of fixation; it is an important landmark in fluorescein angiography. Within the fovea is a central pit known as the *foveola*, a 0.35-mm-diameter region where the cones are slender and densely packed. Within the foveola is a small depression known as the *umbo*. Surrounding the fovea is a ring 0.5 mm in diameter, called the *parafoveal area*, where the ganglion cell layer, inner nuclear layer, and outer plexiform layer are thickest. Surrounding this zone, a ring approximately 1.5 mm wide is termed the *perifoveal zone* (Table 1-1).

The retina outside of the macula is commonly divided into a few general regions. The retina around the equator logically enough is called the *equatorial retina*, and the region anterior to this is called the *anterior*, or *peripheral*, *retina*. In the far periphery, the border between the retina and the pars plana is called the *ora serrata*. Periodic jetties of retinal tissue into the pars plana, called *dentate processes*, are more prominent in the nasal peripheral fundus. *Ora bays* are the extensions of the pars plana onto the retinal side. On occasion, dentate processes may wrap around a portion of ora bay to form an

Table 1-1 Anatomic Terminology of the Macula

Term	Synonym	Histologic Definition	Clinical Observation (Size)
Macula	Posterior pole Macula lutea Central retina Area centralis	Peripheral limit at the site where the ganglion cells are reduced to a single layer; contains two or more ganglion cell layers	Ill-defined area 5.5 mm in diameter (3.5 DD* or 18° of visual angle) centered 4.0 mm temporal and 0.8 mm inferior to the center of the optic disc
Fovea	Fovea centralis	A depression in the inner retinal surface, the photoreceptor layer of which is entirely cones	A concave central retinal depression seen on slit-lamp examination 1.5 mm in diameter (1.0 DD or 5°)
Foveola		The central floor of the fovea where the inner nuclear layer and ganglion cell layer are absent	Ill-defined area 0.35 mm in diameter (0.3–0.4 DD); approximately equal to the capillary-free (foveal avascular) zone of the retina
Umbo	Clivus Light reflex	Small central concavity of the floor of the foveola	Observed point corresponding to the normal light reflex but not solely responsible for this light reflex
Parafoveal zone		Outermost limit where the ganglion cell layer, inner nuclear layer, and Henle's layer are thickest (i.e., the retina is thickest)	0.5-mm-diameter ring surrounding the fovea
Perifoveal zone		From the outermost limit of the parafovea to the outer limit of the macula	1.5-mm-diameter ring surrounding the parafoveal zone

* DD = Disc diameter

enclosed ora bay. This may create the false impression of a peripheral retinal hole. A *meridional fold* is a radially oriented, prominent thickening of retinal tissue extending into the pars plana. These meridional folds look like exaggerated dentate processes. When oriented with a ciliary process, they are known as a *meridional complex*.

The layers of the retina can be seen easily in cross-sectional histologic preparations. In Figure 1-2, the layers are listed in order from the outer to inner retina:

- rod and cone inner and outer segments
- external limiting membrane (ELM)
- outer nuclear layer (the nuclei of the photoreceptors)
- outer plexiform layer
- inner nuclear layer
- inner plexiform layer
- ganglion cell layer
- nerve fiber layer (the axons of the ganglion cell layer)
- internal limiting membrane (ILM)

Light striking the retina must travel through the full thickness of the retina to reach the photoreceptors. The density and distribution of photoreceptors vary with topographic

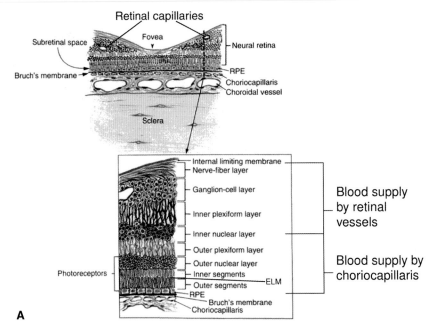

Figure 1-2 A, Schematic cross section of retina demonstrating layers of retina and approximate location of blood supply to these layers. *(Modified with permission from D'Amico DJ. Diseases of the retina. N Engl J Med. 1994;331:95–106.)* *(Continues on next page.)*

location within the retina. In the fovea is a densely packed arrangement of cones, predominantly red- and green-sensitive, with a density exceeding 140,000 cones per square millimeter. The central fovea has no rods; it contains only cones and supporting Müller cells, which optimize the transmission of light by limiting the number of intervening layers. The number of cones decreases rapidly away from the center; the periphery contains almost no cones. The rods have their greatest density about 20° from fixation, where they reach a peak density of about 160,000 rods per square millimeter. Although the rod density is high, the visual acuity of this region is decreased because of summation of multiple rod responses in each receptive field. The density of rods also decreases toward the periphery. The light-sensitive molecules in rods and cones are derived from vitamin A bound to an apoprotein known as an opsin. In rods, the resultant molecule is known as rhodopsin. Cones have 3 different opsins that selectively confer sensitivity to red, green, and blue light.

Whereas in most nerve cells, a transient depolarization generates an action potential "spike," in photoreceptors, the response is graded, with changes in membrane polarization being proportional to the amount of stimulating light. The response is modified, to a certain extent, by horizontal cells synapsed to adjacent photoreceptors.

The photoreceptors also synapse with bipolar cells. Cone photoreceptors have a 1-to-1 synapse with a type of bipolar cell known as a midget bipolar. Other types of bipolar cells also synapse with each cone. On the other hand, more than 1 rod—and sometimes more than 100 rods—converges on each bipolar cell. Like photoreceptors, bipolar cells have a graded response with a change in polarization. Bipolar cells synapse with ganglion

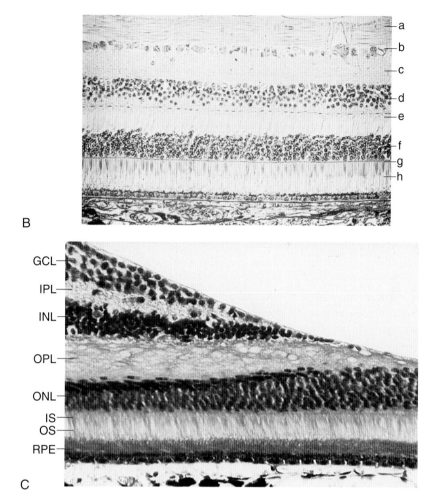

Figure 1-2 *(Continued)* **B,** Normal retinal layers. From vitreous to choroid: *a,* nerve fiber layer; *b,* ganglion cell layer; *c,* inner plexiform layer; *d,* inner nuclear layer; *e,* outer plexiform layer; *f,* outer nuclear layer; *g,* external limiting membrane; *h,* photoreceptors of rods and cones. The internal limiting membrane is not shown. **C,** In the region of the foveola, the inner cellular layers are absent, with an increased density of pigment in the RPE. The incident light falls directly on the photoreceptor outer segments, reducing the potential for distortion of light by overlying tissue elements. GCL = ganglion cell layer; IPL = inner plexiform layer; INL = inner nuclear layer; OPL = outer plexiform layer; ONL = outer nuclear layer; IS = inner segment of photoreceptors; OS = outer segment of photoreceptors. *(Photographs courtesy of David J. Wilson, MD.)*

cells. The ganglion cells summate responses from bipolar and amacrine cells and develop action potentials that are conducted to the dorsolateral geniculate nucleus in the brain. Amacrine cells help in primitive signal processing by responding to specific alterations in retinal stimuli such as sudden changes in light intensity or when certain sizes of stimuli are present. The nerve fiber layer, an extension of the ganglion cell layer, courses along the inner portion of the retina to aggregate in the posterior portion of the globe to form the optic nerve. The ILM, which is formed by the footplates of Müller cells, is contiguous with the most posterior aspect of the vitreous. Two additional "membranes" have been identified by histologists, but in actuality these are not true membranes. At the outer extent of the Müller cells, alterations in the plasma membrane coincide with similar alterations in the photoreceptor cell bodies. Zonular attachment between photoreceptors and Müller cells at this level creates the ELM, a structure visible by light microscopy. Thus, the Müller cells course through almost the entire thickness of the retina. The inner third of the outer plexiform layer has a linear density where a synaptic connection between the photoreceptors and the processes of the bipolar cells occurs. This linear density has been called the middle limiting membrane, but it is actually not a membrane.

The central retinal artery (derived from the ophthalmic artery) and its branches are located in the inner retina and supply circulation to all of the inner retinal layers, extending as posteriorly as the inner portion of the inner nuclear layer. The retinal vasculature, including its capillaries, retains the blood–brain barrier with tight junctions between capillary endothelial cells. Occasionally, a cilioretinal artery, branching from the ciliary circulation, will supply circulation to a portion of the inner retina between the optic nerve and the center of the macula. The metabolic needs of the outer retina, extending from the outer portion of the inner nuclear layer through the RPE, are met by the choriocapillaris, a capillary system of the choroidal arteries that branch from the ciliary arteries. See also Part I, Anatomy, of BCSC Section 2, *Fundamentals and Principles of Ophthalmology.*

Retinal Pigment Epithelium

The retinal pigment epithelium (RPE) is a single layer of hexagonally shaped cuboidal cells of neuroectodermal origin lying between Bruch's membrane and the retina (Fig 1-3). This layer extends from the margin of the optic disc to the ora serrata and is continuous with the pigment epithelium of the ciliary body. The apical portion of the RPE lies adjacent and is intimately related to the photoreceptor cell layer. Each RPE cell has an apical portion with villous processes that envelop the outer segments of the photoreceptor cells (see the top part of Figure 4-1). RPE cells are low, cuboidal cells approximately 16 μm in diameter. In the macula, however, the cells are taller and denser than they are in the peripheral regions. The lateral surfaces of adjacent cells are closely apposed and joined by tight junctional complexes (zonulae occludentes) near the apices. These junctional complexes form the outer retinal blood–ocular barrier. The basal surface of the cells shows a rich infolding of the plasma membrane. The RPE contributes to retinal function in several ways; it

- absorbs light
- maintains the subretinal space
- phagocytizes rod and cone outer segments
- participates in retinal and polyunsaturated fatty acid metabolism
- forms the outer blood–ocular barrier
- heals and forms scar tissue

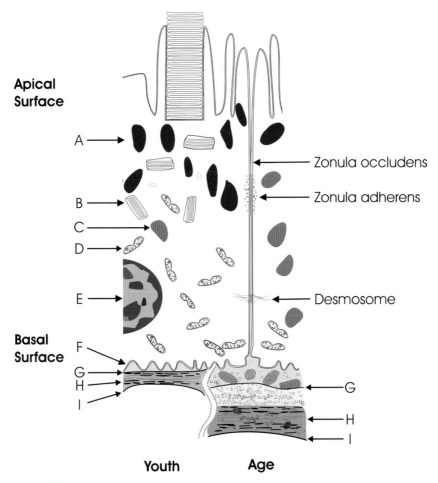

Apical Surface

A ⟶

B ⟶

C ⟶

D ⟶

E ⟶

Basal Surface

F

G
H
I

⟵ Zonula occludens

⟵ Zonula adherens

⟵ Desmosome

⟵ G

⟵ H

⟵ I

Youth   **Age**

Figure 1-3 RPE and Bruch's membrane. *A,* melanosomes; *B,* phagolysosome; *C,* lipofuscin; *D,* mitochondria; *E,* nucleus; *F,* plasma membrane; *G,* basement membrane; *H,* trilaminar core of Bruch's membrane; *I,* basement membrane of choriocapillaris. What is referred to as Bruch's membrane is a 5-layered structure composed of *G, H,* and *I.* Bruch's membrane and associated structures undergo a number of changes with aging *(right)*. Between the plasma membrane and the basement membrane, material called *basal laminar deposit,* which includes wide-spaced collagen, accumulates. External to the basement membrane, a material called *basal linear deposit* accumulates. This material has a high lipid content with membranous debris. Mounds of this material are visible as soft drusen. With age there is also an increased amount of lipofuscin in the RPE cell, as well as thickening of Bruch's membrane. Lateral attachment among adjacent RPE cells is accomplished through desmosomes, zonulae occludentes, and zonulae adherentes. *(Drawing by Richard Spaide, MD.)*

The typical RPE cell has a number of melanosomes, each designed to be a biologic light absorber. A melanosome has a spheroid shape, with melanin distributed on protein fibers. Although melanin has a neutral gray color, light entering a melanosome reflects off innumerable melanin molecules within the structure of the melanosome. Because of Rayleigh absorption, which affects shorter wavelengths more than longer wavelengths, blue light is absorbed much more than red light.

RPE cells serve a phagocytic function, continually ingesting the membranes, or disks, shed by the outer segments of the photoreceptor cells. This process of shedding, phagocytosis, and photoreceptor renewal follows a daily rhythm. Rods shed disks at dawn and cones shed them at dusk. The ingested outer segments are digested gradually through the action of enzymes produced from cytoplasmic organelles. The retinal and polyunsaturated fatty acids found in the outer segment disks are recycled. Oxidatively damaged molecules, particularly those derived from retinoids and lipids, can build up in RPE cells and are converted into lipofuscin.

Visual pigments contain 11-cis-retinaldehyde that is converted to the 11-trans-retinaldehyde. Most of the steps of regeneration of the 11-cis configuration occur in the RPE. A variety of pathologic changes may develop if this process of phagocytosis and renewal is impaired by genetic defects, drugs, dietary insufficiency (vitamin A), or senescence. The barrier function of the RPE prevents diffusion of metabolites between the choroid and the subretinal space. Because of this barrier, the environment of the photoreceptors is largely regulated by the selective transport properties of the RPE. Because the RPE has a high capacity for water transport, fluid does not accumulate in the subretinal space under normal circumstances. This RPE-mediated dehydration of the subretinal space also modulates the bonding properties of the interphotoreceptor matrix, which bridges between the RPE and photoreceptors and helps to bond the neurosensory retina with the RPE. In response to trauma, inflammation, or other stimuli, the RPE may proliferate, migrate, atrophy, or undergo metaplasia. These changes are often responsible for the many of the ophthalmoscopic features of chorioretinal lesions.

Hypertrophy is caused by the enlargement of cells. Hypertrophy of the RPE cells may result from a variety of causes, including trauma. Congenital hypertrophy of the RPE (CHRPE) produces slate gray to black flat lesions, usually in the periphery. They often have depigmented lacunae, particularly in older individuals, and are often surrounded by a depigmented halo. These lesions may be confused with a melanoma, which is generally thick and elevated. A modified form of CHRPE that causes fish-shaped figures of altered pigmentation is found in Gardner syndrome, a dominantly inherited disorder marked by intestinal polyposis.

Hyperplasia is caused by an increased number of cells. RPE cells may proliferate in response to a number of stimuli. They frequently migrate, particularly into the retina, and often show a penchant for enveloping retinal vessels. When this occurs, it produces the bone spicule appearance seen in retinitis pigmentosa, syphilitic infections, and a number of other inflammatory conditions. Hyperplasia of the RPE may contribute to membrane formation in either preretinal locations (eg, as in macular pucker or proliferative vitreoretinopathy following rhegmatogenous retinal detachment) or subretinal sites. Atrophy of the RPE is marked by the thinning and senescence of RPE cells. Death may result from necrosis or apoptosis. With loss of the RPE, there is often corresponding atrophy of the overlying photoreceptors and underlying choriocapillaris.

Bruch's Membrane

The basal portion of the RPE is attached to Bruch's membrane, which has 5 layers. Starting with the innermost, these are

- basement membrane of the RPE
- inner loose collagenous zone
- middle layer of elastic fibers
- outer loose collagenous zone
- basement membrane of the endothelium of the choriocapillaris

Throughout life, lipids and oxidatively damaged materials build up within Bruch's membrane. Some disease states, such as pseudoxanthoma elasticum, are associated with increased fragility of Bruch's membrane, presumably due to abnormalities within its collagen or elastic portions. Patients with pseudoxanthoma elasticum may develop breaks or cracks within Bruch's membrane that radiate from the optic nerve and form angioid streaks, named after their vessellike appearance.

Choroid

Blood enters the choroid through the short posterior ciliary arteries. The outer layer of choroidal vessels, known as Haller's layer, is relatively large. The choroidal vessels in this layer merge with a layer of smaller diameter vessels known as Sattler's layer. These vessels distribute the blood arriving from the short posterior ciliary arteries over the extent of the choroid. In the process, they help reduce arterial pressure to the relatively low pressure found in the choriocapillaris. The choroid has a maximal thickness posteriorly, where it is 0.22 mm thick. It becomes progressively thinner anteriorly; at the ora serrata, it is 0.1 mm thick. In the posterior pole, the choriocapillaris is a plexus of capillaries that functionally act as lobules, although the capillaries themselves are not arranged strictly into lobules. The capillary arrangement becomes looser as one moves toward the periphery, where the capillaries are arranged in a radial orientation.

After reaching the choriocapillaris, the blood is collected into venules, which coalesce into ampullae, which are collecting channels leading to the vortex veins. Most eyes have 4 or 5 vortex veins, which leave the eye at the equator. The vortex veins drain into the superior ophthalmic vein. The retina has one of the highest metabolic rates per gram of tissue in the body; it is served by the choroid, which has the highest blood flow of any tissue. Although the flow rate is high within the choriocapillaris, the blood does not flow uniformly throughout the cardiac cycle. High-speed indocyanine green angiography of the choriocapillaris suggests that there is a pulsatile flow that occurs chiefly during systole. The venous blood exiting the choroid still has a very high oxygen tension. Interspersed between the vessels of the choroid are loose connective tissue, fibroblasts, and melanocytes. The melanocytes help absorb excessive light transmitted through the retina and RPE. The rapid flow of the choroid acts as a heat sink to remove thermal energy from the light absorption. The melanocytes may undergo malignant transformation, possibly induced by light damage, to create a melanoma, the most common intraocular tumor in adults.

Green WR. Retina. In: Spencer WH, ed. *Ophthalmic Pathology: An Atlas and Textbook.* 4th ed. Philadelphia: Saunders; 1996:vol 2, chap 8.

Marmor MF, Wolfensberger TJ, eds. *The Retinal Pigment Epithelium: Function and Disease.* New York: Oxford University Press; 1998.

Spaide RF, Miller-Rivero NE. Anatomy. In Spaide RF, ed. *Diseases of the Retina and Vitreous.* Philadelphia: Saunders; 1999.

CHAPTER 2

Diagnostic Approach to Retinal Disease

Techniques of Examination

Diagnosing retinal disease requires a combination of careful clinical examination and diagnostic imaging techniques. An essential component in the evaluation of the retina is a well-dilated pupil. Pupil dilation is accomplished through a variety of pharmacologic agents, including 1% tropicamide, 2.5% phenylephrine, or 1% cyclopentalate. The simplest examination technique for viewing the retina is using the direct ophthalmoscope, which provides an upright monocular image of the retina. However, the instrument's lack of stereopsis, its small field of view, and its poor view of the retinal periphery have limited its use. These shortcomings are overcome by using the binocular indirect ophthalmoscope (BIO) in combination with a hand-held magnifying lens. The inverted, binocular image of the retina allows examination of most of the retina; however, to see the entire retina, the BIO examination needs to be combined with scleral depression. In general, 20, 28, and 30 diopter (D) lenses are used to view the retina. Because the field of view is inversely proportional to the power of the lens, the 30 D lens has the widest field of view and lowest magnification.

Magnification of even the lowest power BIO lens is insufficient to evaluate subtle retinal changes or abnormalities of the vitreous body. To evaluate these structures, slit-lamp biomicroscopy is required. A variety of lenses is available for viewing the retina with the slit lamp. Contact lenses offer the advantage of better stereopsis and higher resolution. They require topical corneal anesthesia and are placed directly on the cornea to eliminate its power and the cornea–air interface. Fluids used range from contact lens wetting solutions to viscous clear gel solutions. The more viscous the solution, however, the more it interferes with the quality of any photography or angiography performed shortly after the examination. In contrast, non–contact lenses use the power of the lens in combination with the cornea to produce an inverted image with a wider field of view. The biconvex indirect lenses used with the slit lamp do not touch the cornea, and thus topical anesthesia is not necessary. In general, high-plus optical power lenses such as the 60, 78, and 90 D lenses are used; however, more specialized lenses have been developed. Non–contact lenses are easier to use and offer more rapid evaluation of the retina. Finally, a Hruby lens, an external planoconcave lens with high negative optical power attached to the slit-lamp frame, is another option if a contact or non–contact lens is not available.

Like the biconvex indirect lenses, it does not require topical anesthesia or placement of other drops on the cornea. However, the Hruby lens does not give an inverted image and may be less versatile than the biconvex indirect lenses for viewing outside the fovea.

Detection of retinal thickening in macular edema, cystic spaces in cystoid macular edema, or subretinal fluid in choroidal neovascularization (CNV) is enhanced by using a thin slit beam, ideally at a 45° angle, and a biomicroscopic lens with high magnification. The inner aspect of the beam is directed at the surface of the retina and retinal vessels, the outer aspect at the retinal pigment epithelium (RPE). The distance between the inner and outer aspect is recognized as the thickness of the retina. Once the normal thickness of the retina is known for a given location within the macula, abnormal thicknesses may be evaluated in other areas. The same technique is useful to determine the level of hemorrhage—preretinal, intraretinal, or subretinal. Careful examination of the beam as it hits the retina can differentiate between elevation or depression of a retinal lesion. Transillumination is another technique that may help highlight cystic changes of the neurosensory retina or help detect pigment epithelial detachments where the edge of the beam appears to glow. Red-free (green) light may be used to assist detection of small vessels (such as intraretinal microvascular abnormalities or retinal neovascularization) or dots of hemorrhage that may be difficult to see against an orange background when viewed with the normal slit beam. A lighter color to the retina on red-free light may correspond to the presence of fluid, fibrin, or fibrous tissue associated with CNV.

Friberg TR. Examination of the retina: ophthalmoscopy and fundus biomicroscopy. In: Albert DM, Jakobiec FA, eds. *Principles and Practice of Ophthalmology*. 2nd ed. Philadelphia: Saunders; 2000: 1820–1830.

Retinal Angiography Techniques

Fluorescein Angiography

Fluorescein angiography permits study of the circulation of the retina and choroid in normal and diseased states. Photographs of the retina are taken after intravenous injection of sodium fluorescein. Sodium fluorescein is an orange-red crystalline hydrocarbon with a molecular weight of 376 daltons that diffuses through most of the body fluids. It is eliminated through the liver and kidneys within 24 hours. Eighty percent of the fluorescein is protein-bound and not available for fluorescence; the remaining 20% circulates in the vasculature and tissues of the retina and choroid. Fluorescein is injected in a peripheral vein and enters the ocular circulation 8–12 seconds later. The peak fluorescence usually occurs approximately 1 minute after injection.

To image the fluorescein in the eye, special excitation and barrier filters are required. Sodium fluorescein is a hydrocarbon that fluoresces at a wavelength of 520–530 nm after excitation by a light of 465–490 nm. To obtain a fluorescein angiogram, white light from the camera flash unit passes through a blue (excitatory) filter, and blue light enters the eye. The blue light, with its wavelength of 490–645 nm, excites the unbound fluorescein molecules circulating in the retinal and choroidal layers or that have leaked out of the vasculature, and stimulates them to emit a longer wavelength yellow-green light (520–

530 nm). Both the emitted yellow-green fluorescence and some degree of reflected blue light from structures that do not contain fluorescein exit the eye and return to the camera. A yellow-green (barrier) filter on the camera lens blocks the reflected blue light, permitting only the yellow-green light, which has originated from the fluorescein molecules, into the camera.

The image formed by the emitted fluorescence, originating from the retina and choroid, is recorded on black-and-white, high-contrast 35-mm film, on videotape, or on a digital system. The 35-mm film permits higher-resolution images of the retinal vessels and choroid and is generally easier to use for capturing stereoscopic frames and stereoscopic viewing than videotape. Newer digital systems offer high-resolution images rivaling those of 35-mm film and can adjust contrast and brightness to highlight certain details; they can also zoom in on areas of concern, which is not possible with film-based images.

Fluorescein particles that are not bound to protein can pass through the spaces between the endothelial cells of the capillaries of the choriocapillaris, but normally they cannot leak through the RPE or zonulae occludentes between adjacent RPE cells to gain access into the subretinal space. Therefore, fluorescein from the choroid cannot enter the neurosensory retina unless the RPE has a defect. Normally, the retinal vessels respect the blood–brain barrier and hyperfluoresce during the transit phases of the angiogram but do not leak fluorescein. Although the fluorescence in the choroid is partially blocked by the pigment in the RPE, it is visible as deep, diffuse background fluorescence.

Fluorescein can leak out of retinal capillaries into the retina only when the capillary endothelium is damaged, as in diabetic retinopathy. Similarly, fluorescein can leak from the choriocapillaris through pigment epithelial cells into the subretinal space and the retinal interstitium only when the latter are abnormal, as in central serous chorioretinopathy. Thus, patterns of hyperfluorescence and stereoscopic images yield valuable information about leakage from retinal vessels or through abnormal pigment epithelium. Abnormalities seen with fluorescein angiography can be grouped into 2 categories, associated with one of the following:

- hypofluorescence
- hyperfluorescence

*Hypo*fluorescence occurs when there is reduction or absence of normal fluorescence; it is present in 2 major patterns:

- vascular filling defect
- blocked fluorescence

Vascular filling defects occur where the retinal or choroidal vessels do not fill properly, as in nonperfusion of an artery, vein, or capillary in the retina or choroid. These defects produce either a delay or a complete absence in filling the involved vessels. *Blocked fluorescence* occurs when the stimulation or visualization of the fluorescein is blocked by fibrous tissue or other barrier such as pigment or blood, producing an absence of normal retinal or choroidal fluorescence in the area.

Blocked fluorescence is most easily differentiated from hypofluorescence due to hypoperfusion by evaluating the ophthalmoscopic view where a lesion is usually visible that corresponds to the area of blocked fluorescence. If no corresponding area is visible clinically, then it is likely an area of vascular filling defect and not blocked fluorescence. By evaluating the level of the blocked fluorescence in relation to the retinal circulation, one can determine how deep the lesion resides. For example, when lesions block the choroidal circulation but retinal vessels are present over this blocking defect, it indicates that the lesions are above the choroid and below the retinal vessels.

*Hyper*fluorescence occurs when there is an excess of normal fluorescence; it is seen in several major patterns:

- leakage
- staining
- pooling
- transmission defect
- autofluorescence

Leakage refers to the gradual, marked increase in fluorescence throughout the angiogram when fluorescein molecules seep through the pigment epithelium into the subretinal space or neurosensory retina, out of retinal blood vessels into the retinal interstitium, or from retinal neovascularization into the vitreous. The borders of hyperfluorescence become increasingly blurred, and the greatest intensity of hyperfluorescence is appreciated in the late phases of the study, when the only significant fluorescein dye remaining in the eye is extravascular. Examples include choroidal neovascularization (Fig 2-1), microaneurysms and telangiectatic capillaries in diabetic macular edema, or neovascularization of the disc.

Staining refers to a pattern of hyperfluorescence where the fluorescence gradually increases in intensity through transit views and persists in late views, but its borders

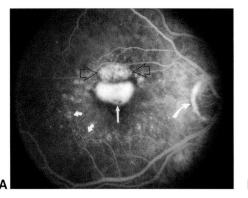 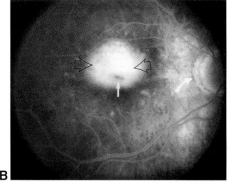

A   B

Figure 2-1 Classic and occult CNV in age-related macular degeneration. **A,** Early-phase angiogram demonstrates classic CNV *(straight arrow)* and boundaries of occult CNV *(open arrows)*. Small curved arrows show slight transmission of fluorescence (window defect) from drusen. Large curved arrow shows transmission resulting from RPE atrophy around optic nerve. **B,** Late-phase angiogram demonstrates leakage of dye from classic CNV *(straight arrow)* and occult CNV *(open arrows)*. Transmission of fluorescence from drusen *(see small curved arrows in A)* has faded. Large curved arrow shows staining of sclera around optic nerve. *(Reproduced with permission from Bressler SB. Management of a small area of choroidal neovascularization in an eye with age-related macular degeneration [AMD] and relatively good visual acuity. The Wilmer Retina Update. 1995;1:3–7.)*

remain fixed throughout the angiogram process. Staining results from fluorescein entry into a solid tissue or similar material that retains the fluorescein, such as a scar, drusen, optic nerve tissue, or sclera (see Fig 2-1B).

Pooling refers to the accumulation of fluorescein in a fluid-filled space in the retina or choroid. The margins of the space trapping the fluorescein are usually distinct, as seen in an RPE detachment in central serous chorioretinopathy (Fig 2-2D).

A *transmission defect,* or *window defect,* of fluorescence refers to a view of the normal choroidal fluorescence through a defect in the pigment or loss of pigment in the RPE, such as shown in Figures 2-1A and 2-1B. In a transmission defect, the hyperfluorescence occurs early, corresponding to filling of the choroidal circulation, and reaches its greatest intensity with the peak of choroidal filling. The fluorescence does not increase in size or shape and usually fades in the late phases of the angiogram, as the choroidal fluorescence becomes diluted by blood that does not contain fluorescein. The fluorescein remains in the choroid and does not enter the retina.

Autofluorescence describes the appearance of fluorescence from the fundus captured on film or videotape *prior* to intravenous fluorescein injection. It is seen with structures that naturally fluoresce, such as optic nerve drusen and lipofuscin.

Side effects of fluorescein angiography

Fluorescein is a relatively safe, injectable drug. All patients injected with fluorescein have temporary yellowing of the skin and conjunctiva lasting from 6 to 12 hours after injection, as well as orange-yellow discoloration of the urine that lasts from 24 to 36 hours. Other side effects include:

- nausea, vomiting, or vasovagal reactions in approximately 10% of injections; more severe vasovagal reactions, including bradycardia, hypotension, shock, and syncope are rarer
- extravasation with subcutaneous granuloma, toxic neuritis, or local tissue necrosis—these are extremely rare
- urticarial *(anaphylactoid)* reactions in about 1% of cases
- *anaphylactic* reactions (cardiovascular shock) at a rate of probably less than 1 in 100,000 injections

Prior urticarial reactions increase a patient's risk of having a similar reaction on subsequent injections; however, premedicating the individual with antihistamines and/or corticosteroids decreases the risk.

If the dye extravasates into the skin during injection, local pain may develop. Ice-cold compresses should be placed on the affected area for 5–10 minutes. The patient may be reassessed over hours or days as necessary until the edema, pain, and redness resolve. Although teratogenic effects have not been identified, many ophthalmologists try to avoid fluorescein angiography in pregnant women unless absolutely necessary. Also of note, the fluorescein will be transmitted to breast milk in lactating women.

Berkow JW, Flower RW, Orth DH, et al. *Fluorescein and Indocyanine Green Angiography: Technique and Interpretation.* 2nd ed. Ophthalmology Monograph 5. San Francisco: American Academy of Ophthalmology; 1997.

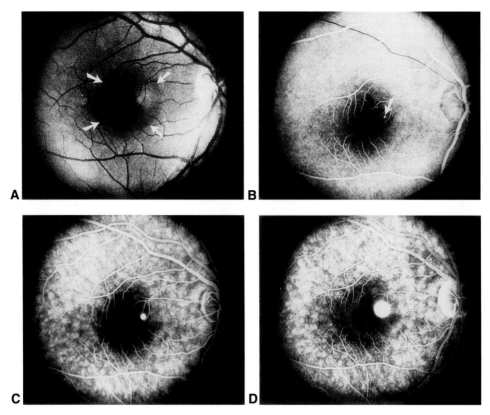

Figure 2-2 Typical central serous chorioretinopathy. **A,** The red-free black-and-white photograph of the right macula reveals a well-demarcated serous detachment of the sensory retina *(arrows)*. **B,** Early transit frame of the angiogram reveals pinpoint focus of hyperfluorescence, indicating early fluorescein leakage *(arrow)* through the RPE, nasal to the foveal avascular zone. **C,** A late venous phase frame of the angiogram reveals increasing fluorescence from continuing leakage. **D,** A later frame of the angiogram demonstrates pooling of fluorescein in a pigment epithelial detachment. Also note mild hyperfluoresence caused by generalized staining of the serous fluid beneath the sensory retina. The RPE outside the fovea typically is mottled and hyperfluorescent.

Kwiterovich KA, Maguire MG, Murphy RP, et al. Frequency of adverse systemic reactions after fluorescein angiography: results of a prospective study. *Ophthalmology.* 1991;98:1139–1142.

Rabb MF, Burton TC, Schatz H, et al. Fluorescein angiography of the fundus: a schematic approach to interpretation. *Surv Ophthalmol.* 1978;22:387–403.

Indocyanine Green Angiography

Indocyanine green (ICG) is a water-soluble tricarbocyanine dye with a molecular weight of 775 daltons that is almost completely protein-bound (98%) after intravenous injection. Because it is protein-bound, diffusion through the small fenestrations of the choriocapillaris is limited. The retention of ICG in the choroidal circulation, coupled with low permeability, makes ICG angiography ideal for imaging of the choroidal circulation.

ICG fluoresces in the near-infrared range (790–805 nm). Because its fluorescence efficacy is only 4% that of fluorescein dye, it can be detected only with specialized infrared video angiography using modified fundus cameras, a digital imaging system, or a scanning laser ophthalmoscope (SLO). With advances in computer technology, high-speed ICG angiography can produce up to 30 frames per second in a continuous recording of the angiogram. This system has been used to help visualize structures that appear only briefly on traditional systems, such as feeder vessels of CNV.

A theoretical advantage of ICG is its ability to fluoresce better through pigment, fluid, lipid, and hemorrhage than fluorescein dye, thereby increasing the possibility of detecting abnormalities such as CNV that may be blocked by an overlying thin, subretinal hemorrhage or hyperplastic RPE on a fluorescein angiogram. Choroidal neovascularization appears on ICG angiography as a plaque, focal spot, or a combination of both. However, ICG used in eyes with these features has not consistently produced images of well-defined CNV that looks like traditional CNV on fluorescein angiography. Whether the theoretical advantages of ICG will yield clinical benefits in the management of patients with CNV awaits confirmation by well-designed, randomized controlled clinical trials.

Indocyanine green is also useful in delineating the abnormal aneurysmal outpouchings of the inner choroidal vascular network seen in idiopathic polypoidal choroidal vasculopathy, the focal areas of choroidal hyperpermeability in central serous chorioretinopathy, and the abnormal fluorescence patterns seen in choroidal inflammatory conditions such as birdshot retinochoroidopathy and multifocal choroiditis. Future investigation will likely continue to study ICG as a means of evaluating choroidal circulation in normal and diseased states.

Side effects of indocyanine green

Indocyanine green appears to have a lower rate of side effects than fluorescein dye. Unlike fluorescein dye, nausea and vomiting are rare with ICG. Mild adverse events are seen in less than 1% of patients. Allergic reactions are no more common with ICG than with fluorescein, but the dye should be used with caution in individuals with a history of allergy to iodides and shellfish because ICG contains 5% iodide. Angiographic facilities should develop an emergency plan and establish a protocol to minimize risks and manage complications associated with either fluorescein or ICG administration.

American Academy of Ophthalmology. Indocyanine green angiography. *Ophthalmology.* 1998;105:1564–1569.

Hope-Ross M, Yannuzzi LA, Gragoudas ES, et al. Adverse reactions due to indocyanine green. *Ophthalmology.* 1994;101:529–533.

Other Imaging Techniques

More recent advances in posterior segment imaging have employed noncontact techniques that do not require the use of imaging dyes. Additional studies using each of these modalities will be needed to clarify their place in the routine clinical care of patients.

Optical Coherence Tomography

Optical coherence tomography (OCT) is a noninvasive, noncontact imaging modality that produces micron-resolution, cross-sectional images of ocular tissue. OCT produces a 2-dimensional, false color image of the backscattered light from different layers in the retina analogous to ultrasonic B-scan and radar imaging. The only difference is that the OCT device, using the principle of low-coherence interferometry, measures optical rather than acoustic or radio wave reflectivity. By using light instead of sound, the resolution is enhanced and the speed is much greater. First- and second-generation OCT scanners produced cross-sectional images of the retina with an axial (depth) resolution of approximately 12–15 μm; current commercial OCT scanners offer a resolution of 8–10 μm. Because axial resolution depends on the "coherence length" of the light source, with titanium sapphire laser light sources, experimental scanners offer a resolution of 2–3 μm or even better.

OCT single-scan tomograms offer a cross-sectional view of the retina similar to that of a histopathologic specimen. Tissues with higher reflectivity, such as the RPE, appear in brighter colors (red-white), and less dense structures, such as the vitreous and intra-retinal fluid, appear in darker colors (blue-black). OCT is useful for differentiating lamellar from pseudo- and full-thickness macular holes, diagnosing vitreomacular traction syndrome, differentiating traction-related diabetic macular edema, monitoring the course of central serous chorioretinopathy, and evaluating for subtle subretinal fluid that is not visible on fluorescein angiography. OCT can also produce a retinal thickness map from 6 radial scans that looks like a topographic map, with areas of increased thickening in brighter colors and areas of lower levels of thickening in darker colors. An assessment of macular volume can also be obtained from the retinal thickness map to follow treatment regimens.

Hee MR, Puliafito CA, Wong C, et al. Optical coherence tomography of macular holes. *Ophthalmology.* 1995;102:748–756.

Hee MR, Puliafito CA, Wong C, et al. Quantitative assessment of macular edema with optical coherence tomography. *Arch Ophthalmol.* 1995;113:1019–1029.

Huang D, Swanson EA, Lin CP, et al. Optical coherence tomography. *Science.* 1991;254:1178–1181.

Scanning Laser Ophthalmoscopy

A confocal scanning laser ophthalmoscope (SLO) uses a laser beam that rapidly scans the posterior pole in a raster fashion—similar to how a television creates an image on a monitor. The reflected light is detected by a photodiode and the digitized image is stored in a computer. Stereoscopic high-contrast images can be produced with and without fluorescein or ICG, and altering the laser wavelength permits selective examination of different tissue depths. The SLO is capable of imaging structures at very high magnification and high frame rate, allowing accurate diagnosis of retinal structures poorly seen by ordinary fundus cameras, using low levels of light exposure and improved contrast. In addition, a topographic 3-dimensional map with optical slices can be made digitally from 32 consecutive and equidistant optical section images obtained from the SLO. From this topographic map, retinal thickness can be estimated. One historic disadvantage of the SLO was the fact that it produced only a monochromatic image because a single wavelength laser was used; however, true color representation of the fundus with an SLO is now possible by combining images taken using blue, green, and red lasers, as well as simultaneous ICG and fluorescein angiography by using an argon laser (488 nm) and a diode laser (795 nm) from an external source delivered by single-mode fibers. Present clinical applications include high-resolution ICG and fluorescein angiography, wide-field imaging of the retina through small pupils, microperimetry, and noninvasive assessment of retinal blood flow. In addition, SLO has also been combined with OCT in a single experimental unit that may offer even greater diagnostic capabilities in the future.

Freeman WR, Bartsch DU, Mueller AJ, et al. Simultaneous indocyanine green and fluorescein angiography using a confocal scanning laser ophthalmoscope. *Arch Ophthalmol.* 1998;116:455–463.

Ip MS, Duker JS. Advances in posterior segment imaging techniques. *Focal Points: Clinical Modules for Ophthalmologists.* San Francisco: American Academy of Ophthalmology; 1999, module 7.

Retinal Thickness Analyzer

The retinal thickness analyzer (RTA) is a multipurpose system that combines a digital fundus camera, computerized scanning slit lamp, and retinal thickness analyzer. The RTA enables acquisition, display, and analysis of retinal optical cross sections and provides registered maps of retinal thickness by projecting a helium-neon (HeNe) (543-nm) laser beam at an angle onto the retina across the central 20° of the macula and measuring the backscattering of the reflected light. The RTA's software identifies the location of the nerve fiber layer and the RPE at each point in the scanned area and calculates the difference to determine the retinal thickness. The system's software analyzes the optical cross sections of the retina, and the information is displayed as a deviation map from a normative database as a color-coded, 2- or 3-dimensional retinal thickness map that can be overlaid on a fundus image to facilitate accurate localization of the findings (Fig 2-3).

Asrani S, Zeimer R, Goldberg MF, et al. Application of rapid scanning retinal thickness analysis in retinal disease. *Ophthalmology.* 1997;104:1145–1151.

Shahidi M, Ogura Y, Blair NP, et al. Retinal thickness analysis for quantitative assessment of diabetic macular edema. *Arch Ophthalmol.* 1991;109:1115–1119.

Common Uses of Imaging Technology

Common uses of diagnostic imaging technology include the following:

- choroidal neovascularization
- chorioretinal inflammatory conditions
- subretinal fluid accumulation
- retinal perfusion abnormalities
- macular edema
- vitreomacular interface changes

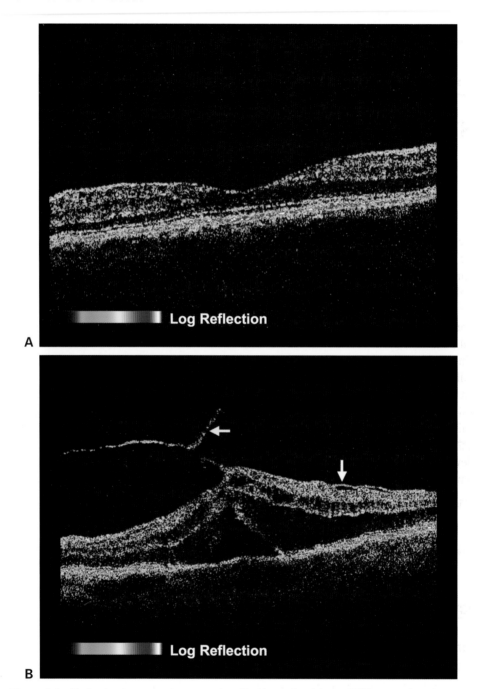

Figure 2-3 Optical coherence tomography. **A,** Normal subject. OCT scan showing normal foveal depression and retinal thickness. Note the retinal pigment epithelium/Bruch's membrane appears red and the vitreous appears dark. **B,** Patient with diabetic macular edema and vitreous traction. Note the posterior hyaloid *(yellow arrow)* pulling on the retina, a fine epiretinal membrane *(white arrow)* on the retinal surface, and the increased retinal thickness. *(OCT scans courtesy of Peter K. Kaiser, MD.)*

CHAPTER 3

Retinal Physiology and Psychophysics

Clinical electrophysiologic and psychophysical testing allows an assessment of nearly the entire length of the visual pathway. Most electrophysiologic tests are evoked responses. A representation of the sequence of events along the visual pathway, from changes in the retinal pigment epithelium (RPE) to cortical potentials of the occipital lobes, can be made by adjusting stimulus conditions and techniques of recording. However, because an abnormality at a proximal source usually gives an abnormal signal farther along the visual pathway, test results can be misleading if interpreted in isolation from the clinical findings or tests specific to other areas of the visual pathway. For instance, an abnormal visually evoked response might be found in macular degeneration or a cone dystrophy, but it could be misinterpreted as a central pathway conduction defect unless a fundus examination or an electroretinogram (ERG) is also performed. A careful history and eye examination before electrophysiologic and psychophysical tests are ordered will help the clinician determine the appropriate tests and thus increase their usefulness in diagnosing the level of dysfunction. BCSC Section 5, *Neuro-Ophthalmology,* discusses and illustrates the entire visual pathway.

> Fishman GA, Birch GA, Holder GE, et al. *Electrophysiologic Testing in Disorders of the Retina, Optic Nerve, and Visual Pathway.* Ophthalmology Monograph 2. 2nd ed. San Francisco: American Academy of Ophthalmology; 2001.
>
> Van Boemel GB, Ogden TE. Clinical electrophysiology. In: Ryan SJ, ed. *Retina.* 3rd ed. St Louis: Mosby; 2001.

Electroretinogram

Recording and Interpreting the Response

The clinical electroretinogram is a mass response evoked from the entire retina by a brief flash of light. Five different responses are basic to most clinical evaluations and are standardized internationally so that ERG results can be interpreted easily at different medical centers (Fig 3-1):

- "rod response" (dark-adapted)
- maximal combined response (dark-adapted)
- oscillatory potentials (dark-adapted)

DARK ADAPTED   **LIGHT ADAPTED**

"Rod response"   Single-flash "cone response"

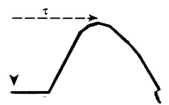

Maximal combined response

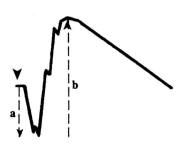

Approximate Calibrations

	rod/cone responses	oscillatory potentials	
	100	30	μV
	20	10	ms

Oscillatory potentials   30-Hz flicker responses

              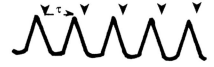

Figure 3-1 Diagram of the 5 basic ERG responses defined by the International Standard for Electroretinography. These waveforms and calibrations are exemplary only, as there is a moderate range of normal values. The large arrowheads indicate the stimulus flash, and the dashed lines show how to measure a-wave and b-wave amplitude and time-to-peak (implicit time, τ). The implicit time of a flicker response is normally less than the distance between peaks for stimulation at 30 Hz. *(Reprinted by permission of Kluwer Academic Publishers from Marmor MF, Zrenner E. Standard for clinical electroretinography [1994 update]. Doc Ophthalmol. 1995;89:199–210.)*

- single-flash "cone response" (light-adapted)
- 30-hertz (-Hz) flicker responses (light-adapted)

In general, the ERG is characterized by a negative waveform *(a-wave)* that represents the response of the photoreceptors, followed by a positive waveform *(b-wave)* generated by a combination of cells in the Müller and bipolar cell layer. The duration of the entire response is usually less than 150 msec. A-wave amplitude is measured from baseline to the a-wave trough; b-wave amplitude is measured from the a-wave trough to the b-wave peak. The implicit time (τ), the time to reach a peak, is measured from the onset of the stimulus to the trough of the a-wave or the peak of the b-wave. Figure 3-1 shows typical response amplitudes and durations, but normal values vary with recording technique and should be provided by each laboratory. The use of standardized conditions is essential for meaningful interpretation of the ERG, because variations in lighting and recording conditions, in the intensity of flashes, or in the degree of light and dark adaptation can all greatly affect the test results.

Use of a corneal contact lens electrode to record the ERG gives the most accurate and reproducible results. The pupils should be dilated and light flashes presented full-field to the entire retina. A bowl similar to that of a perimeter is used to illuminate the entire retina. Signals are evoked either by a single flash or by repetitive flashes (with computer averaging if desired). To record light-adapted (photopic) ERGs, a uniform background light is projected in the bowl. It is important diagnostically, especially in evaluating hereditary and other retinal degenerations, to test the rod and cone systems separately.

Dark-adapted testing

Rods are 1000 times more sensitive to light than cones. The *rod response,* or *scotopic,* ERG shown in Figure 3-1 is produced by dark-adapting the patient for at least 20 minutes and stimulating the retina with a dim white flash that is below the cone threshold. The resulting waveform has a prominent b-wave but almost no detectable a-wave. A larger waveform *(maximal combined response)* is generated by using a bright flash in the dark-adapted state, which maximally stimulates both cones and rods and results in large a- and b-wave amplitudes with oscillatory potentials superimposed on the ascending b-wave. The *oscillatory potentials* can be isolated by filtering out the slower ERG components. Oscillatory potentials are believed to be the result of feedback interactions among the integrative cells of the proximal retina. They are reduced in retinal ischemic states and in some forms of congenital stationary night blindness.

Light-adapted testing

The *single-flash cone response,* or *photopic,* ERG is obtained by maintaining the patient in a light-adapted state and stimulating the retina with a bright white flash. The rods are suppressed by light adaptation and do not contribute to the waveform. Cone responses can also be elicited with a flickering stimulus light. In theory, rods can respond to a stimulus up to 20 Hz, or cycles per second, although in most clinical situations 8 Hz is their practical limit. Thus, a stimulus rate of 30 Hz is used to screen out the rod response and measure cone responses *(30-Hz flicker response)*.

ERG interpretation

Some examples of ERG changes in specific diseases are illustrated in Figure 3-2. The ERG evoked by a full-field (Ganzfeld) stimulus measures the response of the entire retina, but retinal cells are unevenly distributed; the density of cones is very high in the fovea and macula, whereas rods are most populous about 15° away from the fovea. It might seem intuitive that the ERG would distinguish between macular and peripheral lesions on the basis of cone and rod signals. However, this is *not* true. Even though cones are more populous in the fovea, fully 90% of them lie beyond the macula.

In a patient with a large atrophic macular lesion and an otherwise normal retina, the photopic (cone) ERG b-wave amplitude would be reduced only about 10%. This degree of loss is not recognizable clinically because the range of normal values for the ERG is fairly wide. Conversely, when a patient with a macular lesion has a reduced photopic ERG, the patient must have a diffuse degeneration affecting cones beyond the macula. Because the ERG measures a panretinal response, it does not necessarily correlate with visual acuity, which is a function of the fovea.

A number of factors may influence the amplitude and timing of the normal electro-retinogram. The intensity of the stimulus, pupil size, and the area of retina stimulated all have effects. The ERG is relatively insensitive to refractive error, except in eyes with

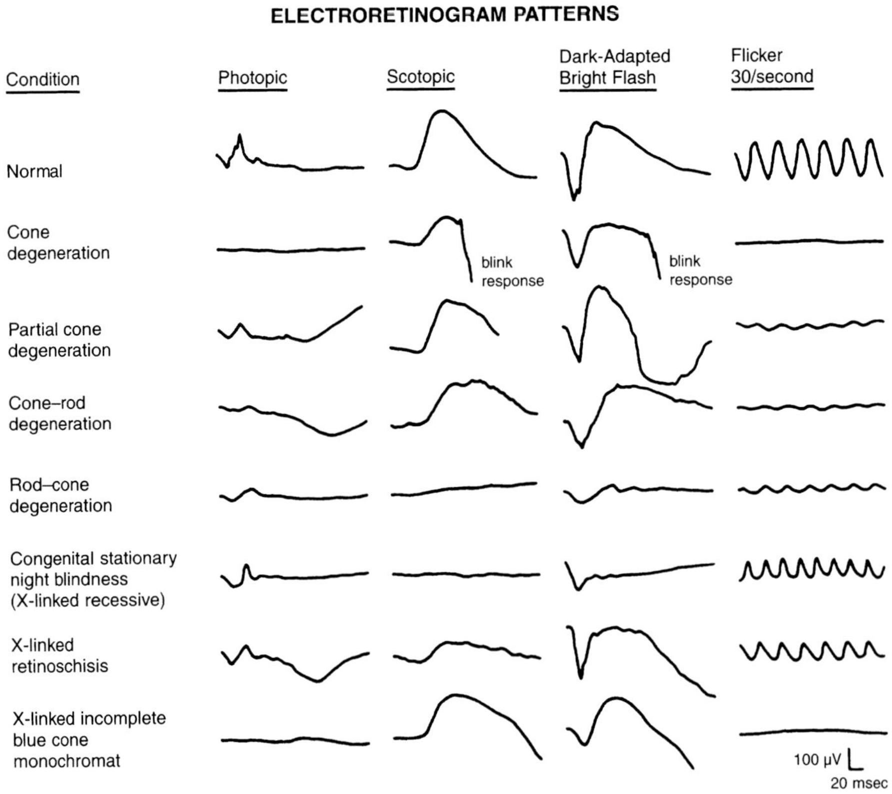

ELECTRORETINOGRAM PATTERNS

Figure 3-2 Examples of ERG changes in retinal diseases. Note that some diseases are selective for the cone system, the rod system, or the inner retina (b-wave).

high myopia, which can have somewhat reduced signals but generally not to the extent seen in patients with hereditary retinal degeneration. Elderly individuals often show signals that are slightly reduced in amplitude compared with signals from a younger population. Newborn infants have a small ERG signal, but it rises rapidly in the first few months of life to a magnitude that allows most clinical distinctions to be made. Debate continues as to whether optic nerve lesions occasionally enhance the ERG, possibly because centrifugal inhibitory signals are interrupted.

Marmor MF, Zrenner E. Standard for clinical electroretinography (1994 update). *Doc Ophthalmol.* 1995;89:199–210.

Specialized Types of ERG

Early receptor potentials and c-wave

The *early receptor potential (ERP)* is a small response that occurs with no detectable latency before the a-wave (Fig 3-3). It is evoked by an intense stimulus flash and has been, in part, correlated with electrical changes in the cell membrane that occur during the conversion of lumirhodopsin to metarhodopsin. (This process is discussed and illustrated in Chapter 16, Retina, of BCSC Section 2, *Fundamentals and Principles of Ophthalmology.*) In humans, 60%–80% of the ERP amplitude is generated by cones. The ERP has been used primarily in research settings to measure visual pigment bleaching and regeneration.

The *c-wave* is a late positive response occurring 2–4 seconds after the stimulus and is generated by the RPE. It is discussed later in this chapter in conjunction with other RPE responses (see Figure 3-11).

Focal and multifocal ERG testing

It is possible to stimulate only the foveal or the parafoveal cones while presenting a bright light on the rest of the retina to suppress the rod system and prevent interference. A rapidly flickering stimulus is typically used so that several hundred small ERG responses

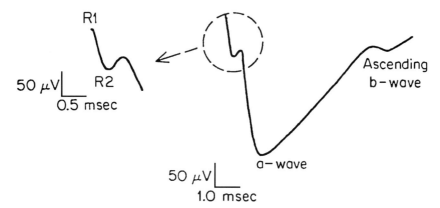

Figure 3-3 Early receptor potential (ERP). The response is very small and occurs before the a-wave. *(Redrawn from Berson EL, Goldstein EB. Early receptor potential in dominantly inherited retinitis pigmentosa. Arch Ophthalmol. 1970;83:412–420.)*

can be summated. Foveal ERG testing is used primarily for cases in which the physical findings do not correlate clearly with a patient's loss of acuity. The foveal ERG can provide objective information about the presence or absence of organic disease in the macula.

It is now possible to produce a topographic ERG map of the retina using a specialized technology. This is referred to as *multifocal ERG*. Multifocal ERG tests cone-generated responses that subtend 25° radially from fixation. In patients with stable and accurate fixation, this test can determine objectively whether or not macular dysfunction is present (Fig 3-4). It also may hold the potential to evaluate or compare treatment responses in various macular conditions.

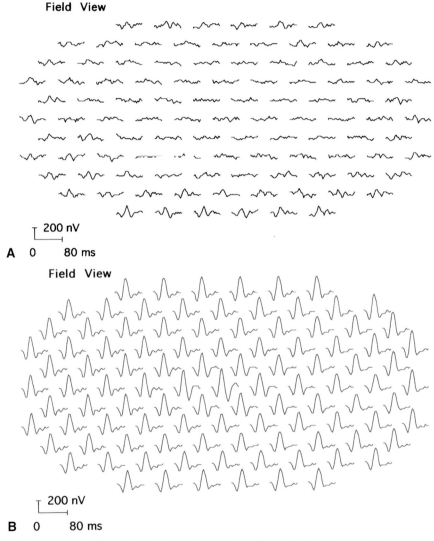

Figure 3-4 Multifocal ERG tracings of the right eye of a patient with unexplained decreased visual acuity. The central macular region has marked decreased waveform amplitudes **(A)** compared to the reference traces **(B).** *(Photographs courtesy of Carl Regillo, MD.)*

Bright-flash ERG

The ability to perform vitrectomies and repair retinal trauma has led to active interest in judging retinal function in eyes with opaque media. The bright-flash ERG is performed with a flash stimulus that is brighter than usual, such as a high-intensity photographic strobe. An unrecordable ERG indicates a poor prognosis due to widespread retinal damage, whereas a moderate signal (eg, 50 μV) suggests that some salvageable retina does exist. The test gives no direct information about visual acuity or possible damage to the optic nerve.

Pattern ERG

The pattern ERG (PERG) can be elicited from the retina by an alternating checkerboard stimulus presented to the central retina. The responses to several hundred stimuli (alternations) are averaged to obtain a measurable signal (Fig 3-5). The PERG has been shown to correlate with integrity of the optic nerve and thus gives information about the ganglion cells and their retinal interactions. Initial work suggested that comparison of the focal ERG and PERG might distinguish between outer and inner retinal pathology and that the PERG could be a specific test for the recognition of early glaucoma. In practice, however, the PERG has proven difficult to record reproducibly, and the signals are very sensitive to confounding factors such as blurred vision (including cataract) and maculopathy. PERGs are typically recorded with a conductive fiber or foil electrode touching the cornea.

Fishman GA, Birch GA, Holder GE, et al. *Electrophysiologic Testing in Disorders of the Retina, Optic Nerve, and Visual Pathway.* Ophthalmology Monograph 2. 2nd ed. San Francisco: American Academy of Ophthalmology; 2001.

Marmor MF, Holder GE, Porciatti V, et al. Guidelines for basic pattern electroretinography: recommendations by the International Society for Clinical Electrophysiology of Vision. *Doc Ophthalmol.* 1995–96;91:291–298.

Scholl HP, Zrenner E. Electrophysiology in the investigation of acquired retinal disorders. *Surv Ophthalmol.* 2000;47:29–47.

Applications and Cautions

The ERG is important for diagnosing and following retinal dystrophies and degenerations. Although not a direct test of macular function (because it is a mass response), it

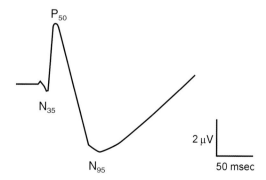

Figure 3-5 Diagram of the pattern ERG, elicited by alternation of a checkerboard pattern. The major negative and positive waves are labeled according to their typical latencies. *(Reprinted by permission of Kluwer Academic Publishers from Marmor MF, Holder GE, Porciatti V, et al. Guidelines for basic pattern electroretinography: recommendations by the International Society for Clinical Electrophysiology of Vision. Doc Ophthalmol. 1995– 96;91:291–298.)*

can be invaluable nevertheless in the evaluation of macular diseases to confirm whether pathology is limited to the macula. Macular disorders with peripheral involvement have more serious visual implications for the patient. The ERG is also useful in assessing disorders of dark adaptation, color vision, and visual acuity, and it may be a part of the evaluation of hysteria or malingering.

The ERG can often help to distinguish between retinal damage caused by diffuse disease, such as a hereditary dystrophy or drug toxicity, as opposed to focal disease, such as branch vascular occlusion or regional uveitic damage. Panretinal disorders not only reduce ERG amplitude but also cause delayed and abnormal waveforms that reflect the malfunction of cells throughout the retina (Fig 3-6). Focal disease, which typically has a better long-term prognosis, reduces ERG amplitude in proportion to the area of damaged retina, but the remaining signal from healthy areas of retina shows normal waveform and timing. ERG timing is most easily assessed using the 30-Hz flicker response, which normally shows a b-wave implicit time (stimulus-to-peak interval) of less than 32 msec.

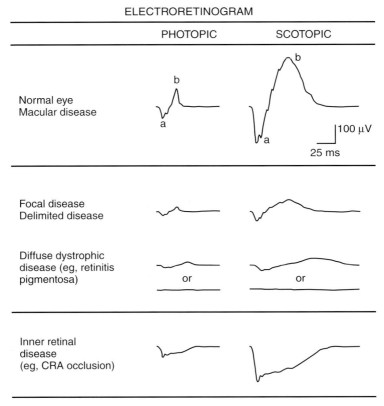

Figure 3-6 Characteristics of the ERG with different types of retinal damage. Disease that damages only parts of the retina reduces the ERG amplitude, but the unaffected areas of retina produce a normal waveform. Diffuse disease leads to responses that are delayed as well as reduced in amplitude. Inner retinal disease may selectively diminish the b-wave. *(Reprinted with permission from Marmor MF. The management of retinitis pigmentosa and allied diseases. Ophthalmology Digest. 1979;41:13–29.)*

The ERG can be useful in the evaluation of chronic ischemic damage from vascular disease. Retinal capillary loss or vascular insufficiency causes abnormalities of the b-wave and oscillatory potentials such as a delay in the implicit time and/or a reduction of amplitude (Fig 3-7). Normally, the b-wave is larger in amplitude than the a-wave, and inversion of the b/a–wave ratio or a delay in the 30-Hz cone flicker responses is a potentially ominous sign in eyes with central retinal vein occlusion.

The ERG may aid in the detection of certain hereditary diseases in affected family members. In X-linked conditions particularly, such as choroideremia, the fundus in female carriers is often a mosaic of normal and abnormal areas, and the ERG will typically show subtle abnormalities. The ERG may reveal retinal abnormalities in children long before symptoms or clear-cut ophthalmoscopic signs become evident. ERGs can be recorded in children of all ages, although interpretation can be difficult in the first few months of life before adult waveforms have developed. Pediatric ERGs can be performed without general anesthesia, although oral sedation is sometimes necessary (Fig 3-8). Anesthesia can depress the ERG responses.

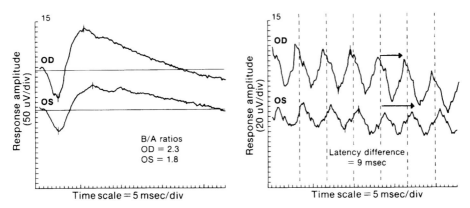

Figure 3-7 ERG in central retinal vein occlusion. The right eye is normal. The left eye shows a mild reduction in b-wave amplitude but a striking delay in the latency of the flicker responses. The implicit time (arrows) of the responses from the left eye is longer than the interval between peaks, a sign that is strongly suggestive of diffuse damage to the retina. *(Reprinted with permission from Breton ME, Quinn GE, Keene SS, et al. Electroretinogram parameters at presentation as predictors of rubeosis in central retinal vein occlusion patients. Ophthalmology. 1989;96:1343–1352.)*

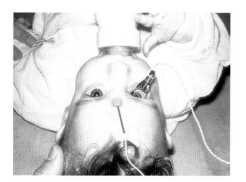

Figure 3-8 A 5-month-old infant with a contact lens electrode in place for ERG recording. The child was quite comfortable and required little restraint until the bottle ran out. *(Reprinted with permission from Marmor MF. Corneal electroretinograms in children without sedation. J Ped Ophthalmol. 1976;13:112–116.)*

The ERG can be used to estimate the extent of damage from trauma or from drug toxicity. A reasonable ERG signal behind opaque media, especially when a bright flash is used, indicates that the retina is attached and functional. Cataracts do not appreciably affect the ERG, but the bright-flash technique is necessary for eyes filled with blood. The ERG can help to judge whether a retained foreign body is causing siderosis or other toxic damage and can document damage from drugs such as thioridazine or chloroquine. A series of follow-up recordings may be needed to determine whether the damage is continuing and (in cases of trauma) to differentiate the toxic effects of a foreign body from the physical effects of the injury.

Johnson MA, Marcus S, Elman MJ, et al. Neovascularization in central retinal vein occlusion: electroretinographic findings. *Arch Ophthalmol.* 1988;106:348–352.

Electrooculogram and RPE Responses

Electrooculogram

As described in Chapter 1, the RPE is a monolayer of cells that are linked by tight junctions near the apical surface. These junctions separate the apical and basal membranes of the pigment epithelium, which have different ionic permeability characteristics that lead to the generation of a voltage across the cell (Fig 3-9). This voltage, called the *standing potential,* is positive at the cornea and measures 6–10 mV.

Although the RPE itself is not a light receptor, activation of the photoreceptors in the neurosensory retina can lead to changes in the ionic composition of the extracellular (subretinal) space or to the release of transmitter substances that produce an electrical response in the RPE. For example, when a dark-adapted eye is exposed to steady light, the standing potential across the RPE rises very slowly and reaches a peak 5–10 *minutes* after the onset of light. The voltage change of this *light response* has been shown to originate across the basal membrane of the RPE. We still do not know what substances mediate between the capture of light by the photoreceptors and the slow voltage changes in the RPE, although current evidence suggests that the messenger substance may be derived from the photoreceptors.

The light response of the standing potential develops so slowly that it is hard to measure directly without artifacts from movement or electrical drift. To resolve this problem, clinics use the indirect technique of electrooculography, in which electrodes are placed at either side of the eye (usually on the skin at the canthi), and the voltage between them is recorded as the patient looks back and forth (Fig 3-10). The amplitude of these voltage shifts is proportional to the actual voltage across the eye. An international standard technique for recording the electrooculogram (EOG) defines the optimal placement of electrodes, the time of adaptation, and the intensity of the light stimulus, which depends on whether the pupils are dilated.

Arden proposed that, for clinical purposes, a ratio be derived from the highest point of the light peak and the lowest point of the baseline in the dark. This light–dark ratio, or Arden ratio, is normally 1.85 or above, although variation among individuals is considerable. Values below 1.85 are generally termed subnormal, and those less than about

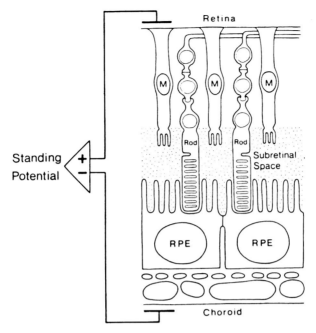

Figure 3-9 Electrical circuit of the standing potential. The RPE cells generate a voltage from apex to base because of the different ionic permeability characteristics on each surface and the presence of impermeable tight junctions between the cells. Changes in the voltage across the apical or basal RPE membrane are reflected in the standing potential and are measurable clinically as the c-wave on ERG or with EOG. M = Müller cells. *(Reprinted with permission from Steinberg RH. Monitoring communications between photoreceptors and pigment epithelial cells: effects of "mild" systemic hypoxia. Friedenwald Lecture.* Invest Ophthalmol Vis Sci. *1987;28:1888–1904.)*

1.30 are severely subnormal or nearly extinguished. The amplitude of the EOG is dominated by the rod system, and, like the ERG, it is a mass response.

Arden GB, Fojas MR. Electrophysiological abnormalities in pigmentary degenerations of the retina. *Arch Ophthalmol.* 1962;68:369–389.

Marmor MF, Zrenner E. Standard for clinical electro-oculography. International Society for Clinical Electrophysiology of Vision. *Arch Ophthalmol.* 1993;111:601–604.

Uses and limitations of EOG

The major limitation of the EOG as a clinical tool is that the origin and meaning of this electrical response are not well understood. The EOG depends not only on the integrity of the RPE but also on the activity of the photoreceptors and possibly of the inner retinal layers. Thus, the EOG is not a useful test for most disorders in which the retina itself is significantly damaged; it is most specific for involvement of the RPE when other studies have shown the retina to be normal.

The relationship of the EOG to physiologic functions of the RPE is unclear because it does not correlate closely with either pigmentary changes in the RPE or with visual function. For example, the EOG light–dark ratio is normal or only mildly subnormal in some diseases (eg, diffuse fundus flavimaculatus or pattern dystrophy) in which the RPE seems to be primarily involved. However, it is severely reduced in Best disease, in which

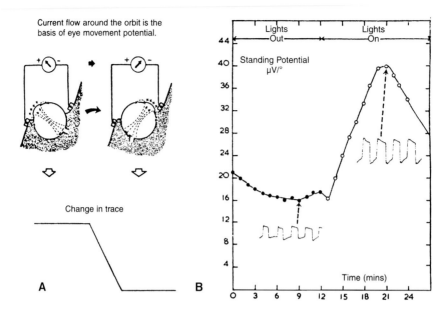

Figure 3-10 The clinical EOG. **A,** The voltage between skin electrodes at either side of an eye varies as the eye turns, in proportion to the size of the standing potential. **B,** Plot of the amplitude of the oscillations, showing how the standing potential diminishes to a trough in the dark and then rises to a peak after light is turned on. In clinical practice, the EOG is often evaluated as the ratio between this peak and trough. *(Reprinted with permission from Arden GB, Fojas MR. Electrophysiological abnormalities in pigmentary degenerations of the retina: assessment of value and basis. Arch Ophthalmol. 1962;68:369–389.)*

most of the retina appears and functions normally. In rubella retinopathy, the RPE can be diffusely altered, but the EOG is normal.

The EOG is most specific as a test for Best vitelliform dystrophy and thus is useful in the evaluation of any yellow lesions or macular scars that might be manifestations of vitelliform dystrophy. Its use in the evaluation of diffuse RPE diseases is less clear, because patients who show an abnormal EOG usually show obvious fundus changes that are the main basis for the diagnosis. Some authors feel the EOG is a sensitive indicator of early chloroquine toxicity, but others argue that mass electrical responses like the EOG or ERG are not sensitive to early toxicity. Serial testing may show progressive changes.

Other RPE Tests

The *c-wave* of the ERG is a cornea-positive wave that appears 1–5 seconds after the onset of the light stimulus (Fig 3-11). It represents a hyperpolarization of the apical RPE membrane in response to the light-induced decrease of potassium concentration in the subretinal space. It is difficult to record clinically because it is too fast for electrooculography but too slow to avoid artifacts. The c-wave seems to correlate clinically with the EOG, but it has not been used extensively.

The *fast oscillation* is a cornea-negative wave that appears 1–2 minutes after the onset of light, as shown in Figure 3-11, and represents a delayed effect from potassium changes in the subretinal space. It is actually generated across the basal RPE membrane and

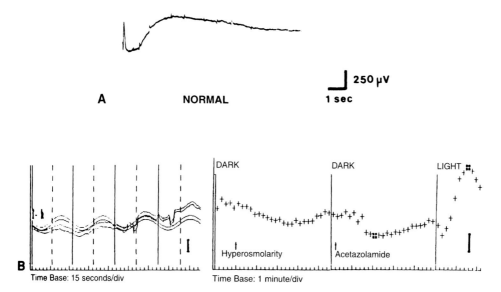

Figure 3-11 Other RPE responses. **A,** C-wave recorded from the human eye. **B,** Fast oscil-lation (on the left) generated by alternating light and dark (beginning at each solid and dashed line), respectively. *Hyperosmolarity* and *acetazolamide* responses (on the right) do not depend on light and are generated by a direct chemical effect on the RPE cell membranes. *(Part A reproduced with permission from Hock PA, Marmor MF. Variability of the human c-wave. Doc Ophthalmol Proc Ser. 1983;37:151–157. Part B reproduced with permission of Kluwer Academic Publishers from Gupta LY, Marmor MF. Sequential recording of photic and nonphotic electro-oculogram responses in patients with extensive extramacular drusen. Doc Ophthalmol. 1994;88:49–55.)*

probably involves chloride conductance pathways. It does not always mirror the EOG in disease, and its clinical value is uncertain. It may show changes in cystic fibrosis, a disorder involving chloride conductance.

Changes in the standing potential can be induced by chemicals as well as by light (see Fig 3-11). Intravenous injections of hyperosmolar solution, acetazolamide, or sodium bicarbonate all lead to a depolarization of the basal RPE membrane that can be recorded with electrooculography. The clinical significance of these *nonphotic responses* is uncertain, but they give information about the RPE independent of photoreceptor activity.

Marmor MF. Clinical electrophysiology of the retinal pigment epithelium. *Doc Ophthalmol.* 1991;76:301–313.

Cortical Evoked Potentials

Visually Evoked Potentials

The *visually evoked cortical potential* (VECP, but also abbreviated VEP or VER, for visually evoked potential or response) is an electrical signal generated by the occipital visual cortex in response to stimulation of the retina by either light flashes or patterned stimuli (typically alternating checkerboards or stripes on a TV monitor). The response to many alternations (or flashes) is recorded and averaged. The use of a checkerboard stimulus is preferable when the eye is optically correctable, because the occipital cortex is very sensitive to sharp edges and contrast, whereas it is relatively insensitive to diffuse light.

Because most of the visual cortex represents the macular area of the eye, the VECP is primarily a method of determining macular function. There is some peripheral retinal input, but it is minimal. It should be noted that the VECP represents the endpoint of the visual process and can therefore reflect an abnormality anywhere from the retina to the cortex.

A normal pattern-evoked VECP is represented in Figure 3-12. The signal is recorded with electroencephalogram electrodes; often the inion (back of the occiput) is compared to locations to the right and left of the inion, although different recording sites have been used by different laboratories. The VECP is characterized by 2 negative (N) and 2 positive (P) peaks, whose amplitude and implicit times depend on the check size, contrast, and alternation frequencies of the stimulus. Although absolute amplitudes of the VECP can be measured, using them as a clinical measure is difficult because of variability among normal individuals. The temporal aspect of the VECP is less variable and more reliable as a clinical measure.

VECPs have mainly been used clinically to confirm the diagnosis of optic neuropathy and other demyelinating disease. They also have the following uses:

- to assess misprojection of optic nerve fibers, such as may be found in albinism, which produces asymmetric VECPs between left and right recording positions
- to estimate visual acuity in infants and nonverbal children by using a checkerboard stimulus of decreasing size, where increased visual acuity corresponds to responses to decreased stimuli
- to detect and locate visual field defects by comparing the response to stimuli in different locations

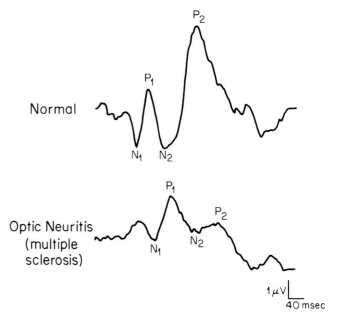

Figure 3-12 Visually evoked cortical responses from a normal individual *(top)* and a patient with optic neuropathy from multiple sclerosis *(bottom)*, who shows not only a reduced amplitude but a marked delay in the appearance of the peaks.

- to evaluate the potential for reasonable visual acuity in patients with opacities of the ocular media

The VECP can also be an important tool in the detection of malingering.

Electrically Evoked Potentials

Responses in the visual system can be evoked by mechanical and electrical stimuli as well as by light. Passage of a small, brief electric current (roughly 0.5 mA) through the eye generates a neural signal that is transmitted to the visual cortex and causes a sensation of light (phosphene). The cortical response is recorded in a manner similar to that used with the VECP and is an indicator of the integrity of the retina as well as the subsequent visual pathway. The primary clinical use of the electrically evoked response is to evaluate the condition and salvageability of traumatized eyes with hemorrhage and possible retinal detachment in which even the bright-flash ERG is unrecordable.

Psychophysical Testing

Although electrophysiologic testing objectively measures cell layers and cell types in the visual pathway, it does not always allow testing of localized responses, and it may not be sensitive to small degrees of visual dysfunction. Psychophysical tests can be exceedingly sensitive, but they are always subjective and are usually not tissue-specific because perception represents an integration of information processing by different parts of the visual pathway. Psychophysical tests relevant to retinal disease include

- visual acuity
- visual field
- dark adaptation
- color vision
- contrast sensitivity

The last three tests are discussed in this chapter. See BCSC Section 10, *Glaucoma,* for extensive discussion of visual field testing.

Pokorny J, Smith VC. Color vision and night vision. In: Ryan SJ, ed. *Retina.* 3rd ed. St Louis: Mosby; 2001:171–187.

Walsh TJ, ed. *Visual Fields: Examination and Interpretation.* Ophthalmology Monograph 3. 2nd ed. San Francisco: American Academy of Ophthalmology; 1996.

Dark Adaptation

The sensitivity of the human eye extends over a range of 10–11 log units. Our cones and rods adapt to different levels of background light through neural mechanisms and through the bleaching and regeneration of visual pigments. Clinical dark adaptometry primarily measures the absolute thresholds of cone and rod sensitivity.

Dark adaptation is most often tested on an instrument such as the *Goldmann-Weekers adaptometer* (Fig 3-13). The patient is first light-adapted to a bright background light. This light is then extinguished, and the patient, now in the dark, is presented with a

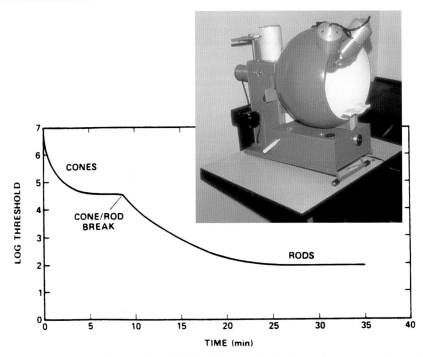

Figure 3-13 Dark adaptation testing with the Goldmann-Weekers adaptometer *(inset)* yields a biphasic curve after preadaptation to bright light. *(Reprinted with permission from Marmor MF. Clinical physiology of the retina. In: Peyman GA, Sanders DR, Goldberg MF. Principles and Practice of Ophthalmology. Philadelphia: Saunders; 1980:823–856.)*

series of dim light targets approximately 11° below fixation. The intensity of the test lights is controlled by neutral-density filters, and the threshold at which the test light is perceived is plotted against time. Under these conditions, the dark adaptation curve illustrated in Figure 3-13 shows two plateaus: the first represents the cone threshold, which is usually reached in 5–10 minutes, and the second represents the rod threshold, which is reached after about 30 minutes. If the clinical interest is limited to rod sensitivity in the dark, the test can be shortened by eliminating the first step of adaptation to bright light and recording only an endpoint rod threshold, which is normally reached within about 10 minutes of dark adaptation.

Dark adaptometry is useful in the evaluation of night blindness. Although the test is subjective, poor cooperation or malingering is easily recognized. A record of dark adaptation is complementary to the electroretinogram because adaptometry is a *focal test* (a point to remember in interpreting results from patients with patchy disease), and thus it may in some instances be more sensitive than the ERG as an indicator of pathologic conditions. Dark adaptometry can also help in the evaluation of cone dysfunction syndromes by demonstrating the degree of cone adaptation.

Color Vision

The perception of color is a response to electromagnetic energy at wavelengths between 400 and 700 nm, which is absorbed by cone outer segment visual pigments. Each cone contains one of 3 types of photolabile pigments. Blue-sensitive (short wavelength), green-sensitive (middle wavelength), and red-sensitive (long wavelength) cones are commonly referred to as the initiators of color vision. However, the integrative cells in the retina and higher visual centers are organized primarily to recognize *contrasts* between light or colors, and the receptive fields of color-sensitive cells typically have regions that compare the intensity of red versus green or blue versus yellow.

The classification and the testing of dysfunctional color vision are rooted in this contrast-recognition physiology. Red-green color deficiency, which occurs commonly on the basis of X-linked inheritance in males, has traditionally been separated into protan and deutan categories, referring to absent or defective red-sensitive pigment or green-sensitive pigment, respectively. These distinctions have some clinical value in terms of what patients perceive, even though normal individuals often have a duplication of pigment genes, and color-deficient individuals do not necessarily have single or simple gene defects (see Figure 8-1 and the accompanying discussion). Blue-yellow color deficiency, exceedingly rare on a congenital basis, is frequently found in acquired diseases and thus can be an important marker for them. The inherited color vision defects are described in Chapter 8.

The most accurate instrument for classifying congenital red-green color defects is the *anomaloscope*, but it is not widely used. The patient views a split screen and is asked to match the yellow appearance of one half by mixing varying proportions of red and green light in the other half. Individuals with red-green color deficiency use abnormal proportions of red and green to make the match.

Tests of color vision

The most common tests for color vision use colored tablets or diagrams. These color tests are accurate only in proper lighting, usually blue-white illumination that mimics sunlight. Pseudoisochromatic plates such as the *Ishihara* and *Hardy-Rand-Rittler plates* depict colored numbers or figures that stand out from a background of colored dots (Fig 3-14). The colors of the test figure and background are purposely pale and are carefully chosen from hues that are difficult for a color-deficient patient to distinguish. Individuals with defective color vision see either no pattern at all or an alternative pattern based on brightness rather than hue. The pseudoisochromatic plate tests can be done quickly and are sufficiently sensitive for screening color-deficient people, but they are not effective in classifying deficiency.

The panel tests, including the Farnsworth Panel D-15 and Farnsworth-Munsell 100-hue tests, are much more accurate in classifying color deficiency. The *Farnsworth-Munsell 100-hue test* is very sensitive because the difference in hues between adjacent tablets approximates the minimum that a normal observer is able to distinguish (1–4 nm). The spectrum is divided into 4 parts during testing and the patient is asked to discriminate between subtle shades of similar colors. However, the test is fatiguing and time-consuming.

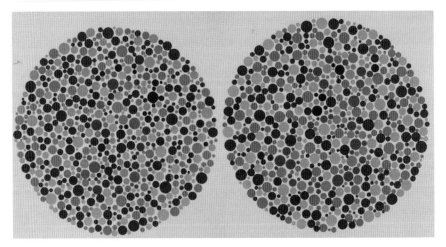

Figure 3-14 Pseudoisochromatic plates. *(Photographs courtesy of Carl Regillo, MD.)*

The *Farnsworth Panel D-15* (Fig 3-15) is a considerably quicker and more convenient test for routine clinical use because it consists of only a single box of 15 colored tablets. The hues are more saturated, and they cover the spectrum so that patients will confuse colors for which they have deficient perception (such as red and green). The patient is asked to arrange the tablets in sequence, and errors can be plotted very quickly on a simple circular diagram to define the nature of the color deficiency (Fig 3-16). The D-15 test is not very sensitive and may miss mildly affected individuals, but its speed and accuracy make it useful. The relative insensitivity can also be an asset in judging the practical significance of mild degrees of color deficiency. For example, individuals who fail the Ishihara plates but pass the D-15 panel will probably not have color discrimination problems under most circumstances and in most jobs. Desaturated versions of the D-15 test, which recognize more subtle degrees of color deficiency, are also available.

The Panel D-15 is probably the most useful color test in assessing retinal diseases because it discriminates well between congenital and acquired defects. Individuals with major congenital color deficiencies typically make errors that show a very precise protan or deutan pattern on the D-15 scoring graph, whereas those with acquired optic nerve or retinal disease show an irregular pattern of errors (see Fig 3-16). The D-15 test shows tritan (blue-yellow confusion) errors very clearly; these almost always signify acquired disease. The blue cones are few in number relative to the red and green cones and seem to be preferentially affected in many diseases. Although it is sometimes written that optic nerve disease usually causes red-green defects and retinal disease blue-yellow defects, this distinction is not reliable.

Green DG. Visual acuity, color vision, and adaptation. In: Albert DM, Jakobiec FA, eds. *Principles and Practice of Ophthalmology.* 2nd ed. Philadelphia: Saunders; 2000:1673– 1689.

Nathans J, Piantanida TP, Eddy RL, et al. Molecular genetics of inherited variation in human color vision. *Science.* 1986;232:203–210.

Nathans J, Thomas D, Hogness DS. Molecular genetics of human color vision: the genes encoding blue, green, and red pigments. *Science.* 1986;232:193–202.

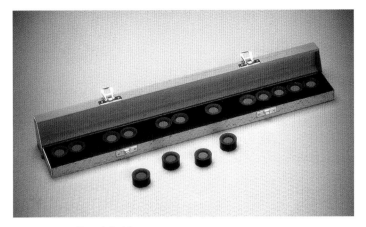

Figure 3-15 Panel D-15 test. *(Photograph courtesy of Luneau Ophtamologie.)*

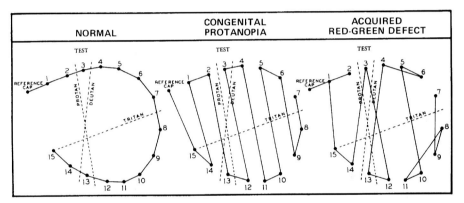

Figure 3-16 Graphed results of the Farnsworth Panel D-15 test. Individuals with congenital red-green defects make errors that show a well-defined axis of confusion. Individuals with acquired defects tend to make irregular errors. *(Reprinted with permission from Marmor MF. The management of retinitis pigmentosa and allied diseases.* Ophthalmology Digest. *1979;41:13–29.)*

Contrast Sensitivity

Visual acuity measures only one component of the visual process. Our visual system codes most of what we see on the basis of *contrast* rather than spatial resolution. Subtleties of light and dark provide much of the richness of visual perception. When dusk, fog, or smoke reduces contrast, it becomes very difficult to resolve ordinary objects. Patients with retinal disease may have poor contrast sensitivity, which causes them to complain of dim vision or show poor object recognition even though they can still read small letters under ideal test conditions. Thus, contrast sensitivity is an independent test of visual function.

Testing of contrast sensitivity

Several clinical contrast sensitivity tests are now on the market, and most of them relate contrast sensitivity to *spatial frequency*, which refers to the size of the light–dark cycles.

We are normally most sensitive to contrast for objects having a spatial frequency between 2 and 5 cycles per degree (Fig 3-17), but this can change in disease. Some contrast sensitivity tests are based on letters or optotypes of varying dimness and size to provide a more clinical context.

Contrast sensitivity testing shows clearly why some patients with nominal good acuity have subjective visual difficulties. The vast majority of patients with retinitis pigmentosa, for example, show reduced contrast sensitivity even when their visual acuity is good (20/25 or better). However, this is also true in patients with media opacities, optic nerve disease, and ill-defined age-related eye disease. Because disease-specific diagnostic pat-

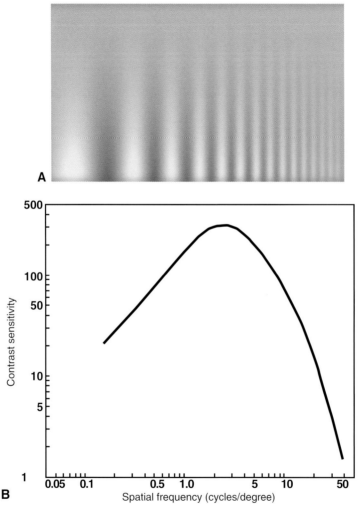

Figure 3-17 Contrast sensitivity. **A,** Grating in which the contrast diminishes from bottom to top, and the spatial frequency of the pattern increases from left to right. The pattern appears to have a hump in the middle at the frequencies for which the human eye is most sensitive to contrast. **B,** Plot of the contrast sensitivity function. *(Part A courtesy of Brian Wandell, PhD.)*

terns of contrast deficiency have not yet emerged, the main value of contrast sensitivity testing is to demonstrate or corroborate visual disability rather than to diagnose disease.

Contrast sensitivity testing is discussed further in BCSC Section 3, *Clinical Optics*, and in Section 5, *Neuro-Ophthalmology*.

Marmor MF. Contrast sensitivity versus visual acuity in retinal disease. *Br J Ophthalmol.* 1986;70:553–559.

Nadler MP, Miller D, Nadler DJ, eds. *Glare and Contrast Sensitivity for Clinicians.* New York: Springer-Verlag; 1990.

PART II

Disorders of the Retina and Vitreous

CHAPTER 4

Acquired Diseases Affecting the Macula

This chapter reviews a variety of common, acquired conditions affecting the macula, including central serous chorioretinopathy, age-related macular degeneration and other diseases commonly associated with choroidal neovascularization, and retinal interface disorders (epiretinal membranes, macular cysts, and macular holes). Acquired maculopathies related to systemic or ocular medications are discussed in Chapters 5 and 10.

Central Serous Chorioretinopathy

Central serous chorioretinopathy (CSC), also called *central serous retinopathy (CSR)* or *choroidopathy*, is an idiopathic condition characterized by the development of a well-circumscribed, serous detachment of the sensory retina (neuroepithelium) resulting from altered barrier and deficient pumping functions at the level of the retinal pigment epithelium (RPE), although the primary pathology may involve the choriocapillaris. Some cases may also show serous detachments of the RPE, usually under the superior half of the serous retinal detachment. Often, small, whitish subretinal precipitates or gray-white subretinal sheets may be noted, probably indicating the presence of fibrin. In many patients, evidence of previous episodes is indicated by extramacular RPE atrophic areas.

CSC occurs preferentially in healthy men between 25 and 55 years of age. Most patients are asymptomatic unless the central macula is affected. CSC is common in Caucasians, Asians, and Hispanics, and rare in African Americans. Symptomatic patients describe the sudden onset of blurred and dim vision, micropsia, metamorphopsia, paracentral scotomata, or decreased color vision. In general, vision ranges from 20/20 to 20/200, but in most patients vision is better than 20/30. The decreased vision can often be corrected with a hyperopic correction. In rare cases, these symptoms are accompanied by a migraine-like headache. Certain personality types, including type A personality; hypochondria; hysteria; conversional neurosis; and psychiatric medication use have been associated with CSC. Patients with elevated levels of steroids due to either steroid administration (inhaled, topical, or systemic) or Cushing syndrome are at an increased risk of developing CSC. Finally, stress has also been implicated as an etiologic factor, but no conclusive proof has been presented.

Carvalho-Recchia CA, Yannuzzi LA, Negrao S, et al. Corticosteroids and central serous cho-rioretinopathy. *Ophthalmology.* 2002;109:1834–1837.

Fluorescein Angiography of CSC

Three characteristic fluorescein angiographic patterns are seen in CSC:

- expansile dot pattern
- smokestack pattern
- diffuse pattern

An *expansile dot* of hyperfluorescence is the most common presentation. The dot represents a small, focal hyperfluorescent leak from the choroid through the RPE that appears in the early phase of the angiogram and increases in size and intensity as the angiogram progresses (see Fig 2-2 in Chapter 2). Fluorescein dye also slowly pools into the subretinal detachment as the angiogram progresses. Late-phase frames of the angiogram at 10 or 15 minutes are often required to detect very slow leaks or to discern the extent of fluorescein pooling in the subsensory retinal space. In some patients, several leaking expansile dots may be present. If no expansile dot is seen in the macula, the extramacular space, especially superiorly, should be evaluated.

Occasionally, fluorescein leakage into the subretinal fluid pocket produces a pattern of subretinal pooling referred to as a *smokestack.* The fluorescein starts with a central spot of hyperfluorescence that spreads vertically and, finally, laterally, in a configuration evocative of a plume of smoke. This unique pattern is felt to be secondary to convection currents and a pressure gradient between the protein concentration of the subretinal fluid and the fluorescein dye entering the detachment. Although dramatic, this angiographic presentation is uncommon, occurring in approximately 10% of cases.

In rare cases, an extensive, often gravity-dependent, serous detachment of the retina may develop from one or more leak points outside the posterior pole. This situation produces a *diffuse pattern* of fluorescein leakage, often without any obvious leakage point. Patients with this condition often have large areas of serous detachment and extensive RPE changes. Thus, CSC must be considered in the differential diagnosis of nonrhegmatogenous serous retinal detachment. Indolent cases also occur, in which fluid moves chronically from the choroid to the subretinal space and causes areas of abnormal RPE to expand.

Leakage should not be interpreted as the only reason for accumulation of subretinal fluid. Although a leak is necessary for fluid to enter the subretinal space, this fluid would normally be removed promptly by the RPE/choroid. In CSC, however, the fluid continues to accumulate because the primary disease is probably a diffuse abnormality of the RPE/choroid that impairs fluid removal. Thus, a localized serous detachment of the RPE without overlying neurosensory elevation can be seen.

Other Imaging Modalities for CSC

Optical coherence tomography (OCT) is an excellent, noninvasive method to use for diagnosing and following the resolution of the subretinal fluid in CSC. Subtle fluid accumulation beneath the sensory retina and the RPE not evident on fluorescein angiography and clinical examination can often be picked up by OCT.

Indocyanine green (ICG) angiography can be used to show characteristic multifocal choroidal hyperfluorescent patches that appear early in the angiogram. These areas slowly enlarge during the angiogram but are less prominent in late views. ICG can be useful in helping to distinguish atypical diffuse CSC in older patients from occult choroidal neovascularization (CNV) in exudative age-related macular degeneration (AMD) and idiopathic polypoidal choroidal vasculopathy.

Differential Diagnosis

The presence of subretinal fluid in older patients with CSC requires the physician to also consider a diagnosis of CNV associated with AMD, optic nerve pits, idiopathic polypoidal choroidal vasculopathy, and idiopathic uveal effusion syndrome (IUES). Features that help to differentiate CSC from these other entities include the following:

- A pinpoint leak relative to a large area of subretinal fluid most likely represents CSC, whereas the area of subretinal fluid associated with CNV and idiopathic polypoidal choroidal vasculopathy usually corresponds closely to the area of leakage on angiography. The leakage in IUES is usually diffuse.
- Optic nerve pits are often visible on the nerve and are contiguous with the subretinal fluid accumulation. No pinpoint leakage is seen.
- Multifocal RPE abnormalities, including small serous pigment epithelial detachments (PED) in one or both eyes, more likely represent CSC, whereas the presence of large drusen more likely represents AMD.
- Saccular outpouchings are characteristic of idiopathic polypoidal choroidal vasculopathy; these can be differentiated from the multifocal hyperfluorescent patches of CSC through ICG angiography.
- Absence of blood or significant lipid is more likely to represent CSC, whereas their presence is more likely to represent CNV or idiopathic polypoidal choroidal vasculopathy.

Older patients presenting with CNV occasionally may show evidence suggestive of previous CSC.

Natural Course and Management

The visual prognosis of CSC is usually good except in chronic, recurrent cases and in cases of bullous CSC. Most eyes with CSC (80%–90%) undergo spontaneous resorption of subretinal fluid within 3 to 4 months; recovery of visual acuity usually follows, but can take up to a year. Mild metamorphopsia, faint scotomata, abnormalities in contrast sensitivity, and mild color vision deficits frequently persist. Some eyes suffer permanently diminished visual acuity, and many (40%–50%) experience one or more recurrences. A small subset of patients has poor visual outcomes.

Laser photocoagulation at the site of fluorescein leakage can induce rapid remission; resorption of subretinal fluid may occur within several weeks of the photocoagulation therapy. A randomized, controlled clinical study by Watzke and colleagues in 1974 of ruby laser photocoagulation in eyes with active CSC showed a significantly more rapid resorption of subretinal fluid in treated eyes (5-week median duration from laser treatment to remission) than in untreated eyes (23-week median duration from examination to spontaneous remission). However, this study did not find that the final Snellen visual acuity was any better in the treated eyes despite the shorter duration of the disease; nor was there any evidence that treatment altered the recurrence rate. Because no patients in this study were treated earlier than 8 weeks following the onset of symptoms, it is uncertain whether earlier treatment would have improved the visual prognosis. Furthermore, the number of patients evaluated was too small to rule out a small or moderate difference between treated and untreated eyes; follow-up was limited; and standardized protocol refractions and visual acuity testing were not performed.

Until the value of early photocoagulation has been tested further, current treatment guidelines suggest that patients may be observed for at least 3–4 months (average time for spontaneous recovery) in most first episodes of unilateral CSC. Laser photocoagulation may be considered in the following instances:

- The serous detachment persists beyond 3–4 months.
- The disease recurs in eyes with visual deficits from previous episodes.
- A permanent visual deficit is present from previous episodes in the fellow eye.
- Chronic signs develop, such as cystic changes in the neurosensory retina or widespread RPE abnormalities.
- Occupational or other patient needs require prompt restoration of vision or stereopsis.

If laser photocoagulation is performed, follow-up within 3–4 weeks may assist in detecting the rare complication of postlaser CNV. However, even without laser treatment, patients with typical CSC may, rarely, develop CNV.

According to some case reports, when the leakage site was too close to the center of the fovea for laser photocoagulation, CSC was resolved by photodynamic therapy (PDT) treatment.

Gass JD. Bullous retinal detachment: an unusual manifestation of idiopathic central serous choroidopathy. *Am J Ophthalmol*. 1973;75:810–821.

Loo RH, Scott IU, Flynn HW Jr, et al. Factors associated with reduced visual acuity during long-term follow-up of patients with idiopathic central serous chorioretinopathy. *Retina*. 2002;22:19–24.

Marmor MF. Control of subretinal fluid: experimental and clinical studies. *Eye*. 1990;4(pt 2):340–344.

Watzke RC, Burton TC, Leaverton PE. Ruby laser photocoagulation therapy of central serous retinopathy. I. A controlled clinical study. II. Factors affecting prognosis. *Trans Am Acad Ophthalmol Otolaryngol*. 1974;78:205–211.

Watzke RC, Burton TC, Woolson RF. Direct and indirect laser photocoagulation of central serous choroidopathy. *Am J Ophthalmol*. 1979;88:914–918.

Age-Related Macular Degeneration

Age-related macular degeneration (AMD), previously called *age-related maculopathy* or *senile macular degeneration,* is the leading cause of severe central visual acuity loss in one or both eyes in people over 50 years of age in the United States. Although the term *macular degeneration* may be used to describe any degenerative abnormality in the macula, the words *age-related* should probably be added only for eyes that demonstrate the nonneovascular or neovascular abnormalities described in the following discussion.

Normal aging results in a spectrum of changes in the macula, many clinically undetected, that affect the outer retina, RPE, Bruch's membrane, and choriocapillaris:

- Photoreceptors are reduced in density and distribution.
- Ultrastructural aging changes occur in the pigment epithelium, including loss of melanin granules, formation of lipofuscin granules, and accumulation of residual bodies.
- Basal laminar deposits accumulate; these consist of granular lipid-rich material and widely spaced collagen fibers collecting between the basal lamina (plasma membrane) of the RPE cell and the inner aspect of the basement membrane of the RPE (Fig 4-1).
- Progressive involutional changes occur in the choriocapillaris.

All of these changes represent aging but may not be part of AMD. Abnormalities associated with AMD that are not necessarily part of normal aging may be classified into nonneovascular and neovascular abnormalities.

Population-based studies have shown that most patients with AMD have only nonneovascular abnormalities such as drusen, focal hyperpigmentation, or geographic atrophy (RPE degeneration). These patients are usually asymptomatic or may have a mild decrease in vision and/or metamorphopsia. The advanced atrophic form may have central or pericentral scotomata. Severe visual loss from AMD usually occurs in individuals with neovascular abnormalities or subfoveal geographic atrophy of the RPE.

The risk of AMD increases with age. In the Framingham Eye Study, 6.4% of patients aged 65–74 years old and 19.7% of patients older than 75 years had signs of AMD. Other risk factors for AMD include positive family history, cigarette smoking, hyperopia, light iris color, hypertension, hypercholesterolemia, female gender, and cardiovascular disease.

Nonneovascular Abnormalities in AMD

The hallmark of the nonneovascular (nonexudative) form of AMD is drusen; other indicators are abnormalities of the RPE, including geographic atrophy and areas of hyperpigmentation.

Drusen

Clinically, drusen are small, round, yellow lesions located at the level of the RPE within the macula (Fig 4-2). Histologically, this material corresponds to the abnormal thickening of the inner aspect of Bruch's membrane shown in Figure 4-1. Ultrastructurally, the material includes basal *laminar* deposits (granular lipid-rich material and widely spaced collagen fibers) and basal *linear* deposits (phospholipid vesicles and electron-dense granules *within* the inner aspect of Bruch's membrane). Both are illustrated in Figure 4-1.

The thickened inner aspect of Bruch's membrane, along with the RPE, may separate from the rest of Bruch's membrane, resulting in a pigment epithelial detachment. When

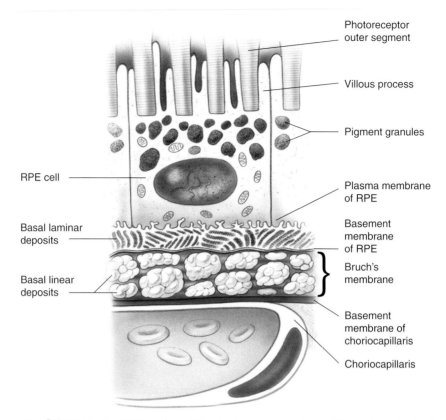

Photoreceptor outer segment

Villous process

Pigment granules

RPE cell

Plasma membrane of RPE

Basement membrane of RPE

Basal laminar deposits

Bruch's membrane

Basal linear deposits

Basement membrane of choriocapillaris

Choriocapillaris

Figure 4-1 Schematic illustration of basal laminar deposits and basal linear deposits that result in a thickened inner aspect of Bruch's membrane. *(Illustration by Christine Gralapp.)*

small, such a detachment may be identified as a large druse. When the detachment covers a relatively large area, it may be recognized as a detachment of the RPE. Whether small or large, these areas of detachment may fill rapidly with fluorescein as the dye leaks out of the choriocapillaris and pools within the area of detached RPE.

Because drusen seldom affect the photoreceptors overlying the area of abnormal material, they typically do not cause symptoms. However, some patients may have some

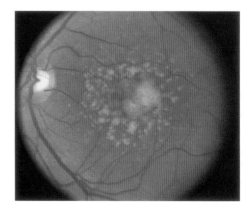

Figure 4-2 Soft, confluent drusen in AMD.

minimal photoreceptor loss, causing a reduction in vision or difficulties with dark adaptation.

When fundus photographs are obtained of entire populations over the age of 50, the vast majority of participants show tiny yellow deposits—drusen—at the level of the outer retina. Because many of these patients will not actually progress to visual loss from subsequent atrophy or CNV, various classifications have been developed in an attempt to distinguish the yellow deposits that will likely lead to atrophy or CNV from those that will not. Drusen have been categorized as

- *small* (usually <64 μm in diameter)
- *intermediate* (usually 64–124 μm in diameter)
- *large* (usually ≥125 μm in diameter)

Small drusen are well-defined focal areas of lipidization in the RPE or accumulations of hyaline material in Bruch's membrane. Small, hard drusen occur with aging and may be a precursor to AMD, but alone they are not enough to make the diagnosis of AMD. In the Age-Related Eye Disease Study (AREDS), the risk of progression to advanced AMD over a 5-year period for patients with early AMD (many small drusen or few intermediate drusen) was 1.3%. In contrast, the risk in patients with many intermediate or larger drusen was 18%. Patients in the latter group are also more likely to develop RPE abnormalities and geographic atrophy or CNV compared to patients with a few small or medium drusen. The presence of many intermediate or larger drusen is enough to diagnose nonneovascular AMD.

In addition, the boundaries of drusen have been described as

- *hard* (discrete and well demarcated)
- *soft* (amorphous and poorly demarcated; see Fig 4-2)
- *confluent* (contiguous boundaries between drusen)

Soft drusen are associated with the presence of diffuse thickening of the inner aspects of Bruch's membrane. An eye with soft, and perhaps *confluent*, drusen is more likely to progress to atrophy or CNV than an eye with only *hard* drusen.

On fluorescein angiography, drusen will stain in late views, or fluorescein may pool in areas of diffuse thickening.

Abnormalities of the RPE

Several patterns of RPE abnormalities characterize nonneovascular AMD:

- geographic atrophy
- nongeographic atrophy
- focal hyperpigmentation

Characteristic abnormalities Spontaneous flattening of RPE detachments or regression of soft, confluent drusen may lead to attenuation or atrophy of RPE cells. When the area in which the RPE is either absent or attenuated is contiguous, the condition is known as *geographic atrophy* of the RPE. In areas of geographic atrophy, the underlying choroidal vessels are more readily visible and the overlying outer retina may appear thin (Fig 4-3). Often, the underlying choriocapillaris will be attenuated or atrophied as well. These areas of atrophy can coalesce and enlarge, often ringing the fovea. On fluorescein angiography,

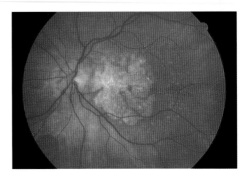

Figure 4-3 A well-demarcated area of geographic atrophy of the RPE; choroidal vessels can be easily seen within the atrophied area. *(Photograph courtesy of Neil M. Bressler, MD.)*

geographic atrophy shows a characteristic window defect. If the atrophy does not cover a contiguous area, it may appear as a mottled area of depigmentation called *nongeographic atrophy*, or RPE degeneration.

Photoreceptors cannot be seen by biomicroscopy, but they are usually attenuated or absent in areas overlying atrophied RPE. Consequently, RPE atrophy in AMD may be associated with visual loss, depending on the extent of the atrophy and its location relative to the foveal center. Although not everyone with drusen will develop atrophy, the incidence of atrophy appears to increase with age. Moreover, eyes with geographic atrophy are at risk of visual loss with enlargement of the atrophic areas and progressive foveal involvement. The incidence of legal blindness due to central geographic atrophy is 12%–20%.

Increased pigmentation at the level of the outer retina leads to *focal hyperpigmentation* of the RPE. On fluorescein angiography, these areas often show blockage. The incidence of focal hyperpigmentation increases with age, and patients with focal clumps of hyperpigmentation are at an increased risk of progressing to the more advanced forms of AMD.

Other abnormalities As atrophy develops, other abnormalities of the RPE may become recognizable. For example, the material that makes up the drusen may begin to disappear, a condition sometimes referred to as *regressed drusen*. In addition, dystrophic calcification may occur, resulting in pinpoint glistening within the atrophy or remaining drusen material, sometimes called *calcified drusen*. Furthermore, pigment or pigment-laden cells (either RPE cells or macrophages that have ingested the pigment) may migrate to the photoreceptor level, resulting in focal clumps or a reticulated pattern of hyperpigmentation.

Fluorescein angiogram patterns of AMD

The fluorescein patterns of AMD are varied and can be categorized into hyper- and hypofluorescent lesions:

Hyperfluorescent lesions:

- hard and soft drusen
- RPE atrophy
- RPE tear
- CNV (discussed further later in the chapter)
- serous pigment epithelial detachment

- subretinal fibrosis
- laser scars

Hypofluorescent lesions:

- hemorrhage at any level
- lipid
- pigment proliferation

Bressler SB, Bressler NM, Gragoudas ES. Age-related macular degeneration: drusen and geographic atrophy. In: Albert DM, Jakobiec FA, eds. *Principles and Practice of Ophthalmology.* 2nd ed. Philadelphia: Saunders; 2000:1982–1991.

Sarks JP, Sarks SH, Killingsworth MC. Evolution of geographic atrophy of the retinal pigment epithelium. *Eye.* 1988;2(pt 5):552–577.

Differential diagnosis for nonneovascular AMD

A variety of conditions may have abnormalities of the RPE that mimic the nonneovascular changes in AMD. *Central serous chorioretinopathy (CSC)* (discussed earlier) may cause RPE changes similar to those in AMD; the diagnosis may not be difficult in individuals under 50 years of age. In individuals over 50 years of age, the absence of drusen, mottled RPE atrophy, and/or multiple small serous detachments of the RPE may help differentiate CSC from nonneovascular changes in AMD. *Pattern dystrophy* of the RPE may include one or more areas of focal pinpoint or reticular hyperpigmentation surrounded by a yellowish abnormality (vitelliform detachment) of the outer retina. Fluorescein angiography depicts early blocked fluorescence with a surrounding zone of hyperfluorescence. Late staining of the yellow material may occur and helps distinguish these cases of pattern dystrophy from AMD. These features may occur in individuals younger than those who would normally be suspected of having AMD. Alternatively, these changes may be seen in older individuals who have developed the more typical drusen and abnormalities of the RPE seen in AMD. *Basal laminar,* or *cuticular, drusen,* a clinical syndrome that may be seen in patients in their 30s or 40s, consists of innumerable and homogeneous round small or large drusen, more apparent on angiography ("starry-night" appearance) than biomicroscopy, often with a vitelliform accumulation of yellow material in the central macula. The retinal signs of *drug toxicity,* such as the mottled hypopigmentation that may develop in chloroquine toxicity, may resemble nongeographic atrophy (RPE degeneration); a history of specific drug ingestion and lack of large drusen may help to differentiate these abnormalities from AMD (see Chapter 10).

Bressler NM, Bressler SB, Gragoudas ES. Age-related macular degeneration: RPE detachment and subretinal neovascularization. In: Albert DM, Jakobiec FA, eds. *Principles and Practice of Ophthalmology.* 2nd ed. Philadelphia: Saunders; 2000.

Management of nonneovascular form of AMD

Education and follow-up Eyes with soft drusen and RPE hyperpigmentation are at increased risk of developing geographic atrophy and CNV. Patients with drusen or abnormalities of the RPE in one or both eyes should be taught how to recognize symptoms of advanced AMD and instructed to contact an ophthalmologist promptly if such symptoms are noted. Office staff should be educated to respond promptly to these new symptoms. Each eye is tested *individually* for any new metamorphopsia, scotoma, or other significant change in central vision. If visual loss is found to be caused by geographic atrophy in both eyes, a low vision evaluation should be considered. Periodic examinations are advised to monitor for intercurrent treatable eye disease (eg, cataract) and to reevaluate progressive low vision needs.

Micronutrients Patients often inquire about the role of micronutrients in preventing either the development or the progression of AMD. Ophthalmologists should counsel patients that several epidemiologic studies have demonstrated positive associations between certain micronutrients and decreased risk of AMD, although only some micronutrients have been studied.

The Age-Related Eye Disease Study (AREDS; Clinical Trial 4-1) enrolled 4753 patients at 11 clinical centers and evaluated the effect of high-dose micronutrient supplements consisting of antioxidants and vitamins (500 mg vitamin C, 400 IU vitamin E, and 15 mg beta carotene) and zinc (80 mg zinc oxide and 2 mg cupric oxide to prevent zinc-induced anemia) on AMD and vision loss. The results showed that individuals with intermediate AMD (few intermediate or at least one large druse, or nonsubfoveal geographic atrophy) or advanced unilateral AMD (vision loss due to AMD in one eye) who had been randomly assigned to the combination supplement group had a 25% reduction of risk for progression to advanced AMD and a 19% risk reduction in rates of moderate vision loss ($\geq$3 lines of visual acuity) by 5 years. Subjects with no AMD or only early AMD (few small drusen) did not derive any benefit.

CLINICAL TRIAL 4-1

Age-Related Eye Disease Study (AREDS)

Objectives: (1) Evaluate incidence of age-related cataract and age-related macular degeneration. (2) Evaluate risk factors associated with these two age-related eye diseases. (3) Evaluate whether antioxidants or zinc supplements can reduce development or progression of cataract or AMD.

Participants: 4757 men and women, age 55–80 at time of enrollment (1992–1995) at 11 tertiary care centers or retina referral private practices. Study eyes have either no evidence of AMD or varying levels of drusen or RPE abnormalities, with visual acuity of $\geq$20/32.

Intervention: Participants without AMD randomly assigned (1:1) to placebo or antioxidants. Participants with early or intermediate AMD or unilateral advanced AMD randomly assigned (1:1:1:1) to placebo, antioxidants, zinc, or a combination of antioxidants and zinc.

Outcome Measure: Doubling of the visual angle or development of advanced AMD.

Present Status: Participants examined at 6-month intervals through fall 2001, then annually through 2006. See discussion under Management of Nonneovascular Form of AMD for results announced in fall 2001.

Recommendations of the AREDS include the following:

- Identify individuals at high risk of AMD progression and vision loss, including those with
  - extensive intermediate drusen
  - at least 1 large druse
  - noncentral geographic atrophy
  - advanced AMD in 1 eye
- Consider supplementation for these patients with a combined antioxidant and mineral formulation to decrease rates of disease progression and vision loss. (Supplementation without beta carotene is preferable for patients who smoke because beta carotene has been shown to increase the risk of lung cancer in smokers.)
- In patients with early AMD or those at high risk of AMD (including family members), supplementation was not shown to be beneficial; however, these patients should maintain a balanced diet and avoid smoking.
- The benefits of lutein and other micronutrients are not known, and thus such micronutrients are not recommended until the results of additional studies are positive.

Age-Related Eye Disease Study Research Group. A randomized, placebo-controlled, clinical trial of high-dose supplementation with vitamins C and E, beta carotene, and zinc for age-related macular degeneration and vision loss: AREDS report no. 8. *Arch Ophthalmol.* 2001;119:1417–1436.

Avoiding UV light Although a small correlation has been seen between increased exposure to visible light over a 20-year period and the development of geographic atrophy or disciform scarring, no studies have proven a relationship between ultraviolet light and AMD. Several epidemiologic studies have suggested that light toxicity might have a role in the development or progression of AMD, but the data have not shown *consistent* associations across studies, and the associations do not *prove* a cause-and-effect relationship. Nevertheless, the use of sunglasses or a hat outdoors, which may block out some visible light with little expense and no known side effects, certainly should not be discouraged.

Laser photocoagulation The Choroidal Neovascularization Prevention Trial (CNVPT) was a multicenter randomized pilot study determining the feasibility of a large-scale trial to evaluate prophylactic photocoagulation in eyes with high-risk nonneovascular AMD. Results from the Fellow Eye Study Group demonstrated a higher incidence of CNV among treated eyes (15% vs 3%) compared to observed eyes. However, despite the increased risk of CNV with prophylactic laser, there was no detrimental effect on visual acuity. Similarly, in the pilot study of the Prophylactic Treatment of AMD (PTAMD) Trial, treated patients were more likely to have a CNV event (21% vs 14%; $P = .02$) compared to the observed eyes at 18 months. Although another large study, the Bilateral Drusen Study Group, did not demonstrate a significant difference in the incidence of CNV between the 2 groups, the recommendation of the PTAMD is that prophylactic laser is of no benefit in preventing CNV if the fellow eye has already suffered a neovascular event. Currently, 2 large, nationwide randomized trials are evaluating the use of lower-power laser photocoagulation in a grid pattern to decrease the risk of visual loss in nonexudative AMD:

- Complications of Age-Related Macular Degeneration Prevention Trial (CAPT; Clinical Trial 4-2): 1052 patients were enrolled in a study (mean age 71 years; 99.3% Caucasian) to determine if macular grid argon photocoagulation in one eye of an individual with bilateral nonneovascular AMD reduces vision loss from advancing AMD.
- Prophylactic Treatment of AMD Trial: 635 patients were enrolled in this study to determine if a grid of 48 spots using subthreshold treatment with an 810-nm diode laser in 1 eye of an individual with bilateral nonneovascular AMD reduces vision loss from advancing AMD.

Finally, differential membrane filtration or Rheopheresis (OccuLogix Corporation, Clearwater, FL) is a blood filtration system that depletes circulating macromolecules from the blood and is currently being evaluated in a randomized clinical trial. Until the results of this clinical trial are known, Rheopheresis is not recommended for nonexudative AMD.

Bressler NM, Bressler SB. Preventive ophthalmology: age-related macular degeneration. *Ophthalmology*. 1995:102:1206–1211.

Ho AC, Maguire MG, Yoken J, et al. Laser-induced drusen reduction improves visual function at 1 year. Choroidal Neovascularization Prevention Trial Research Group. *Ophthalmology*. 1999;106:1367–1374.

Laser treatment in eyes with large drusen: short-term effects seen in a pilot randomized clinical trial. Choroidal Neovascularization Prevention Trial Research Group. *Ophthalmology*. 1998;105:11–23.

CLINICAL TRIAL 4-2

Complications of Age-Related Macular Degeneration Prevention Trial (CAPT)

Objective: To determine if prophylactic laser treatment in eyes with nonneo-vascular AMD can reduce vision loss from subsequent CNV or geographic atrophy development.

Participants: 1052 individuals, minimum age of 50, with $\geq$10 large ($\geq$125 μm) drusen in each eye.

Intervention: Random assignment of right or left eye to photocoagulation. Treatment consists of 3 concentric rings of 100-μm laser spots placed 1500–2500 μm from the fovea, totaling 60 spots. At 1 year, eyes with inadequate drusen regression are retreated.

Outcome Measures: Vision loss, CNV or geographic atrophy development, change in contrast sensitivity or print size for reading.

Present Status: Enrollment closed March 2001; follow-up of all patients for 5 years planned.

Neovascular AMD

The hallmark of the neovascular form of AMD is the presence of CNV. Any disturbance of Bruch's membrane, such as the presence of drusen, thickening of the inner aspect, or conditions similar to the nonneovascular changes associated with AMD, can increase the likelihood that a break will occur, allowing buds of neovascular tissue from the choriocapillaris to perforate the outer aspect of Bruch's membrane. These new vessels are accompanied by fibroblasts, resulting in a fibrovascular complex that proliferates within the inner aspect of Bruch's membrane (Fig 4-4). This fibrovascular complex can disrupt and destroy the normal architecture of the choriocapillaris, Bruch's membrane, and the RPE. In addition, fibroglial and fibrovascular tissue can also disrupt and destroy the normal architecture of the photoreceptors and remaining outer retina leading to the formation of a disciform scar.

Signs and symptoms of neovascular AMD

Patients who develop neovascular AMD complain of the sudden onset of decreased vision, metamorphopsia, and paracentral scotomata. Clinically, there may be elevation of the RPE; subretinal or intraretinal lipid, fluid, or blood; pigment epithelial detachment (PED); retinal pigment epithelial tears; and occasionally the gray-green CNV lesion itself is seen. The presence of an intraretinal hemorrhage may be an early sign of a retinal angiomatous proliferation (RAP) lesion, with flow from the retinal circulation connecting to the CNV. Fluorescein angiography is the gold standard for diagnosing CNV. In cases with overlying blood or occult CNV, indocyanine green angiography offers clues to help in the decision-making process.

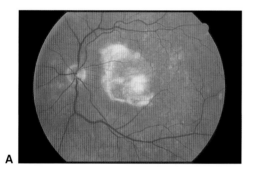

A

Figure 4-4 A, Endstage CNV that has progressed to fibrovascular scar, often called a *disciform scar.* **B,** Schematic cross section of a disciform scar depicting sub-RPE fibrovascular component and subretinal fibrocellular component. Note partial loss of photoreceptor layer overlying the disciform process and disturbance of the RPE and Bruch's membrane. *(Part A reproduced with permission from Bressler NM, Bressler SB, Fine SL. Age-related macular degeneration. Surv Ophthalmol. 1988;32:375–413. Part B illustration by Christine Gralapp.)*

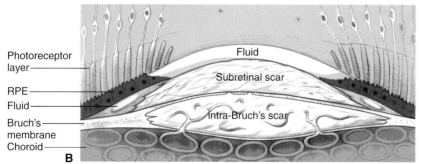

Photoreceptor layer

Fluid

Subretinal scar

RPE

Fluid

Intra-Bruch's scar

Bruch's membrane

Choroid

B

Choroidal neovascularization

CNV in the fovea is the major cause of severe central visual loss in AMD. A variety of clinical symptoms suggests the diagnosis of CNV. Patients often present with an otherwise unexplained, fairly sudden, decrease in visual acuity; central metamorphopsia; or a relative central scotoma. Signs of CNV may include

- the presence of subretinal fluid
- subretinal or sub–pigment epithelial blood
- subretinal or intraretinal lipid
- subretinal pigment ring
- irregular elevation of the pigment epithelium
- subretinal gray-white lesion
- cystoid macular edema
- a sea fan pattern of subretinal small vessels

CNV is an ingrowth of new vessels from the choriocapillaris through a break in the outer aspect of Bruch's membrane into the sub–pigment epithelial space, as shown in Figure 4-5. Within this space, the CNV can leak fluid and blood and may be accompanied by a serous or hemorrhagic detachment of the RPE. The blood may resorb, dissect under the retina, or, rarely, break into the vitreous cavity. In addition to the vascularization from the choroid, fibrous tissue may grow within Bruch's membrane, possibly accompanied by either fibrovascular or fibrocellular tissue between the neurosensory retina and the RPE. Ultimately, this process results in a disciform fibrovascular scar that replaces the normal architecture of the outer retina and leads to permanent loss of central vision (see Fig 4-4).

Fluorescein angiogram patterns of CNV Fluorescein patterns of CNV vary because the CNV lesion may be a complex of several lesion components that may include classic CNV, occult CNV, and features that may obscure CNV. Two major patterns of CNV are seen on fluorescein angiography:

- classic CNV
- occult CNV

Classic CNV is an area of bright, fairly uniform hyperfluorescence identified in the early phase of the angiogram that progressively intensifies throughout the transit phase, with leakage of dye obscuring the boundaries of this area by the late phases of the angiogram (Fig 4-6; see also Fig 2-1).

Occult CNV consists of 2 forms:

- fibrovascular pigment epithelial detachment (PED)
- late leakage of an undetermined source

Fibrovascular PED refers to an irregular elevation of the RPE with stippled or granular irregular fluorescence first seen early in the angiogram, usually by 1–2 minutes after dye injection. The irregular elevation of the RPE is best seen with stereo views on the angiogram. As the study progresses, there is progressive leakage from these regions, with a

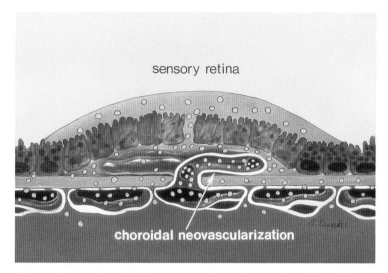

Figure 4-5 Schematic drawing of CNV originating from the choriocapillaris. Neovascularization proliferates within the diffusely thickened inner aspect of Bruch's membrane. Fibrosis accompanies the CNV beneath the RPE, and fibrovascular tissue has replaced normal RPE in some areas. Fibroglial tissue can be seen between the RPE and the photoreceptors, and some of the photoreceptors have been replaced by fibrovascular or fibroglial tissue. *(Reproduced with permission from Bressler NM, Bressler SB, Fine SL. Age-related macular degeneration.* Surv Ophthalmol. *1988;32:375–413.)*

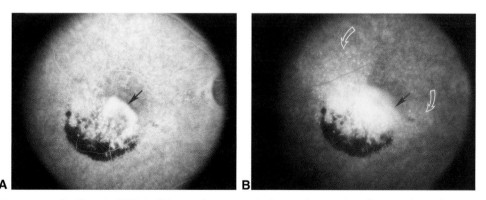

Figure 4-6 A, Classic CNV *(solid arrow)* appears during early transit as intense hyperfluorescence with early leakage manifested as blurred margins. **B,** Occult CNV *(curved arrows)* manifested as late leakage of an undetermined source lies contiguous to the classic CNV component of this lesion. The late leakage marked by the curved arrows creates poorly defined boundaries for the lesion. Furthermore, it does not correspond to classic CNV or to irregular elevation of the RPE in the early or midphase frames of the angiogram. *(Reproduced with permission from Macular Photocoagulation Study Group. Subfoveal neovascular lesions in age-related macular degeneration: guidelines for evaluation and treatment in the macular photocoagulation study.* Arch Ophthalmol. *1991;109:1242–1257.)*

stippled hyperfluorescent pattern that is not as diffuse as seen in classic CNV (see Fig 2-1B). *Late leakage of an undetermined source* refers to regions of fluorescence at the level of the RPE that are best appreciated in the late phases of an angiogram; they do not correspond to classic CNV or to areas of irregular elevation of the RPE during the early or mid phases of the angiogram.

The distinction between classic and occult CNV is important because the benefits of laser treatment have been shown only for cases that have some evidence of classic CNV, and the benefits of photodynamic therapy have presently been established only for those lesions that are *predominantly* classic or purely occult CNV. In addition, the natural course of CNV lesions that consist solely of occult CNV differs from that of CNV lesions that either consist solely of classic CNV or are mixtures of classic and occult CNV.

Lesion components such as contiguous thick blood, pigment, scar tissue, or a serous PED may either block fluorescence or intensify hyperfluorescence and thus obscure underlying CNV. When any of these obscuring features lies contiguous to hyperfluorescence from classic or occult CNV, visualization in that site of hyperfluorescence from underlying CNV may not be possible because of either

- blocked fluorescence, in the case of blood, pigment, or scar
- intense hyperfluorescence, in the case of serous PED

In either case, it is presumed that CNV lies beneath these elements, and they are included as lesion components.

When determining the size of a choroidal neovascular lesion, the examiner must take into account all areas of classic and occult CNV, as well as areas with obscured features. Recognition of blood, pigment, or scar tissue as a lesion component depends on clinical examination and blocked fluorescence during the fluorescein angiogram. Identification of a serous PED as a lesion component requires a smooth or dome-shaped area of RPE elevation with rapid, early, homogeneous, and intense fluorescence, that retains its same boundaries and intensity throughout the study. In contrast to a serous PED, a fibrovascular PED or occult CNV has irregular topography of the RPE elevation, a stippled and nonhomogeneous pattern of fluorescence, and a slow rate of filling with fluorescein. Such areas fluoresce between 1 and 3 minutes rather than between 20 and 60 seconds, and they may either leak or stain in the late phase.

The terms *predominantly classic, minimally classic,* and *occult with no classic* are important to know in order to understand who may benefit from photodynamic therapy. Predominantly classic lesions are lesions where the CNV occupies more than 50% of the lesion, including contiguous blood, pigment, scar, and staining. In addition, the proportion of classic CNV also occupies more than 50% of the entire lesion—not just 50% of the CNV. Minimally classic CNV is present when the proportion of classic CNV occupies between 1% and 49% of the entire lesion. Finally, occult with no classic CNV is present when there is no classic CNV in the lesion—only occult CNV.

The terms *poorly defined* or *poorly demarcated* CNV and *well-defined* or *well-demarcated* CNV should not be used as synonyms for classic and occult CNV, respectively. "Classic" and "occult" describe *fluorescein patterns* of CNV. "Poorly defined" and "well defined" describe how distinct the *boundaries* are between the entire CNV lesion and the uninvolved retina. In poorly defined CNV, the boundaries separating CNV from normal retina cannot be readily distinguished (see Fig 4-6); in well-defined CNV, the boundaries can easily be determined (see Fig 2-1A). Occult CNV can have well-defined borders and classic CNV can have poorly defined boundaries. This distinction is important because laser therapy should be applied to the entire area of CNV, and that area can be identified only when the boundaries of the entire lesion are well demarcated. The distinction is not as important when performing photodynamic therapy.

The appearance, shape, and size of a disciform lesion are related to a variety of factors, including the amount of fibrovascular tissue, the extent of RPE proliferation, and continued leakage from CNV. Massive exudation may occur beneath the neurosensory retina, resulting in an extensive nonrhegmatogenous retinal detachment.

Other imaging modalities, including high-speed angiography, ICG angiography, and ocular coherence tomography (OCT) can also image CNV; however, no randomized trials have proven the usefulness of these images in the management of CNV.

Differential diagnosis of neovascular AMD

A variety of conditions can mimic the neovascular changes of AMD. These clinical entities are listed in Table 4-1.

Retinal arterial macroaneurysms may be associated with preretinal, intraretinal, or subretinal hemorrhage. Because they present with sudden visual loss when blood involves the macula, the clinical appearance may resemble hemorrhage from CNV. In many cases, the subretinal hemorrhage *surrounds* the macroaneurysm, and fluorescein and ICG angiography may demonstrate the dilated lumen of the macroaneurysm along a retinal arteriole (Fig 4-7).

> Levin MR, Gragoudas ES. Retinal arterial macroaneurysms. In: Albert DM, Jakobiec FA, eds. *Principles and Practice of Ophthalmology.* 2nd ed. Philadelphia: Saunders; 2000:1950–1957.

Adult vitelliform dystrophy may resemble a retinal pigment epithelial detachment or a fundus with large confluent drusen. In vitelliform macular dystrophy, the staining of the vitelliform in an eye with *pattern dystrophy of the RPE* or in a patient with *basal laminar drusen* may be mistaken for the leakage seen in CNV. Usually, the staining of the vitelliform material is associated with marked blocked fluorescence in the early phase of the angiogram (Fig 4-8). Furthermore, even though the lesion often involves the foveal center, visual acuity remains relatively good.

> Vine AK, Schatz H. Adult-onset foveomacular pigment epithelial dystrophy. *Am J Ophthalmol.* 1980;89:680–691.

Polypoidal choroidal vasculopathy, also known as *posterior uveal bleeding syndrome,* is characterized by multiple and recurrent serosanguinous RPE detachments, which often

---

Table 4-1 Differential Diagnosis of Neovascular AMD

Macroaneurysms
Vitelliform detachments
Polypoidal choroidal vasculopathy
Central serous chorioretinopathy
Inflammatory conditions
Small tumor such as choroidal melanoma

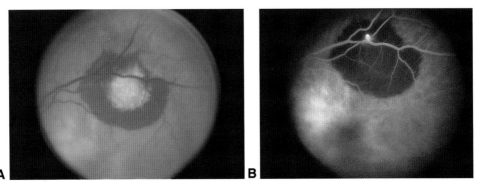

Figure 4-7 Retinal arterial macroaneurysm with subretinal hemorrhage resembling AMD. **A,** Clinical photograph shows subretinal hemorrhage surrounding the macroaneurysm. **B,** Fluorescein angiogram shows a characteristic hyperfluorescence of the macroaneurysm with blockage from the surrounding blood. *(Photographs courtesy of Harry W. Flynn Jr, MD.)*

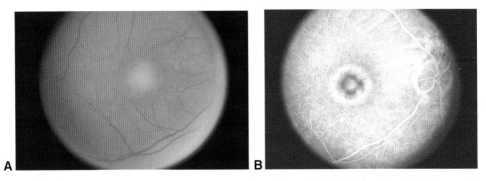

Figure 4-8 Adult vitelliform macular dystrophy. **A,** Patient with 20/50 visual acuity. The macular changes have been present for many years, and yet the patient has maintained relatively good visual acuity. **B,** Fluorescein angiogram shows a hyperfluorescent central lesion surrounded by a halo of retinal pigment epithelial atrophy. *(Photographs courtesy of Harry W. Flynn Jr, MD.)*

resemble hemorrhagic detachment in AMD. The first description of this syndrome was the occurrence of lesions in persons of African American or Asian ancestry and typically occurred in middle-aged females. It is now felt to occur in all races and also in males. The areas of serosanguinous detachment are often peripapillary, multifocal, orange, and nodular. Vitreous hemorrhage may occur more frequently than in AMD, and the typical soft drusen of AMD are not usually present. The natural history and visual acuity outcomes of polypoidal vasculopathy may be better than those of CNV associated with AMD (Fig 4-9).

Yannuzzi LA, Wong DW, Sforzolini BS, et al. Polypoidal choroidal vasculopathy and neovascularized age-related macular degeneration. *Arch Ophthalmol.* 1999;117:1503–1510.

Chronic central serous chorioretinopathy (CSC) with subretinal fluid can occasionally mimic the subretinal fluid seen with CNV and AMD. However, patients with CSC are usually younger and usually do not show a subretinal hemorrhagic process. CSC can be further differentiated by characteristic signs, including patches of mottled RPE atrophy (which sometimes assumes a gutterlike configuration) or multiple PEDs (Fig 4-10). The areas of pigment epithelial atrophy remaining after reabsorption of subretinal fluid are often geographic in their pattern and may extend below the inferior temporal arcade from the gravitational effect.

A variety of *inflammatory conditions* may cause changes in the outer retina with subretinal fluid accumulation in the macula. These include Vogt-Koyanagi-Harada syndrome, posterior scleritis, and systemic lupus erythematosus. These diseases generally have other distinguishing ocular and systemic features.

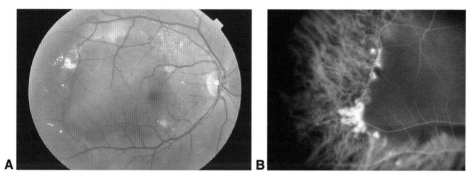

Figure 4-9 Polypoidal choroidal vasculopathy. **A,** Clinical photograph shows a large RPE detachment with multiple yellow-orange nodular lesions temporally. **B,** The ICG angiogram demonstrates the characteristic polypoidal lesions temporally. *(Photographs courtesy of Lawrence A. Yannuzzi, MD.)*

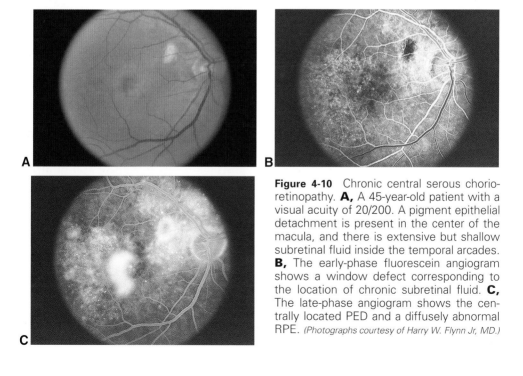

Figure 4-10 Chronic central serous chorioretinopathy. **A,** A 45-year-old patient with a visual acuity of 20/200. A pigment epithelial detachment is present in the center of the macula, and there is extensive but shallow subretinal fluid inside the temporal arcades. **B,** The early-phase fluorescein angiogram shows a window defect corresponding to the location of chronic subretinal fluid. **C,** The late-phase angiogram shows the centrally located PED and a diffusely abnormal RPE. *(Photographs courtesy of Harry W. Flynn Jr, MD.)*

Choroidal tumors, such as a small choroidal melanoma or choroidal hemangioma, may present with a mass effect and, occasionally, CNV on the surface that resembles AMD. Ultrasonography can help to differentiate the low reflectivity of a choroidal melanoma from the moderate to high reflectivity of a disciform scar.

Management of neovascular form of AMD

If neovascular AMD is suspected based on signs or symptoms, fluorescein angiography should be obtained and interpreted promptly. Stereoscopic angiography and late-phase photographs (2, 5, and 10 minutes after dye injection) may facilitate identification of occult CNV. Interpretation of fluorescein angiographic patterns of CNV associated with AMD can be fairly complicated (see Age-Related Macular Degeneration, Neovascular AMD, Choroidal Neovascularization in this chapter), but correct interpretation is crucial to making appropriate management recommendations.

Laser photocoagulation (thermal laser) Laser treatment has been used for classic CNV with well-demarcated boundaries or for lesions with classic and occult CNV components in which the lesion boundary has been well demarcated. Photocoagulation remains a proven therapy for extrafoveal and juxtafoveal lesions in those cases where the treating physician feels the foveal center will not be damaged by the treatment. In patients with subfoveal lesions or juxtafoveal lesions so close to the foveal center that laser treatment may damage the center of vision, treatment preference is shifting toward photodynamic therapy.

The goal of photocoagulation is specifically to decrease the risk of additional severe visual acuity loss beyond what the patient has already experienced (Table 4-2). In the Macular Photocoagulation Study (MPS), *severe visual acuity loss* was defined as the loss of 6 or more lines of vision on the vision chart, or a quadrupling or worse of the visual angle—for example, having visual acuity deteriorate from 20/40 to 20/160 or from 20/200 to 20/800 or worse. In all the MPS trials, treatment (as compared to observation) did not decrease the patient's chance of maintaining good visual acuity or vision within 1.5 lines of the visual acuity measured just prior to treatment. However, by 3–5 years after randomization, the proportion of eyes, treated or untreated, that maintained good visual acuity or vision within 1.5 lines of the initial measurement was very small.

A patient undergoing treatment for an extrafoveal or a juxtafoveal lesion (ie, a lesion that does not involve the foveal center) should understand that this therapy typically will not improve existing vision and will induce a permanent scotoma. Rather, as mentioned earlier, treatment is recommended to decrease the risk of progressive severe visual loss and a larger central scotoma. However, despite photocoagulation, many treated eyes with extrafoveal or juxtafoveal lesions continue to lose vision because of persistent or recurrent CNV, which usually extends into the foveal center and has a major impact on subsequent visual acuity (Fig 4-11). At the time of the MPS trials on extrafoveal and juxtafoveal lesions, the benefits of treating recurrences in the foveal center with any modality were not yet known; therefore, any subfoveal recurrences usually were left untreated. If the subfoveal recurrences that met treatment criteria for either subfoveal photocoagulation or PDT had actually been treated, it is likely that the benefits of extrafoveal or juxtafoveal photocoagulation would have been greater than what was reported (see Table 4-2).

Table 4-2 Management of Choroidal Neovascularization Based on Prospective Clinical Trials

Entity	Lesion Location/ Characteristics	Recommended Treatment Technique	Posttreatment Visual Acuity	Placebo/Untreated Visual Acuity	Retreatment/Recurrence Rates
AMD, extrafoveal	Foveal edge of CNV ≥200 μm from center of FAZ	Laser to cover CNV, contiguous blockage and 100 μm beyond	MPS at 5 years: 46% ≥6 line loss Median: 20/125	MPS at 5 years: 64% ≥6 line loss Median: 20/200	At 5 years: Recurrent CNV in 54% (78% of patients with REC ≥6 line loss vs 17% without REC)
AMD, juxtafoveal	Foveal edge of CNV <200 μm from center of FAZ	Laser to cover CNV, contiguous blockage and 100 μm beyond on nonfoveal side and if >100 μm from fovea, **unless** lesion is so close to the foveal center that laser may damage fovea; then consider ranibizumab, pegaptanib, or photodynamic therapy (PDT)	MPS at 5 years: 55% ≥6 line loss Median: 20/200	MPS at 5 years: 65% ≥6 line loss Median: 20/250	At 5 years: PER 32% REC 47% (69% of patients with REC ≥6 line loss vs 16% without REC)
AMD, subfoveal, predominantly classic CNV	CNV under fovea, CNV >50% of lesion, and classic CNV ≥50% of entire lesion	Ranibizumab, pegaptanib, or PDT	TAP at 2 years: 15% ≥6 line loss 41% ≥3 line loss VISION at 1 year: 32% ≥ 3 line loss	TAP at 2 years: 36% ≥6 line loss 69% ≥3 line loss VISION at 1 year: 43% ≥ 3 line loss	TAP at 2 years: 5.6 treatments needed TAP extension: 1.6 additional treatments over next 3 years
AMD, subfoveal, minimally classic CNV (≤4 MPS DA)	CNV under fovea, CNV >50% of lesion, and classic CNV <50% of entire lesion	Ranibizumab, pegaptanib, or PDT (needs evidence of disease progression)	VIM at 2 years: 13% ≥6 line loss 53% ≥3 line loss	VIM at 2 years: 35% ≥6 line loss 62% ≥3 line loss	
AMD, subfoveal, minimally classic CNV (>4 MPS DA)	CNV under fovea, CNV >50% of lesion, and classic CNV <50% of entire lesion	Ranibizumab or pegaptanib	TAP at 2 years: 52% ≥3 line loss	TAP at 2 years: 56% ≥3 line loss	
AMD, subfoveal, occult only with no classic CNV (≤4 MPS DA)	CNV under fovea, CNV >50% of lesion, and no classic CNV present	If evidence of recent disease progression, then ranibizumab, pegaptanib, or PDT	VIP at 2 years: 21% ≥6 line loss 45% ≥3 line loss	VIP at 2 years: 46% ≥6 line loss 72% ≥3 line loss	VIP at 2 years: 5.0 treatments needed
AMD, subfoveal, occult only with no classic CNV (vision worse than 20/50⁻¹)	CNV under fovea, CNV >50% of lesion, and no classic CNV present	If evidence of recent disease progression, then ranibizumab, pegaptanib, or PDT	VIP at 2 years: 14% ≥6 line loss 42% ≥3 line loss	VIP at 2 years: 42% ≥6 line loss 76% ≥3 line loss	VIP at 2 years: 5.0 treatments needed
AMD, subfoveal, occult only with no classic CNV (>4 MPS DA)	CNV under fovea, CNV >50% of lesion, and no classic CNV present	Ranibizumab or pegaptanib	VISION at 1 year: 34% ≥3 line loss	VISION at 1 year: 43% ≥3 line loss	
Pathologic myopia, extrafoveal	Foveal edge of CNV ≥200 μm from center of FAZ	Laser to cover CNV, contiguous blockage and 100 μm beyond			

(Continues)

Table 4-2 Management of Choroidal Neovascularization Based on Prospective Clinical Trials (Continued)

Entity	Lesion Location/Characteristics	Recommended Treatment Technique	Posttreatment Visual Acuity	Placebo/Untreated Visual Acuity	Retreatment/Recurrence Rates
Pathologic myopia, juxtafoveal	Foveal edge of CNV <200 µm from center of FAZ	Laser to cover CNV, contiguous blockage and 100 µm beyond on nonfoveal side and if >100 µm from fovea, **unless** lesion is so close to the foveal center that laser may damage fovea; then consider PDT (see below)	VIP at 2 years: 21% ≥3 line loss 36% ≥1.5 line loss	VIP at 2 years: 28% ≥3 line loss 51% ≥1.5 line loss	VIP at 2 years: 5.1 treatments needed
Pathologic myopia, subfoveal	CNV under fovea	Photodynamic therapy			
Histoplasmosis, extrafoveal	Foveal edge of CNV ≥200 µm from center of FAZ	Laser to cover CNV, contiguous blockage and 100 µm beyond	MPS at 5 years: 12% ≥6 line loss Median: 20/40	MPS at 5 years: 42% ≥6 line loss Median: 20/80	At 5 years: Recurrent CNV in 26% (36% of patients with REC ≥6 line loss vs 2% without REC)
Histoplasmosis, juxtafoveal	Foveal edge of CNV <200 µm from center of FAZ	Laser to cover CNV, contiguous blockage and 100 µm beyond on nonfoveal side and if >100 µm from fovea, **unless** lesion is so close to the foveal center that laser may damage fovea; then consider PDT (see below)	MFS at 5 years: 12% ≥6 line loss Median: 20/40	MPS at 5 years: 28% ≥6 line loss Median: 20/64	At 5 years: PER 23% REC 10% (30% of patients with REC ≥6 line loss vs 4% without REC)
Histoplasmosis, subfoveal	CNV under fovea	Photodynamic therapy	VOH at 1 year: 8% ≥3 line loss 16% ≥1.5 line loss	No control	VOH at 1 year: 2.9 treatments needed
Idiopathic, extrafoveal	Foveal edge of CNV ≥200 µm from center of FAZ				
Idiopathic, juxtafoveal	Foveal edge of CNV <200 µm from center of FAZ				
Idiopathic, subfoveal	CNV under fovea	Photodynamic therapy			

FAZ = foveal avascular zone; CNV = choroidal neovascularization; MPS = Macular Photocoagulation Study; TAP = Treatment of Age-related Macular Degeneration with Photodynamic Therapy; VIM = Verteporfin in Minimally Classic Trial; VIP = Verteporfin in Photodynamic Therapy Study; VIO = Visudyne in Occult Trial; VOH = Verteporfin in Ocular Histoplasmosis Study; VISION = VEGF Inhibition Study in Ocular Neovascularization; PER = persistent CNV; REC = recurrent CNV; Disease progression = presence of blood from CNV or growth of the lesion (≥10% increase in greatest linear dimension) with past 12 weeks or loss of best-corrected vision (≥1 line). Treatment algorithm presented in this table based on several roundtable discussions of retinal experts and published in *Retina*: Guidelines for using verteporfin (Visudyne) in photodynamic therapy to treat choroidal neovascularization due to age-related macular degeneration and other causes. *Retina*. 2002;22:6–18. Gragoudas ES, Adamis AP, Cunningham ET Jr, et al. Pegaptanib for neovascular age-related macular degeneration. *N Engl J Med*. 2004;351:2805–2816.

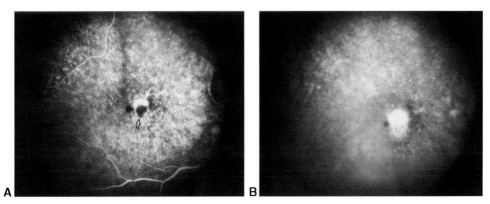

Figure 4-11 **A,** Recurrent subfoveal CNV with staining of prior laser-treated area outside the fovea *(open arrow)* and recurrent CNV extending into the foveal center *(white arrow).* **B,** Late view of the same CNV lesion, showing fluorescein leakage of recurrent CNV. *(Reproduced with permission from Bressler SB. Treatment of subfoveal choroidal neovascularization: decision making when visual acuity is good. The Wilmer Retina Update. 1995;6:9–16.)*

At the time of treatment, patients should be informed of the need to return periodically for follow-up (including visual acuity testing and fluorescein angiography as needed) as well as at any time new symptoms occur. If recurrent CNV is detected, repeat photocoagulation may be considered (if the process remains outside the foveal center), or photodynamic therapy or other treatment modalities may be entertained for subfoveal recurrences.

Other photocoagulation treatment considerations The choice of wavelength for photocoagulation (green or red) appears to have no effect on the treatment benefit. The risk of recurrence appears greatest in the following situations:

- when the fellow eye has evidence of active CNV or scarring
- when treatment fails to cover the neovascular lesion in its entirety
- when photocoagulation is not as intense as a moderately white treatment intensity standard (Fig 4-12)

Currently, various techniques are available for the diagnosis and treatment of CNV. ICG angiography may be used to better identify the boundaries of lesions that are poorly demarcated or that are obscured by extensive hemorrhage or pigmentation on fluorescein angiography.

Photodynamic therapy Photodynamic therapy (PDT) is a 2-step process that entails the systemic administration of a photosensitizing drug followed by an application of light of a particular wavelength to the affected tissue to incite a localized photochemical reaction. This reaction generates reactive oxygen species that can lead to capillary endothelial cell damage and vessel thrombosis. Several photosensitizing drugs are being evaluated in the management of patients with subfoveal CNV and AMD.

The Treatment of AMD with Photodynamic Therapy (TAP) investigation (Clinical Trial 4-3) was conducted at 22 clinical centers and studied 609 patients with new or

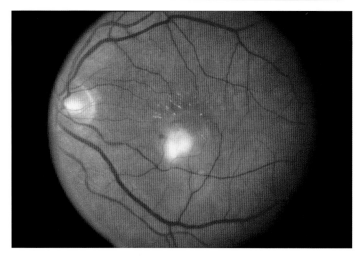

Figure 4-12 The minimal thermal laser treatment intensity standard used in the Macular Photocoagulation Study of juxtafoveal lesions specifies intensity sufficient to produce a uniform whitening of the overlying retina. *(Reproduced with permission from Macular Photocoagulation Study Group. Persistent and recurrent neovascularization after krypton laser photocoagulation for neovascular lesions of ocular histoplasmosis. Arch Ophthalmol. 1989;107:344–352.)*

CLINICAL TRIAL 4-3

Treatment of Age-Related Macular Degeneration with Photodynamic Therapy Study (TAP)

Objective: To determine if photodynamic therapy with verteporfin can reduce the risk of visual loss in patients with subfoveal CNV when compared to placebo-controlled sham treatment.

Participants: Eyes with new or recurrent subfoveal CNV, a classic component, size ≤5400 μm, blood <50% of the lesion, and vision of 20/40 to 20/200 at enrollment at 22 centers throughout North America and Europe.

Outcome Measures: Vision loss of <15 letters at 1 and 2 years. Secondary outcomes include vision loss of <30 letters, contrast threshold function, quality of life, and morphologic outcomes.

Present Status: Results published of 1-, 2-, and 3-year outcomes.

---

recurrent subfoveal CNV demonstrating a classic component on fluorescein angiography. Initial vision ranged from 20/40 to 20/200, and the greatest linear dimension of the lesion was 5400 μm or less. Eyes were randomly assigned in a double-masked fashion to IV infusion with verteporfin or placebo (5% dextrose in water—that is, D5W). The photosensitizing drug was activated by an infared diode laser (689 nm) 15 minutes after initiation of the infusion. Patients assigned to verteporfin were less likely to suffer at least moderate vision loss (≤3 lines of visual acuity) at 1 and 2 years when compared to placebo-assigned patients (the TAP extension study has shown that the benefit persists up to 60 months after initiation of treatment). At 2 years, 59% of verteporfin eyes versus 31% of placebo eyes avoided at least moderate vision loss. Subgroup analysis revealed that participants with predominantly classic CNV (ie, the area of classic CNV occupies ≥50% of the entire lesion) derived the greatest treatment benefit. This treatment effect was sustained up to 5 years after starting treatment, with a reduction in number of treatments required over time (2 treatments in last 3 years). Fluorescein angiographic outcomes provided independent confirmation of a favorable treatment effect in that verteporfin-treated eyes were less likely to demonstrate progression of classic CNV, more likely to demonstrate absence of classic CNV leakage, and less likely to enlarge during 2 years of follow-up. Subgroup analyses did not identify any statistically significant differ-ence in visual acuity outcomes in eyes in which the classic CNV lesion component was more than 0% but less than 50% of the area of the entire lesion (ie, minimally classic lesions) for the entire group of minimally classic lesions; however, subsequent linear regression analysis, as well as the Visudyne in Minimally Classic (VIM) Trial, has sug-gested that smaller minimally classic lesions (<4 MPS disc areas) appeared to benefit from the treatment. In the VIM Trial, smaller minimally classic (<6 MPS DA) lesions showed a statistically significant difference in vision from sham patients. Thus, patients with smaller minimally classic lesions should be considered for verteporfin PDT.

The Verteporfin in Photodynamic Therapy (VIP) study (Clinical Trial 4-4) was con-ducted at 28 clinical centers and evaluated 459 patients with AMD and new or recurrent subfoveal CNV measuring ≤5400 µm in its greatest linear dimension with either (1) oc-cult with no classic CNV, vision ≥20/100, recent disease progression defined as the pres-

CLINICAL TRIAL 4-4

Verteporfin in Photodynamic Therapy Trial (VIP): AMD and Pathologic Myopia

Objective: To determine if photodynamic therapy with verteporfin can reduce the risk of visual loss in patients with subfoveal CNV when compared to pla-cebo-controlled sham treatment.

Participants: Eyes with new or recurrent subfoveal CNV, and AMD with the following stipulations: if classic CNV is present, visual acuity better than 20/40; if occult CNV is present without classic CNV, there must be evidence of either blood or deterioration within the last 3 months. Deterioration defined either *visually* as loss of ≥5 letters (≥1 line) or *anatomically* as a ≥10% in-crease in the lesion's greatest linear dimension. Eyes with subfoveal CNV and pathologic myopia. Lesions ≤5400 µm, blood <50% of the lesion, and vision ≥20/100.

Outcome Measures: Vision loss of <5 letters at 1 and 2 years. For AMD eyes, vision loss of <8 letters at 1 or 2 years for myopic eyes. Secondary outcomes include vision loss of <30 letters, contrast threshold function, quality of life, and morphologic outcomes.

Present Status: Favorable 2-year vision results in AMD and pathologic myo-pia. See text discussion under Photodynamic Therapy for AMD results.

ence of hemorrhage, a recent decrease in vision ≥1 line, or an increase in the size of the lesion ≥10% in greatest linear dimension or (2) classic CNV with or without occult CNV and vision ≥20/40. The treatment and follow-up protocol were the same as for the TAP investigation. At 1 year, rates of at least moderate vision loss were similar between verteporfin-treated and placebo-treated eyes, although a number of secondary visual and angiographic outcomes significantly favored the verteporfin-treated group. However, by the 2-year endpoint, verteporfin-treated eyes were significantly less likely to have either moderate or severe vision loss. The treatment benefit was greatest for eyes with occult CNV without a classic component, particularly if the lesion was relatively small (≤4 disc areas) or associated with relatively lower levels of visual acuity (≤20/50[1]) at baseline. In this subgroup, verteporfin-treated eyes had rates of moderate and severe vision loss of 49% and 21%, respectively, at the 2-year exam compared to 75% and 48% in the placebo-treated group. Additional secondary outcomes (both visual and morphologic) confirmed these beneficial effects. In contrast, lesions that are larger than 4 disc areas in size, with baseline vision better than 20/50, had a worse outcome with verteporfin treatment; these patients should not be treated.

The FDA has approved PDT with verteporfin for eyes with predominantly classic CNV and AMD, as well as for eyes with pathologic myopia and ocular histoplasmosis (see the following major section, Other Causes of Choroidal Neovascularization). Although not FDA approved, PDT with verteporfin should be considered for eyes with occult lesions and no classic component that meet the entry criteria of the VIP study—namely, eyes that have signs of recent disease progression and that are small or associated with poorer levels of vision, as well as smaller, minimally classic lesions. PDT has largely replaced thermal laser photocoagulation in the management of subfoveal lesions. Many eyes with CNV and AMD that were previously untreatable because of larger size or poorly demarcated borders have become candidates for PDT.

See Table 4-3 for a review of ongoing trials for AMD.

Other treatment modalities Other treatment modalities being studied are transpupillary thermotherapy, radiotherapy, submacular surgery to remove subretinal blood and/or the CNV, macular translocation, pneumatic displacement of hemorrhages, and pharmacologic therapies. Macular translocation procedures are undergoing surgical refinement, and safety information is presently being collected to determine if a clinical trial should be recommended in the future. The Submacular Surgery Trials reported no benefit to surgical removal of CNV in age-related macular degeneration, in cases associated with >50% blood and in presumed ocular histoplasmosis or other idiopathic conditions. The Transpupillary Thermotherapy for CNV (TTT4CNV) Trial reported no benefit over sham administration of TTT in occult with no classic CNV measuring <3000 µm in size.

An area of intense research is use of antiangiogenic drugs to prevent neovascular cascade. One such drug, the anti–vascular endothelial growth factor (VEGF) aptamer (pegaptanib [Macugen], Eyetech Pharmaceuticals), blocks the 165 isoform of VEGF. The drug is administered via intravitreal injection every 6 weeks. In a study of 1196 patients worldwide, using a 0.3-mg dose of Macugen, 70% of patients lost less than 3 lines of vision and 10% lost more than 6 lines, compared to 55% and 22%, respectively, in

Table 4-3 Review of Ongoing Clinical Trials for AMD

Study/Sponsor	Testing	Goal	Eligibility	Enrollment/Follow-up Status	Comment
Visudyne in Occult Choroidal Neovascularization Trial (VIO) Novartis Ophthalmics/QLT Inc	Verteporfin (Visudyne) photodynamic therapy	Reduce risk of vision loss; phase 3 study	Subfoveal, occult with no classic CNV, VA 20/50–20/200, ≤6 MPS DA	Enrollment completed 2003; for more information, see www.visudyne.com.	12- and 24-month results missed primary endpoint
Visudyne and Triamcinolone acetonide (VISTA) Trial/Novartis Ophthalmics	Verteporfin (Visudyne) photodynamic therapy alone or in combination with 1- or 4-mg adjunct intravitreal triamcinolone acetonide	Reduce risk of vision loss; phase 3 study	Subfoveal, <50% classic CNV, VA 20/40–20/200, ≤9 MPS DA	Enrollment completed 2006	Results pending 2007
Minimally classic/occult trial of the anti-VEGF antibody rhuFab V2 in treatment of neovascular AMD (MARINA; study ID#FVF2598g) Genentech	300 and 500 µg ranibizumab (Lucentis)	Reduce risk of vision loss; phase 3 study	Subfoveal <50% classic CNV, VA 20/40–20/320, ≤9 MPS DA	Enrollment completed 2003; for more information, see www.gene.com or Robert Kim, MD (650) 225-1044	MARINA at 1 yr Lucentis 95% <3 line loss Control 62% <3 line loss control
Anti-VEGF antibody for treatment of predominantly classic choroidal neovascularization in AMD (ANCHOR; study ID#FVF2587g) Genentech	300 and 500 µg ranibizumab (Lucentis) vs verteporfin (Visudyne) photodynamic therapy	Reduce risk of vision loss; phase 3 study	Subfoveal CNV, ≥50% classic, VA 20/40–20/320, ≤9 MPS DA	Enrollment completed 2004; for more information, see www.gene.com or Robert Kim, MD (650) 225-1044	ANCHOR at 1 yr Lucentis 96% <3 line loss PDT 64% <3 line loss
Anecortave acetate for subfoveal CNV (protocol #C-01-99) Alcon Laboratories	15 mg anecortave acetate (RETAANE) vs verteporfin (Visudyne) photodynamic therapy	Reduce risk of vision loss; phase 3 study	Subfoveal CNV, ≥50% classic, VA 20/40–20/400, ≤5400 µm	Enrollment completed; contact Alcon Laboratories (817) 551-4619	12-month results missed primary endpoint; follow-up planned for 24 months
Anecortave Acetate Risk Reduction Trial (AART)(#C-02-60) Alcon Laboratories	15 and 30 mg anecortave acetate vs sham injection	Reduce the risk of dry AMD progressing to wet AMD in high-risk patients	Patients with CN in fellow eye and study eye with multiple medium or at least 1 large druse with hyperpigmentation	Enrollment completed 2006	

patients who received sham injections at 12 months. The drug appeared safe; however, endophthalmitis was reported in 12 patients (1.3 risk/patient/year). Macugen received FDA approval for treating neovascular AMD in December 2004 and became commercially available for this indication in 2005.

Another drug is a recombinantly produced, humanized Fab fragment of a monoclonal antibody against VEGF called ranibizumab (Lucentis, Genentech). Phase 3 clinical trials (MARINA and ANCHOR) for ranibizumab administered intravitreally at monthly intervals showed excellent visual results with less than 3 lines of visual acuity loss in the ranibizumab-treated arms of over 90% at 1 year. The studies also showed a mean visual acuity improvement of 1–2 lines and 3-line or more visual acuity improvement rates of 30%–40% at month 12. The FDA approved ranibizumab to treat all AMD-related subfoveal CNV in June 2006.

Other management considerations The fellow eye of an individual with unilateral neovascular maculopathy is at high risk of developing CNV, especially if it shows evidence of multiple drusen, large drusen, or focal clumps of hyperpigmentation of the RPE, or if the patient has definite systemic hypertension. If CNV does develop in the second eye, the patient is likely to become legally blind with or without treatment to the second eye. However, if CNV does not develop in the fellow eye, the average visual acuity of the fellow eye is likely to remain 20/40 or better over a 5-year period, even with drusen and abnormalities of the RPE. When central vision in both eyes is significantly affected by AMD, the patient's functional abilities may be improved through low vision rehabilitation and use of optical and nonoptical devices (see BCSC Section 3, *Clinical Optics*).

Summary of clinical trials for AMD

Table 4-3 presents an overview of ongoing clinical trials.

Argon laser photocoagulation for neovascular maculopathy: five-year results from randomized clinical trials. Macular Photocoag. Study Group. *Arch Ophthalmol.* 1991;109:1109–1114.

Bressler NM, Treatment of Age-Related Macular Degeneration with Photodynamic Therapy (TAP) Study Group. Photodynamic therapy of subfoveal choroidal neovascularization in age-related macular degeneration with verteporfin: two-year results of 2 randomized clinical trials—TAP report 2. *Arch Ophthalmol.* 2001;119:198–207.

Choroidal Neovascularization Prevention Trial Research Group. Laser treatment in fellow eyes with large drusen: updated findings from a pilot randomized clinical trial. *Ophthalmology.* 2003;110:971–978.

Eyetech Study Group. Anti-vascular endothelial growth factor therapy for subfoveal choroidal neovascularization secondary to age-related macular degeneration: phase II study results. *Ophthalmology.* 2003;110:979–986.

Fujii GY, de Juan E Jr, Pieramici DJ, et al. Inferior limited macular translocation for subfoveal choroidal neovascularization secondary to age-related macular degeneration: 1-year visual outcome and recurrence report. *Am J Ophthalmol.* 2002;134:69–74.

Gragoudas ES, Adamis AP, Cunningham ET Jr, et al. Pegaptanib for neovascular age-related macular degeneration. *N Engl J Med.* 2004;351:2805–2816.

Laser photocoagulation for juxtafoveal choroidal neovascularization: five-year results from randomized clinical trials. Macular Photocoagulation Study Group. *Arch Ophthalmol.* 1994;112:500–509.

Photodynamic therapy of subfoveal choroidal neovascularization in age-related macular degeneration with verteporfin: one-year results of 2 randomized clinical trials—TAP report. Treatment of Age-Related Macular Degeneration with Photodynamic Therapy (TAP) Study Group. *Arch Ophthalmol.* 1999;117:1329–1345.

Verteporfin Photodynamic Therapy (VIP) Study Group. Verteporfin therapy of subfoveal choroidal neovascularization in age-related macular degeneration: two-year results of a randomized clinical trial including lesions with occult with no classic choroidal neovascularization—Verteporfin in Photodynamic Therapy Report 2. *Am J Ophthalmol.* 2001;131:541–560.

Other Causes of Choroidal Neovascularization

Ocular Histoplasmosis Syndrome (OHS)

Infection with the yeast form of the fungus *Histoplasma capsulatum* is endemic to certain areas of the United States, including states containing the Mississippi and Ohio river valleys. The fungus is carried on the feathers of chickens, pigeons, and blackbirds, as well as in droppings from infected bats. Humans inhale the fungus, which is then disseminated into the bloodstream. The systemic infection eventually subsides, leaving ocular scarring. Most of the visual symptoms occur years after initial infection.

The condition has also been called *presumed ocular histoplasmosis syndrome (POHS)* because the causal relationship between the fungus and the eye disease has been considered tenuous; however, the relationship is supported by epidemiologic and histopathologic data. For example, more than 90% of patients with the typical fundus appearance have a positive skin reaction to intracutaneous histoplasmin, and the highest prevalence of OHS is found where the population has the greatest percentage of positive skin reactors. In one community with endemic histoplasmosis (59% of the total population with positive skin tests), the characteristic peripheral lesions of OHS occurred in 2.6% of the total population surveyed and in 4.4% of the positive responders to the histoplasmin skin test. Only one individual with peripheral lesions showed disciform macular disease. The organism has been identified histologically in the choroid in 5 patients with OHS. Nevertheless, other etiologies besides *H capsulatum* may produce a similar phenotypic picture.

There are 4 signs of OHS:

- punched-out chorioretinal lesions (histo spots)
- juxtapapillary atrophic pigmentary changes
- no vitritis
- choroidal neovascularization

The clinical appearance of OHS includes small, atrophic, punched-out chorioretinal scars in the midperiphery and posterior pole *(histo spots),* linear peripheral atrophic tracks, and *juxtapapillary chorioretinal scarring* with or without *choroidal neovascularization* in the macula (Fig 4-13). The changes are bilateral in over 60% of cases. No vitreous inflammation appears. Most patients with OHS are asymptomatic until they develop CNV. Visual loss, metamorphopsia, and paracentral scotomata are the sequelae of CNV. If CNV

Figure 4-13 Ocular histoplasmosis syndrome with CNV. **A,** Clinical photograph shows peripapillary atrophy and numerous atrophic scars. **B,** Transit frame of the angiogram reveals blocked fluorescence from blood and pigment as well as hyperfluorescence resulting from the CNV *(arrows)* and transmission in areas of atrophy. **C,** Leakage from the choroidal neovascular membrane *(arrows)* late in the angiogram, as well as staining of the sclera beneath atrophic scars.

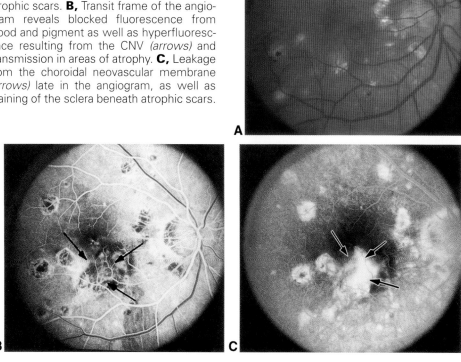

is suspected, patients should undergo fluorescein angiography so the size, location, and characteristics of the CNV can be determined and appropriate treatment begun. Features similar to those of OHS, including the development of CNV, occur in many other types of diseases, including multifocal choroiditis, birdshot choroidopathy, acute posterior multifocal placoid pigment epitheliopathy, and diffuse unilateral subacute neuroretinopathy (DUSN), as discussed in BCSC Section 9, *Intraocular Inflammation and Uveitis.*

Management of OHS

The MPS has shown that untreated eyes with OHS and extrafoveal CNV have a cumulative risk of severe visual loss (losing at least 6 lines of vision) of 44% at 5 years (see Table 4-2). Photocoagulation of the CNV lesion reduces the risk to 9%. The MPS has also shown treatment to be beneficial for juxtafoveal CNV. Although the initial visual acuities at the time of randomization ranged from 20/20 to 20/400, after 5 years the proportion of eyes with severe visual acuity loss was 28% in the untreated group and 12% in the treated group. Even when the CNV originates from a peripapillary scar or when photocoagulation is used in the retina nasal to the fovea or in the papillomacular bundle, treatment is beneficial compared to observation.

As with AMD, recurrent CNV represents a significant ongoing risk to central vision following effective photocoagulation in OHS. Unlike AMD, however, OHS has not been shown to benefit from laser treatment that involves the foveal center in either new or recurrent subfoveal CNV lesions. Because subfoveal CNV in association with OHS may not always progress to severe visual loss, ophthalmologists may not be willing to risk subjecting the foveal center of these eyes to the destructive effects of laser treatment. Although small, short-term, uncontrolled case series of submacular surgery of subfoveal histo CNV lesions have suggested possible benefits in vision outcome, recurrence rates have remained high after surgery and may lead to the loss of any treatment benefit. The Submacular Surgery Trials (SST; Clinical Trials 4-5 and 4-6) evaluated whether surgical removal of these lesions is beneficial compared to observation over a period of 4 years.

CLINICAL TRIAL 4-5

Submacular Surgery Trials (SST)

Objective: Can submacular surgical removal of CNV and blood in eyes with subfoveal CNV associated with AMD stabilize or improve visual outcome when compared to observation?

Participants: Group N: New subfoveal CNV: eyes with subfoveal CNV, a classic component, ≤9 MPS disc areas, blood <50% of lesion area, visual acuity of 20/100 to 20/800 (exclusive of MPS laser-eligible lesions).

Group B: Blood is predominant component of subfoveal CNV lesion (>50% of affected area), ±visualization of classic or occult CNV, ±previous laser treatment outside foveal center, visual acuity of 20/100 to light perception.

Outcome Measures: Stabilization or improvement in visual acuity at 2 and 4 years after enrollment. Surgical complications, contrast sensitivity function, quality of life measures, and morphologic outcomes are secondary endpoints.

Present Status: Enrollment closed September 2001.

CLINICAL TRIAL 4-6

Submacular Surgery Trials (SST)

Objective: To determine if submacular extraction of CNV and blood in eyes with subfoveal CNV associated with ocular histoplasmosis or of idiopathic origin can stabilize or improve vision outcome when compared to observation.

Participants: Group H: New or recurrent subfoveal CNV, a classic component, ≤9 MPS disc areas, ± blood, and visual acuity of 20/50 to 20/800.

Outcome Measures: Stabilization or improvement in visual acuity at 2 and 4 years after enrollment. Surgical complications, contrast sensitivity function, quality of life measures, and morphologic outcomes are secondary endpoints.

Present Status: Recruitment completed September 2001.

An uncontrolled case series of 25 patients treated with photodynamic therapy (PDT) with verteporfin suggests that PDT may limit vision loss in eyes with subfoveal CNV and OHS up to 4 years after initiation of treatment. PDT with verteporfin is approved by the FDA for the treatment of CNV in OHS. Some authors have also reported improved visual results using either systemic or injected steroids either alone or in combination with PDT. Finally, when visual acuity is poor, some authors have noted improved results with submacular surgery and removal of the CNV after PDT. No randomized trials have proven the efficacy of these adjunctive treatments.

If 1 eye has OHS with CNV or disciform scarring, the risk of visual loss in the fellow eye is related to but not limited by the presence or absence of focal macular histo spots. If no findings of OHS are present in the first eye, the risk is 1%. However, when peripapillary atrophy is present, the risk increases to 4%, and if focal macular histo spots are present, the risk rises to 25%. Management of eyes with nonneovascular manifestations of OHS consists of instructing patients to monitor their central vision, often with the assistance of an Amsler grid, and evaluating patients promptly with fluorescein angiography if visual loss or metamorphopsia occurs.

Although eyes without macular lesions have a much better prognosis, new histo spots, which represent an area where CNV may develop later, can develop in either the peripheral or macular region.

Holekamp NM, Thomas MA, Dickinson JD, et al. Surgical removal of subfoveal choroidal neovascularization in presumed ocular histoplasmosis: stability of early visual results. *Ophthalmology.* 1997;104:22–26.

Martidis A, Miller DG, Ciulla TA, et al. Corticosteroids as an antiangiogenic agent for histoplasmosis-related subfoveal choroidal neovascularization. *J Ocul Pharmacol Ther.* 1999;15:425–428.

Saperstein DA, Rosenfeld PJ, Bressler NM, et al. Photodynamic therapy of subfoveal choroidal neovascularization with verteporfin in the ocular histoplasmosis syndrome: one-year results of an uncontrolled, prospective case series. *Ophthalmology.* 2002;109:1499–1505.

Idiopathic CNV

Patients may develop CNV and subsequent disciform scarring in the absence of any other ophthalmoscopic abnormality or disease known to be associated with CNV. Such CNV lesions are termed *idiopathic* and are currently viewed as a distinct group. These patients may represent a number of etiologies, including OHS without histo spots and AMD without characteristic drusen or RPE abnormalities. The MPS showed that the benefits of laser treatment for extrafoveal or juxtafoveal idiopathic CNV are consistent with the results seen in larger samples in the trials studying extrafoveal or juxtafoveal CNV associated with OHS or AMD (see Table 4-2). Likewise, PDT should be considered in cases of idiopathic subfoveal classic CNV. Management of subfoveal CNV of idiopathic origin is also being addressed in Group H of the SST (see Clinical Trial 4-6).

Krypton laser photocoagulation for idiopathic neovascular lesions: results of a randomized clinical trial. Macular Photocoagulation Study Group. *Arch Ophthalmol.* 1990;108:832–837.

Persistent and recurrent neovascularization after krypton laser photocoagulation for neovascular lesions of ocular histoplasmosis. Macular Photocoagulation Study Group. *Arch Ophthalmol.* 1989;107:344–352.

Sickenberg M, Schmidt-Erfurth U, Miller JW, et al. A preliminary study of photodynamic therapy using verteporfin for choroidal neovascularization in pathologic myopia, ocular histoplasmosis syndrome, angioid streaks, and idiopathic causes. *Arch Ophthalmol.* 2000;118:327–336.

Angioid Streaks

Dark red to brown bands of irregular contour that radiate from the optic nerve head are known as *angioid streaks.* They represent discontinuities or breaks in thickened and calcified Bruch's membrane. It is possible to confuse angioid streaks with retinal vessels until their location deep to the retina is recognized (Fig 4-14).

Because the RPE overlying angioid streaks is often atrophic, the streaks appear hyperfluorescent *(window defect)* in the early phase of fluorescein angiography. As in other conditions with defects in Bruch's membrane, choroidal neovascular ingrowth may occur, resulting in exudative macular detachment and loss of central visual acuity.

The systemic disease most commonly associated with angioid streaks is *pseudoxanthoma elasticum (PXE),* or Grönblad-Strandberg syndrome. An additional fundus finding in this condition is a lighter orange appearance against the darker orange color of the normal RPE and choroid. At the interface between the abnormal light color and the normal darker color, the fundus, shown in Figure 4-14, has a fine, stippled appearance referred to as *peau d'orange* (like "the skin of an orange").

Paget disease of bone and *sickle cell anemia (SS)* also may be associated with angioid streaks, as may a number of other, less common, systemic disorders such as *Ehlers-Danlos syndrome* (this syndrome is discussed in a number of BCSC volumes; consult the *Master Index*). Streaklike changes also appear to develop from degenerative factors alone in some elderly patients. Any patient whose angioid streaks are more extensive than would be seen in such elderly patients should receive a thorough workup for an associated condition; however, some patients with streaks have no demonstrable systemic disease.

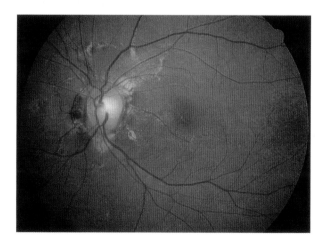

Figure 4-14 Fundus of patient with pseudoxanthoma elasticum shows angioid streaks, "peau d'orange" appearance temporal to the macula, and focal drusen-like lesions (inferotemporal arcade).

The most significant visual complication of angioid streaks is the development of CNV from breaks in Bruch's membrane. No treatment is known to prevent this condition in eyes at risk. Ophthalmologists may wish to extrapolate from the results of the MPS reports for CNV associated with other etiologies in considering laser treatment for CNV associated with angioid streaks. In particular, thermal treatment may not be appropriate for subfoveal lesions. Patients with extrafoveal or juxtafoveal lesions being considered for treatment should understand that results from the MPS reports may or may not apply to their particular circumstances. The results would likely be more similar to CNV in AMD than to that in OHS, because angioid streaks probably resemble a diffuse degenerative process like AMD more closely than they do a focal degenerative process like OHS. PDT may also be considered for eyes with subfoveal CNV, although no prospective clinical study has addressed visual outcome in this setting. In addition, patients should be informed of the risk of recurrence. The use of safety glasses may be advisable for patients with angioid streaks because their eyes are particularly susceptible to choroidal rupture following even minor blunt injury.

Clarkson JG, Altman RD. Angioid streaks. *Surv Ophthalmol.* 1982;26:235–246.

Lim JI, Bressler NM, Marsh MJ, et al. Laser treatment of choroidal neovascularization in patients with angioid streaks. *Am J Ophthalmol.* 1993;116:414–423.

Pathologic Myopia

Myopia is the most common ocular abnormality, with 25% of the population of the United States being myopic. In contrast, *pathologic myopia*, also known as *high myopia* or *degenerative myopia*, is rare, occurring in roughly 2% of the population. Incidence rates are higher in Asians and lower in African Americans. Eyes with pathologic myopia have progressive elongation of the eye, thus creating a propensity for thinning of the RPE and choroid. The spherical equivalents of an eye with high myopia is more than -6.00 D, or an axial length greater than 26.5 mm, whereas patients with pathologic myopia are more than -8.00 D, or an axial length greater than 32.5 mm. Fundus manifestations in pathologic myopia may include the following:

- tilting of the optic disc
- peripapillary chorioretinal atrophy
- lacquer cracks—that is, spontaneous focal linear breaks in Bruch's membrane (Fig 4-15)
- isolated subretinal hemorrhages that may clear spontaneously and may not be a result of CNV
- Fuchs spots (RPE hyperplasia presumably developing in response to a small area of CNV that does not progress to significant disciform scarring)
- posterior staphyloma
- elongation and atrophy of the ciliary body
- gyrate areas of atrophy of the RPE and choroid
- cystoid, cobblestone, and lattice degeneration
- thinning or hole formation in the peripheral retina
- thinning and rearrangement of the collagen layers of the sclera
- choroidal neovascularization

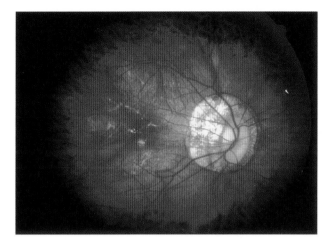

Figure 4-15 Pathologic myopia with tilted disc and peripapillary atrophy of RPE and choroid. Lacquer cracks are visible in the macula. Other features include a scleral crescent and a "blond" fundus allowing visualization of choroidal vessels.

Choroidal neovascularization in myopia

CNV may develop in 5%–10% of eyes with an axial length of more than 26.5 mm, often in conjunction with widespread chorioretinal degeneration and lacquer cracks in the posterior pole. The ophthalmologist considering laser treatment for CNV outside the foveal center that is associated with pathologic myopia may extrapolate with caution from results of the MPS reports for CNV associated with other etiologies. In addition, a small, prospective randomized trial investigating treatment of lesions outside the foveal center, performed in France, documented a short-term benefit of laser treatment in myopic eyes. Treatment may not be appropriate for subfoveal lesions, however, particularly because CNV lesions in myopia tend to remain relatively small. PDT of subfoveal lesions in eyes with pathologic myopia was investigated in the VIP Pathologic Myopia Trial. This randomized trial found a benefit in preventing visual loss with PDT up to 3 years after initiating treatment. PDT is strongly recommended for these eyes and has received FDA approval because this treatment reduces rates of mild and moderate visual loss. PDT should also be considered in patients with juxtafoveal lesions because of scar creep after laser photocoagulation that may involve the fovea months to years after previously successful laser treatment.

Patients who are being considered for extrafoveal (or, with extreme caution in selected cases, juxtafoveal) thermal photocoagulation should understand that results from the MPS reports may not apply to their own circumstances. In general, however, the results might be more similar to those obtained in eyes with CNV associated with AMD than in eyes with CNV associated with OHS because pathologic myopia probably more closely resembles a diffuse degenerative process like AMD than it does a focal degenerative process like OHS. However, unlike AMD and more like OHS, the CNV lesions in pathologic myopia may stabilize without significant visual loss. In addition, patients should be aware of the continuing risk of recurrence, with the understanding that PDT will be strongly considered if subfoveal recurrent disease develops. Finally, it is worth noting that expanding RPE atrophy, which can develop around the laser lesion resulting from any kind of CNV, may occur more frequently and to a greater extent in eyes treated for pathologic myopia. Visual loss may accompany this expanding atrophy.

Blinder KJ, Blumenkranz MS, Bressler NM, et al. Verteporfin therapy of subfoveal choroidal neovascularization in pathologic myopia: 2-year results of a randomized clinical trial—VIP report no. 3. *Ophthalmology.* 2003;110:667–673.

Hampton GR, Kohen D, Bird AC. Visual prognosis of disciform degeneration in myopia. *Ophthalmology.* 1983;90:923–926.

Tabandeh H, Flynn HW Jr, Scott IU, et al. Visual acuity outcomes of patients 50 years of age and older with high myopia and untreated choroidal neovascularization. *Ophthalmology.* 1999;106:2063–2067.

Verteporfin in Photodynamic Therapy Study Group. Photodynamic therapy of subfoveal neo-vascularization in pathologic myopia with verteporfin: 1-year results of a randomized clinical trial. VIP report No 1. *Ophthalmology.* 2001;108:841–852.

Miscellaneous Causes of Choroidal Neovascularization

CNV may complicate a variety of conditions that damage Bruch's membrane, including choroidal rupture, optic disc drusen, and a number of other diseases listed in Table 4-4. In general, the ophthalmologist deciding whether to extend the results of the MPS reports to CNV from these other causes should probably avoid treatment involving the foveal center but consider treating lesions outside the foveal center. The ophthalmologist and

Table 4-4 Conditions Associated With CNV

Degenerative
Age-related macular degeneration
Myopic degeneration
Angioid streaks
Heredodegenerative
Vitelliform macular dystrophy
Fundus flavimaculatus
Optic nerve head drusen
Inflammatory
Ocular histoplasmosis syndrome
Multifocal choroiditis
Serpiginous choroiditis
Toxoplasmosis
Toxocariasis
Rubella
Vogt-Koyanagi-Harada syndrome
Behçet syndrome
Sympathetic ophthalmia
Tumor
Choroidal nevus
Choroidal hemangioma
Metastatic choroidal tumors
Hamartoma of the RPE
Traumatic
Choroidal rupture
Intense photocoagulation
Idiopathic

the patient must understand that because the natural histories are different for CNV of different etiologies, the exact risks and benefits for a particular circumstance may not be analogous to those in the MPS reports. Following laser treatment, all patients must be carefully monitored for recurrent disease.

Vitreoretinal Interface Abnormalities

Epiretinal Membrane

An epiretinal membrane (ERM) is a semitranslucent fibrocellular membrane on the inner retinal surface along the internal limiting membrane (ILM). ERMs can be

- idiopathic and presumably related to an abnormality of the vitreoretinal interface in conjunction with a posterior vitreous detachment
- secondary to a wide variety of conditions, including retinal vascular occlusions, uveitis, trauma, intraocular surgery, and retinal breaks

ERMs are relatively common; at autopsy, they are discovered in 2% of patients over age 50 and in 20% over age 75. Idiopathic epiretinal membranes are most common in patients over age 50, and both sexes are equally affected. The incidence of bilaterality is approximately 10%–20%. Detachment or separation of the posterior vitreous is present in almost all eyes with idiopathic membranes. It is believed that detachment of the posterior vitreous (see Chapter 11) may leave a portion of the posterior cortical vitreous attached to the macular area or may cause dehiscence in the ILM, allowing glial cells from the retina to proliferate along the retinal surface and/or any posterior cortical vitreous remaining on the retinal surface.

Signs and symptoms

Epiretinal proliferation is generally located in the macula—over the fovea, surrounding the fovea, or eccentric to the fovea (Fig 4-16). The membranes usually present with a mild sheen or glint on the retinal surface. Over time, ERMs become highly reflective and, when thickened, they become more opaque, obscuring underlying retinal details. A "pseudohole" may appear if this preretinal membrane has a gap or hole. OCT is useful to differentiate a full-thickness macular hole from a pseudohole. Occasionally, intraretinal hemorrhages or whitened patches of superficial retina representing delayed axoplasmic flow may be present. The cellular origin of ERMs is still under debate. Histologic examination reveals mainly RPE cells and retinal glial cells (astrocytes and Müller cells); however, myofibroblasts, fibroblasts, hyalocytes, and macrophages have also been identified.

Contracture of ERMs produces distortion and wrinkling of the inner surface of the retina, also called *cellophane maculopathy* or *preretinal macular fibrosis* when mild and *surface-wrinkling retinopathy* or *retinal striae* when moderate; in severe cases, it is called *macular pucker*. Greater traction may cause shallow detachment and/or cystic changes of the macula. Furthermore, traction on retinal vessels results in increased vascular tortuosity and straightening of the perimacular vessels. Continued traction can lead to macular edema and cystoid macular edema that is evident clinically and on fluorescein

Figure 4-16 Epiretinal membrane. **A,** Red-free photograph reveals radiating striae of the internal limiting membrane in the macula, caused by this largely transparent membrane. Note the tortuosity of small vessels in this region. **B,** Transit frame of fluorescein angiogram reveals distortion of macular capillaries and some straightening of adjacent vessels. **C,** Late frame shows a small amount of fluorescein leakage in the center of the macula *(arrow)*.

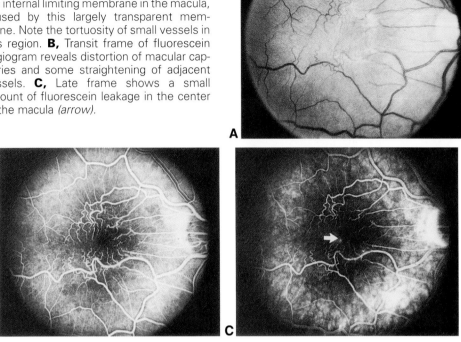

angiography; optic nerve staining may also be seen. OCT scans illustrate the irregular inner retinal surface and the higher reflectivity of the epiretinal membrane.

Affected patients may be asymptomatic when the ERMs are extramacular or thin, or they may present with metamorphopsia, micropsia, monocular diplopia, and a variable degree of loss of visual acuity ranging from 20/20 to 20/200. Retrospective studies suggest that visual acuity and fundus appearance remain remarkably stable in the large majority of patients, with approximately 75% of eyes maintaining acuity of 20/50 or better. Visual acuity in one retrospective study was unchanged in 71% of eyes, decreased 2 lines or more in 26%, and improved in 3%.

Treatment

In rare cases, an ERM can spontaneously detach from the inner retinal surface with a concomitant resolution of retinal distortion and improvement in symptoms and vision. In most cases, the symptoms are mild and surgical treatment is not required. An eye that loses vision to 20/60 or worse and/or has an intolerable level of distortion with better visual acuities may be a candidate for surgical removal of the ERM by vitrectomy techniques. See Chapter 16 for a discussion on vitrectomy for macular disease. After surgical removal, 50%–75% of patients have some degree of improvement in vision; however, return to normal vision is rare.

Capone A Jr. Macular surface disorders. *Focal Points: Clinical Modules for Ophthalmologists.* San Francisco: American Academy of Ophthalmology; 1996, module 4.

Johnson MW. Epiretinal membrane. In Yanoff M, Duker J, eds. *Ophthalmology.* London: CV Mosby; 1999:8/32.1–8/32.4.

Vitreomacular Traction Syndrome

Vitreomacular traction syndrome (VMT) occurs when there is incomplete separation of the posterior vitreous at the macula. The incomplete separation and abnormal adherence of the vitreous that remains attached to the posterior pole leads to traction on the macula. The etiology is unknown. In particular, it is not known whether vitreomacular adhesion is primary or secondary to cellular proliferation induced by partial vitreous detachment. In VMT, abnormal opacities may be present in the vitreous overlying the macular region, usually associated with traction on that region and the optic nerve (Fig 4-17). As with ERMs, the macular region may become distorted, cystic, or tented anteriorly with a shallow detachment, although no ERM is seen (Fig 4-18). Angiography may demonstrate leakage of fluorescein dye from retinal vessels in the macular region as well as from the optic nerve. OCT is useful to demonstrate the vitreoretinal interface abnormalities and the traction of VMT. The condition may be bilateral.

Vitrectomy may be considered if the patient's vision is noted to decrease. Although the long-term risks and benefits of vitrectomy for VMT are unknown, they are believed to be similar to those of surgery for ERMs (see Chapter 16). Spontaneous separation of the focal vitreoretinal adhesion may occur, with resolution of all clinical features.

Features that differentiate VMT from ERM are listed in Table 4-5.

Hikichi T, Yoshida A, Trempe CL. Course of vitreomacular traction syndrome. *Am J Ophthalmol.* 1995;119:55–61.

McDonald HR, Johnson RN, Schatz H. Surgical results in the vitreomacular traction syndrome. *Ophthalmology.* 1994;101:1397–1402.

Smiddy WE, Green WR, Michels RG, et al. Ultrastructural studies of vitreomacular traction syndrome. *Am J Ophthalmol.* 1989;107:177–185.

Idiopathic Macular Hole

Idiopathic macular holes occur primarily in the sixth through eighth decades of life, affect women more frequently than men, and appear at a younger age in myopic eyes. Recent investigations using OCT and ultrasonography suggest that idiopathic macular holes are caused by the tractional forces associated with perifoveal vitreous detachment, an early stage of age-related posterior vitreous detachment (PVD). The observation that an idiopathic macular hole appears to be a complication of the earliest stage of age-related PVD helps explain the age and sex demographics of this condition, which are similar to those of PVD. The following description of the stages of macular hole formation and what OCT reveals at each stage is useful in interpreting biomicroscopic findings and making management decisions (Fig 14-19):

- Patients with *stage 1* macular holes (also known as *impending macular holes*) have visual symptoms that typically include central vision loss (with visual acuity typically measuring 20/25 to 20/60) and metamorphopsia. On biomicroscopy, there

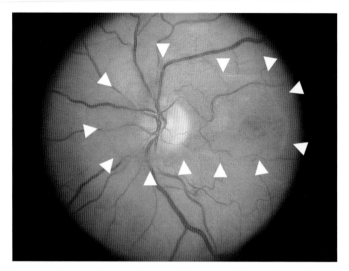

Figure 4-17 Vitreomacular traction syndrome with an ovoid area of persistent attachment extending from the nasal aspect of the optic nerve head to a crescent-shaped area of attachment along the temporal macula *(arrowheads)*. *(Reproduced with permission from Capone A Jr. Macular surface disorders. Focal Points: Clinical Modules for Ophthalmologists. San Francisco: American Academy of Ophthalmology; 1996, module 4.)*

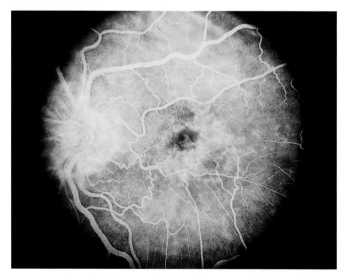

Figure 4-18 Mid–venous phase angiographic image of the eye shown in Figure 4-17, demonstrating disc leakage, vascular distortion, early CME, and diffuse accumulation of dye in the subsensory space as a result of broad, shallow tractional detachment of the posterior pole. *(Reproduced with permission from Capone A Jr. Macular surface disorders. Focal Points: Clinical Modules for Ophthalmologists. San Francisco: American Academy of Ophthalmology; 1996, module 4.)*

Table 4-5 Differential Features of Macular Epiretinal Membrane (ERM) versus Vitreomacular Traction Syndrome (VMT)

Features	ERM	VMT
Posterior/peripheral vitreous separation	Yes/Yes	No/Yes
Traction vector(s)	Tangential	Anteroposterior and tangential
Retinal striae	Yes	Common
Vascular straightening	Common	Common
Tractional retinal detachment outside arcades	No	Yes
CME	Common	Common
Disk leakage on fluorescein angiography	No	Yes

(Modified with permission from Capone A Jr. Macular surface disorders. *Focal Points: Clinical Modules for Ophthalmologists*. San Francisco: American Academy of Ophthalmology; 1996, module 4.)

is loss of the foveal depression associated with a small yellow spot (stage 1A) or yellow ring (stage 1B) in the center of the fovea. OCT examination reveals that a stage 1A hole is a foveal "pseudocyst," or horizonal splitting associated with a vitreous detachment from the perifoveal retina but not from the foveal center. In stage 1B holes, there is progression of the pseudocyst posteriorly to include a break in the outer foveal layer, the margins of which constitute the yellow ring seen clinically. As many as 50% of stage 1 holes resolve spontaneously following separation of the vitreofoveal adhesion and spontaneous relief of tractional forces.

- A *stage 2* macular hole represents the progression of a foveal pseudocyst to a full-thickness dehiscence, as a tractional break develops in the "roof" (inner layer) of the pseudocyst. The small opening in the inner layer (<400 µm diameter) may be either centrally or eccentrically located. Progression to stage 2 typically occurs over several weeks or months and usually involves a further decline in visual acuity. OCT demonstrates that the posterior hyaloid typically remains attached to the foveal center in stage 2 holes.
- A *stage 3* macular hole is a fully developed hole (≥400 µm diameter), typically accompanied by a rim of thickened and slightly elevated retina. Visual acuity may range from 20/40 to 5/200, but it is generally around 20/200. The posterior hyaloid remains attached to the optic disc, but it is detached from the macular region. An operculum may or may not be present, suspended on the posterior hyaloid overlying the hole.
- A *stage 4* macular hole is a fully developed hole with a complete posterior vitreous detachment signified by a Weiss ring.

Fluorescein angiography in eyes with stage 2, 3, and 4 holes demonstrates a circular transmission defect as a result of the loss of xanthophyll at the site of the hole and because of RPE depigmentation and atrophy in the base of the hole. The gold standard in the diagnosis of the various stages of macular holes is OCT examination.

Retrospective studies estimate the incidence of bilaterality in macular holes to be 1%–25%, but this figure is difficult to establish from the current literature because of loss to follow-up or short follow-up. Patients who present with a full-thickness macular hole in one eye and are symptomatic, with loss of foveal depression or stage 1A

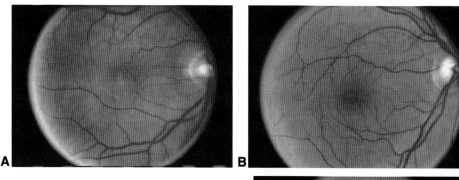

Figure 4-19 Macular holes. **A,** A stage 1A macular hole has a small yellow spot at the fovea. **B,** A stage 1B macular hole has a yellow ring at the fovea. **C,** A stage 2 macular hole is <400 µm in size.

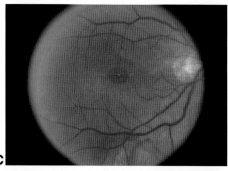

D, Red-free photograph of a full-thickness stage 3 macular hole with a visible central operculum that is smaller than the hole. **E,** A stage 4 macular hole is ≥400 µm in size and has a definite posterior vitreous detachment. *(Parts A, B, C, and E courtesy of Harry W. Flynn, Jr, MD. Part D reproduced with permission from Capone A Jr. Macular surface disorders.* Focal Points: Clinical Modules for Ophthalmologists. *San Francisco: American Academy of Ophthalmology; 1996, module 4.)*

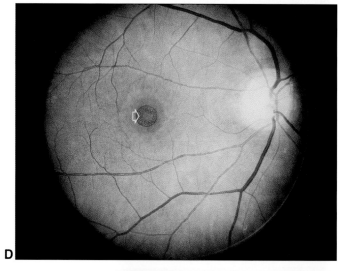

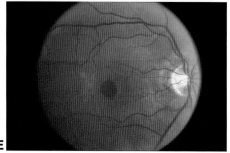

abnormalities in the second eye, have a substantial risk of progressing to a stage 2 hole in the second eye. Patients with a full-thickness macular hole in one eye and a normal retina with a vitreomacular separation in the other eye are at minimal if any risk of developing a macular hole in the second eye. Finally, patients presenting with a full-thickness macular hole in one eye and a normal fellow eye with an attached posterior vitreous probably have an intermediate risk of developing vitreomacular interface abnormalities in the second eye over their lifetimes.

Management options

Investigators in a collaborative multicenter trial that was set up to assess the benefit of vitrectomy in preventing macular holes suggest that surgery should probably not be recommended for stage 1 macular holes because of the high rate of spontaneous resolution (approximately 50%) and the failure of surgery to demonstrate a benefit. The study was limited by a small sample size and the difficulty, in the absence of OCT, of documenting stage 1 holes to ensure that investigators adhered to the eligibility criteria. Spontaneous resolution of more advanced stages of macular holes (stages 2–4) secondary to fibroglial tissue proliferation on the retinal surface or as a result of RPE hyperplasia occurs rarely (in 5% or less of cases). Most cases do not spontaneously resolve and should be considered for vitrectomy surgery. The first series of patients undergoing vitrectomy for idiopathic macular hole was reported in 1991. In 58% of eyes the hole was closed; in 42% visual acuity improved by 2 lines or more. Subsequent series have reported hole closure rates after vitrectomy as high as 92%–100%. See Chapter 16 for discussion of vitrectomy for macular holes.

Chew EY, Sperduto RD, Hiller R, et al. Clinical course of macular holes: the Eye Disease Case-Control Study. *Arch Ophthalmol.* 1999;117:242–246.

de Bustros S. Vitrectomy for prevention of macular holes: results of a randomized multicenter clinical trial. Vitrectomy for Prevention of Macular Hole Study Group. *Ophthalmology.* 1994;101:1055–1060.

Haouchine B, Massin P, Gaudric A. Foveal pseudocyst as the first step in macular hole formation: a prospective study by optical coherence tomography. *Ophthalmology.* 2001;108:15–22.

Johnson MW, Van Newkirk MR, Meyer KA. Perifoveal vitreous detachment is the primary pathogenic event in idiopathic macular hole formation. *Arch Ophthalmol.* 2001;119:215–222.

Spaide RF. Closure of an outer lamellar macular hole by vitrectomy: hypothesis for one mechanism of macular hole formation. *Retina.* 2000;20:587–590.

Valsalva Retinopathy

A sudden rise in intrathoracic or intraabdominal pressure (such as accompanies coughing, vomiting, lifting, or straining for a bowel movement) may raise intraocular venous pressure sufficiently to rupture small superficial capillaries in the macula. The hemorrhage is typically located under the internal limiting membrane (ILM), where it may create a hemorrhagic detachment of the ILM. Vitreous hemorrhage and subretinal hemorrhage may be present. The vision is usually only mildly reduced and the prognosis is excellent, with spontaneous resolution usually occurring within months after onset. The differential diagnosis of Valsalva retinopathy includes posterior vitreous separation, which may cause an identical hemorrhage or a macroaneurysm. Therefore, in all cases, a peripheral retinal tear or an aneurysm along an arteriole must be ruled out.

Purtscher Retinopathy and Purtscher-Like Retinopathy

Following acute compression injuries to the thorax or head, a patient may experience visual loss associated with Purtscher retinopathy in one or both eyes. Large cotton-wool spots, hemorrhages, and retinal edema are found most commonly surrounding the optic disc, and fluorescein angiography shows evidence of arteriolar obstruction and leakage (Fig 4-20). Occasionally, patients will present with disc edema and an afferent pupillary defect. Vision may be permanently lost from this infarction, and optic atrophy may develop.

Systemic and local factors can play a part in the development of Purtscher retinopathy. Injury may activate complement, which causes granulocyte aggregation and leukoembolization. This process in turn may occlude small arterioles such as those found in the peripapillary retina. In addition, local retinal vascular injury can also cause complement-mediated leukostasis and obstruction.

Even in the absence of trauma, various other conditions may activate complement and produce a similar fundus appearance. Because Purtscher's original description involved trauma, cases with similar fundus findings are termed *Purtscher-like retinopathy* (Table 4-6). For example, the retinopathy associated with acute pancreatitis, which appears identical to traumatic Purtscher retinopathy, is probably also caused by complement-mediated leukoembolization. Other conditions that may cause these changes in-

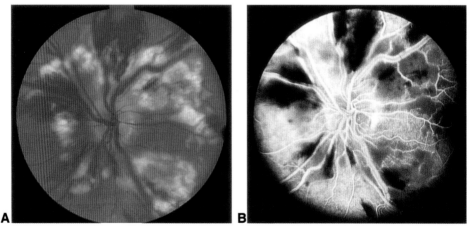

Figure 4-20 Purtscher retinopathy following trauma to head and face. **A,** Extensive cotton-wool spots and hemorrhage of retina. **B,** Fluorescein angiogram; capillary nonperfusion in areas of cotton-wool spots. *(Reproduced from Burton TC. Unilateral Purtscher's retinopathy. Ophthalmology. 1980;87:1096–1105.)*

Table 4-6 Conditions Associated With Purtscher or Purtscher-Like Retinopathy

Trauma
    Head injury
    Chest compression
    Long-bone fractures (fat embolism syndrome)
Acute pancreatitis
Chronic renal failure
Autoimmune diseases
    Systemic lupus erythematosus
    Thrombotic thrombocytopenic purpura
    Scleroderma
    Dermatomyositis
    Sjögren syndrome
Amniotic fluid embolism
Retrobulbar anesthesia
Orbital steroid injection

(Modified from Regillo CD. Posterior segment manifestations of systemic trauma. In: Regillo CD, Brown GC, Flynn HW Jr, eds. *Vitreoretinal Disease: The Essentials.* New York: Thieme; 1999:538.)

clude collagen-vascular diseases (such as systemic lupus erythematosus), child birth, and amniotic fluid embolism.

Fat embolism following crushing injuries or fractures of long bones may cause similar retinal findings. Usually, intraretinal hemorrhages will be scattered in the paramacular area, and the cotton-wool spots of fat embolism are generally smaller and situated more peripherally in the retina than in Purtscher retinopathy.

Terson Syndrome

Terson syndrome is recognized as vitreous and sub-ILM or subhyaloid hemorrhage caused by an abrupt intracranial hemorrhage. Although the exact mechanism is not known, it is suspected that the acute intracranial hemorrhage causes an acute rise in the intraocular venous pressure, resulting in a rupture of peripapillary and retinal vessels. Approximately one third of patients with subarachnoid or subdural hemorrhage have associated intraocular hemorrhage, which may include intraretinal and subretinal bleeding. Terson syndrome occurs mostly in individuals between 30 and 50 years old, but it can occur at any age. In most cases, visual function is unaffected once the hemorrhage clears. Spontaneous improvement generally occurs, although vitrectomy is occasionally required to clear the ocular media.

Gass JD. *Stereoscopic Atlas of Macular Diseases: Diagnosis and Treatment.* 4th ed. St Louis: Mosby; 1997:452–455.

CHAPTER 5

Retinal Vascular Disease

Systemic Arterial Hypertension

Systemic arterial hypertension, which is defined as a minimum diastolic pressure of 90 mm Hg or a minimum systolic pressure of 140 mm Hg, affects more than 50 million Americans. The ocular effects of hypertension can be observed and classified with ophthalmoscopy and angiography. Posterior segment changes in hypertension may occur in the retina, choroid, and optic nerve. Recognition of these posterior segment vascular changes by the ophthalmologist may prompt the initial diagnosis of hypertension and alert the patient to potential complications from this condition. BCSC Section 1, *Update on General Medicine,* discusses hypertension in detail, including several tables that describe drugs and drug interactions with antihypertensive therapy.

Hyman BN, Moser M. Hypertension update. *Surv Ophthalmol.* 1996;41:79–89.

Kim SK, Christlieb AR, Mieler WF, et al. Hypertension and its ocular manifestations. In: Albert DM, Jakobiec FA, eds. *Principles and Practice of Ophthalmology.* 2nd ed. Philadelphia: Saunders; 2000:4506–4524.

Hypertensive Retinopathy

The relationship between hypertensive vascular changes and the changes of arteriosclerotic vascular disease is complex, with great variation in the expression of these disease processes. Hence, classification of retinal vascular changes caused strictly by hypertension is difficult. Following is one commonly used system, the Modified Scheie Classification of Hypertensive Retinopathy:

Grade 0	No changes
Grade 1	Barely detectable arterial narrowing
Grade 2	Obvious arterial narrowing with focal irregularities
Grade 3	Grade 2 plus retinal hemorrhages and/or exudate
Grade 4	Grade 3 plus disc swelling

Mandava N, Yannuzzi LA. Hypertensive retinopathy. In: Regillo CD, Brown GC, Flynn HW Jr, eds. *Vitreoretinal Disease: The Essentials.* New York: Thieme; 1999:193–196.

The most common retinal findings in chronic systemic hypertension include focal or generalized constriction of retinal arterioles. Hypertension is also associated with intraretinal hemorrhages, branch retinal artery occlusion (BRAO), branch retinal vein occlusion (BRVO), central retinal vein occlusion (CRVO), and retinal arterial macroaneurysms. Ischemia secondary to BRVO may result in neovascularization of the retina, preretinal and vitreous hemorrhage, epiretinal membrane formation, and tractional retinal detachment. The coexistence of hypertension and diabetes mellitus may result in more severe diabetic retinopathy.

Klein R, Klein BE, Moss SE, et al. Blood pressure, hypertension and retinopathy in a population. *Trans Am Ophthalmol Soc.* 1993;91:207–226.

Murphy RP, Chew EY. Hypertension. In: Ryan SJ, ed. *Retina.* 3rd ed. St Louis: Mosby; 2001.

Hypertensive Choroidopathy

Hypertensive choroidopathy typically occurs in young patients experiencing acute hypertension, such as patients with preeclampsia, eclampsia, pheochromocytoma, or accelerated hypertension. Zones of nonperfusion of the choriocapillaris may occur initially and result in hyperpigmented patches with a margin of hypopigmentation known as *Elschnig spots* (Fig 5-1). Linear configurations of hyperpigmentation that develop over choroidal arteries in patients with acute uncontrolled hypertension are known as *Siegrist streaks.* Fluorescein angiography shows focal choroidal hypoperfusion in early phases and multiple subretinal areas of leakage in late phases (Fig 5-2). Focal RPE detachments may occur, and extensive exudative retinal detachment may develop on rare occasions.

Hypertensive Optic Neuropathy

Depending on the degree and chronicity of the hypertension, hypertensive optic neuropathy has a variable presentation. Patients with severe hypertension may have linear flame-shaped hemorrhages at the margin of the optic disc, blurring of the disc margins, congestion of associated retinal veins, florid disc edema, and secondary macular exudates

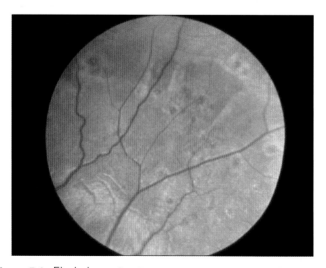

Figure 5-1 Elschnig spots. *(Photograph courtesy of Harry W. Flynn, Jr, MD.)*

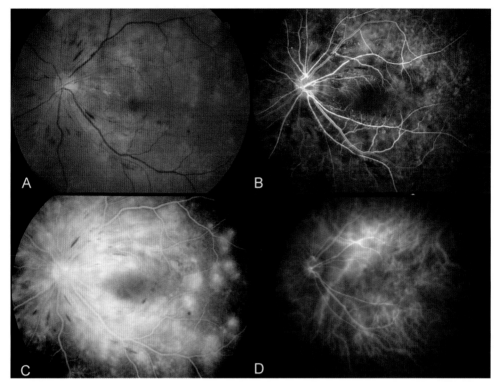

Figure 5-2 Malignant hypertension. **A,** The color fundus photograph shows a shallow detachment of the macula with striae of the inner limiting membrane (ILM). There are splinter hemorrhages in the retina, slight hyperemia of the optic nerve, and a few flecks of lipid in the macula. Also evident are multiple yellowish patches at the level of the RPE and inner choroid. The fluorescein angiogram shows multiple abnormalities of the retinal and choroidal circulation. **B,** In the early phases, areas of retinal capillary nonperfusion and microaneurysm formation are present, as well as a dendritic pattern of choroidal filling defects. **C,** In the later phases of the fluorescein angiogram, there is intense leakage of dye from the retinal vessels as well as from some, but not all, of the yellowish patches seen in part A. **D,** An early phase of the corresponding ICG angiogram shows a moth-eaten appearance of the choriocapillaris. *(Photographs courtesy of Richard Spaide, MD.)*

(Fig 5-3). The differential diagnosis in patients with this clinical appearance includes diabetic papillopathy, radiation retinopathy, CRVO, anterior ischemic optic neuropathy, and neuroretinitis. Treatment of systemic arterial hypertension is essential in reducing or reversing these ocular manifestations of the disease.

Diabetic Retinopathy

A frequent cause of blindness in the United States, diabetic retinopathy is the leading cause in patients aged 20–64 years. For additional information concerning evaluation and treatment of diabetic retinopathy, see the following selected Academy materials.

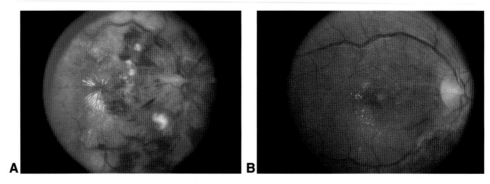

Figure 5-3 **A,** This 25-year-old patient had severe hypertension (210/140) with visual loss to the 2/200 level. Note the disc edema, macular exudates, intraretinal hemorrhage with nerve fiber layer infarct, and venous congestion. **B,** Fundus photograph of same patient taken 10 weeks later, after treatment of hypertension and normalization of blood pressure. The optic disc is now normal, and minimal residual macular exudates are present. The visual acuity has returned to 20/50. *(Photographs courtesy of Harry W. Flynn, Jr, MD.)*

Flynn HW Jr, Smiddy WE, eds. *Diabetes and Ocular Disease: Past, Present, and Future Therapies.* Ophthalmology Monograph 14. San Francisco: American Academy of Ophthalmology; 2000.

Preferred Practice Patterns Committee, Retina Panel. *Diabetic Retinopathy.* San Francisco: American Academy of Ophthalmology; November 2003.

Terminology

The terminology used for types of diabetes is changing and may be confusing. The American Diabetes Association (ADA) has begun using the term *immune-mediated diabetes* instead of *type 1 diabetes,* which has traditionally been known as *insulin-dependent diabetes mellitus (IDDM).* The change in usage is not universal, however. The ADA has also abandoned the use of *non–insulin-dependent diabetes mellitus (NIDDM)* for *type 2 diabetes,* but, again, this change is not yet widespread, and BCSC will continue to use the terminology that is used by individual studies.

Epidemiology

The prevalence of all types of retinopathy in the diabetic population increases with the duration of diabetes and patient age. Diabetic retinopathy is rarely found in children younger than 10 years of age, regardless of the duration of diabetes. The risk of developing retinopathy increases after puberty.

The Wisconsin Epidemiologic Study of Diabetic Retinopathy (WESDR)

This ongoing epidemiologic study of the progression of diabetic retinopathy involves the measurement of visual acuity levels in a large population of patients with diabetes. WESDR is attempting to identify all patients with diabetes treated by physicians in an 11-county area of southern Wisconsin. Between 1979 and 1980, 1210 patients with type 1 diabetes and 1780 patients with type 2 diabetes were entered into the study. Patients underwent several clinical assessments, including 7-field stereoscopic fundus photography, measurements of glycosylated hemoglobin, and recording of visual acuity.

In following this population of patients, WESDR has reported important epidemiologic findings. The duration of diabetes is directly associated with an increased prevalence of diabetic retinopathy in people with both type 1 and type 2 diabetes. After 20 years of diabetes, nearly 99% of patients with type 1 and 60% with type 2 have some degree of diabetic retinopathy, and 3.6% of younger-onset patients (aged <30 years at diagnosis, an operational definition of type 1 diabetes) and 1.6% of older-onset patients (aged ≥30 years at diagnosis, an operational definition of type 2 diabetes) were found to be legally blind. In the younger-onset group, 86% of blindness was attributable to diabetic retinopathy. In the older-onset group, where other eye diseases were more common, one third of the cases of legal blindness were the result of diabetic retinopathy.

WESDR epidemiologic data have been limited primarily to white populations of northern European extraction and may not be applicable to African Americans, populations of Hispanic or Asian descent, or other populations with a higher prevalence of diabetes and retinopathy such as American Indians. The National Health and Nutrition Examination Survey III of type 2 diabetes showed that the frequency of diabetic retinopathy was higher among non-Hispanic blacks (27%) and Mexican Americans (33%) over 40 years of age than in non-Hispanic whites (18%) over 40 years of age.

Harris MI, Klein R, Cowie CC, et al. Is the risk of diabetic retinopathy greater in non-Hispanic blacks and Mexican Americans than in non-Hispanic whites with type 2 diabetes? A U.S. population study. *Diabetes Care.* 1998;21:1230–1235.

Klein R, Klein BE, Moss SE, et al. The Wisconsin Epidemiologic Study of Diabetic Retinopathy. II. Prevalence and risk of diabetic retinopathy when age at diagnosis is less than 30 years. *Arch Ophthalmol.* 1984;102:520–526.

Pathogenesis

The exact cause of diabetic microvascular disease is unknown. It is believed that exposure to hyperglycemia over an extended period results in a number of biochemical and physiologic changes that ultimately cause vascular endothelial damage. Specific retinal vascular changes include the loss of pericytes and basement membrane thickening, which compromises the capillary lumen, as well as decompensation of the endothelial barrier function.

A large number of hematologic and biochemical abnormalities have been correlated with the prevalence and severity of retinopathy:

- increased platelet adhesiveness
- increased erythrocyte aggregation
- abnormal serum lipids
- defective fibrinolysis
- abnormal levels of growth hormone
- upregulation of vascular endothelial growth factor (VEGF)
- abnormalities in serum and whole blood viscosity

However, the precise role of these abnormalities—individually or in combination—in the pathogenesis of retinopathy is not well defined.

Conditions Associated With Potential Visual Loss from Diabetic Retinopathy

The potential for visual loss in patients with diabetic retinopathy can be associated with the following conditions:

- sequelae from ischemia-induced neovascularization
- diabetic macular edema
- ischemic macular changes

Each of these topics will be discussed with specific reference drawn to pertinent related clinical trials. Issues pertaining to medical treatment, laser therapy, and surgical treatment will be addressed.

Ischemia-Induced Neovascularization and Sequelae

Diabetic retinopathy is classified into an early stage, *nonproliferative diabetic retinopathy (NPDR)*, and a more advanced stage, *proliferative diabetic retinopathy (PDR)*. This latter stage is a manifestation of ischemia-induced neovascularization from diabetes. The progression from mild stages of the disease to advanced proliferative changes occurs in a predictable stepwise fashion. The cadence of the progression varies among patients. NPDR, also known as background diabetic retinopathy, is further described as either mild, moderate, severe, or very severe. PDR is described as early, high-risk, or advanced.

Nonproliferative diabetic retinopathy

Retinal microvascular changes that occur in NPDR are limited to the confines of the retina and do not extend beyond the internal limiting membrane (ILM). Characteristic findings in NPDR include microaneurysms, dot-and-blot intraretinal hemorrhages, retinal edema, hard exudates, dilation and beading of retinal veins, intraretinal microvascular abnormalities (IRMA), nerve fiber layer infarcts, arteriolar abnormalities, and areas of capillary nonperfusion. NPDR can affect visual function through 2 mechanisms:

- variable degrees of intraretinal capillary closure, resulting in macular ischemia
- increased retinal vascular permeability, resulting in macular edema

Chew EY, Ferris FL III. Nonproliferative diabetic retinopathy. In: Ryan SJ, ed. *Retina*. 3rd ed. St Louis: Mosby; 2001:1295–1308.

Proliferative diabetic retinopathy

Extraretinal fibrovascular proliferation extends beyond the ILM and is present in varying stages of development in PDR. The new vessels evolve in 3 stages:

1. Fine new vessels with minimal fibrous tissue appear.
2. The new vessels increase in size and extent, with an increased fibrous component.
3. The new vessels regress, leaving residual fibrovascular proliferation along the posterior hyaloid.

Progression to PDR

Severe NPDR, as defined by the Early Treatment Diabetic Retinopathy Study (ETDRS; Clinical Trial 5-1) in the *4:2:1 rule,* is characterized by any one of the following:

Early Treatment Diabetic Retinopathy Study (ETDRS)

Study Questions:

1. Is photocoagulation effective for treating diabetic macular edema?
2. Is photocoagulation effective for treating diabetic retinopathy?
3. Is aspirin effective for preventing progression of diabetic retinopathy?

Eligibility: Mild nonproliferative diabetic retinopathy through early proliferative diabetic retinopathy, with visual acuity 20/200 or better in each eye.

Randomization: 3711 participants: one eye randomly assigned to photocoagulation (scatter and/or focal) and one eye assigned to no photocoagulation; patients randomly assigned to 650 mg/d aspirin or placebo.

Outcome Variables: Visual acuity less than 5/200 for at least 4 months; visual acuity worsening by doubling of initial visual angle (eg, 20/40 to 20/80); retinopathy progression.

Aspirin Use Results:

1. Aspirin use did not alter progression of diabetic retinopathy.
2. Aspirin use did not increase risk of vitreous hemorrhage.
3. Aspirin use did not affect visual acuity.
4. Aspirin use reduced risk of cardiovascular morbidity and mortality.

Early Scatter Photocoagulation Results:

1. Early scatter photocoagulation resulted in small reduction in risk of severe visual loss (<5/200 for at least 4 months).
2. Early scatter photocoagulation is not indicated for eyes with mild to moderate diabetic retinopathy.
3. Early scatter photocoagulation may be most effective in patients with type 2 diabetes.

Macular Edema Results:

1. Focal photocoagulation for diabetic macular edema decreased risk of moderate visual loss (doubling of initial visual angle).
2. Focal photocoagulation for diabetic macular edema increased chance of moderate visual gain (halving of initial visual angle).
3. Focal photocoagulation for diabetic macular edema reduced retinal thickening.

- diffuse intraretinal hemorrhages and microaneurysms in *4* quadrants (Fig 5-4)
- venous beading in *2* quadrants (Fig 5-5)
- intraretinal microvascular abnormalities (IRMA) in *1* quadrant (Fig 5-6)

The ETDRS investigators developed this 4:2:1 rule to help the clinician identify patients at greatest risk for progression to PDR and high-risk PDR. The ETDRS found that severe NPDR had a 15% chance of progression to high-risk PDR within 1 year. Very severe

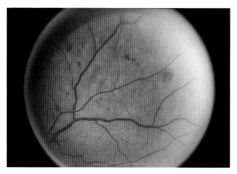

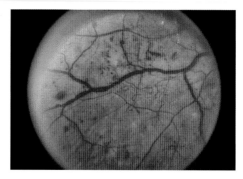

Figure 5-4 Diffuse intraretinal hemorrhages and microaneurysms in NPDR. *(Standard photograph 2A, courtesy of the ETDRS.)*

Figure 5-5 Venous beading in NPDR. *(Standard photograph 6B, courtesy of the ETDRS.)*

Figure 5-6 Intraretinal microvascular abnormalities, or IRMA, in NPDR. *(Standard photograph 8A, courtesy of the ETDRS.)*

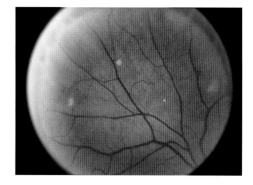

NPDR, defined by the presence of any 2 of the above features, had a 45% chance of progression to high-risk PDR within 1 year.

> Early photocoagulation for diabetic retinopathy. Early Treatment Diabetic Retinopathy Study Research Group. ETDRS report 9. *Ophthalmology.* 1991;98:766–785.

Nerve fiber layer infarcts (also called *cotton-wool spots* or *soft exudates*) also may be present in NPDR. The ETDRS reported that nerve fiber layer infarcts were less helpful in predicting progression to PDR than were other severe NPDR characteristics. Historically, the term *preproliferative diabetic retinopathy* included nerve fiber layer infarcts as well as the features defined by the ETDRS under severe or very severe NPDR. Nerve fiber layer infarcts can be seen easily on clinical examination, and their presence suggests that a careful search for features predicting progression to PDR is called for.

The release of vasoproliferative factors is probably related to the degree of retinal ischemia. One vasoproliferative factor, vascular endothelial growth factor (VEGF), has been isolated from vitrectomy specimens of patients with PDR. This vasoproliferative factor stimulates neovascularization of the retina, optic nerve head, or anterior segment.

> Aiello LP, Avery RL, Arrigg PG, et al. Vascular endothelial growth factor in ocular fluid of patients with diabetic retinopathy and other retinal disorders. *N Engl J Med.* 1994;331: 1480–1487.

Advanced diabetic retinopathy is associated with cardiovascular disease risk factors. Patients with PDR are at increased risk of heart attack, stroke, diabetic nephropathy, amputation, and death.

Medical management of PDR

The principal goal in the medical management of PDR is prevention. This can be achieved by considering both systemic and local measures that influence the progression from NPDR to PDR.

Hypertension, discussed at the beginning of this chapter, is usually associated with a higher risk of progression of diabetic macular edema and diabetic retinopathy in general when poorly controlled over many years. In *asymmetric carotid artery occlusive disease*, the retinopathy may be further influenced by ocular ischemia. Controversy exists as to whether mild or moderate carotid artery occlusive disease has a protective effect on the development and severity of diabetic retinopathy. *Severe carotid artery occlusive disease* may result in advanced PDR as part of the ocular ischemic syndrome. *Advanced diabetic renal disease* and *anemia* also may have an adverse influence on diabetic retinopathy.

Pregnancy is associated with worsening of retinopathy; thus, women with diabetes who become pregnant require more frequent evaluation of the retina. Visual loss may occur from NPDR with diabetic macular edema or from the complications of PDR. Although many of these patients will have some regression of retinopathy after delivery, photocoagulation treatment is generally recommended if high-risk PDR develops during pregnancy.

Brown GC. Arterial occlusive disease. In: Regillo CA, Brown GC, Flynn HW Jr, eds. *Vitreoretinal Diseases: The Essentials.* New York: Thieme; 1999:97–117.

Chew EY, Mills JL, Metzger BE, et al. Metabolic control and progression of retinopathy: The Diabetes in Early Pregnancy Study. National Institute of Child Health and Human Development Diabetes in Early Pregnancy Study. *Diabetes Care.* 1995;18:631–637.

Davis MD, Fisher MR, Gangnon RE, et al. Risk factors for high-risk proliferative diabetic retinopathy and severe visual loss: ETDRS Report 18. *Invest Ophthalmol Vis Sci.* 1998;39:233–252.

One of the most important factors to stress in the medical management of diabetic retinopathy is the need to maintain good glycemic control. The Diabetes Control and Complications Trial (DCCT; Clinical Trial 5-2) and the United Kingdom Prospective Diabetes Study (UKPDS; Clinical Trial 5-3) showed that intensive glycemic control is associated with a reduced risk of newly diagnosed retinopathy and a reduced progression of existing retinopathy in people with diabetes mellitus (type 1 diabetes in DCCT and type 2 diabetes in UKPDS). Furthermore, the DCCT showed that intensive glycemic control (compared to conventional treatment) was associated with reductions in progression to severe nonproliferative and proliferative retinopathy, incidence of macular edema, and need for panretinal and focal photocoagulation. The UKPDS showed that control of hypertension was also beneficial in reducing progression of retinopathy and loss of vision.

Aiello LM, Cavallerano J, Aiello LP. Diagnosis, management, and treatment of nonproliferative diabetic retinopathy and macular edema. In: Albert DM, Jakobiec FA, eds. *Principles and Practice of Ophthalmology.* 2nd ed. Philadelphia: Saunders; 2000:747–759.

CLINICAL TRIAL 5-2

Diabetes Control and Complications Trial (DCCT)

Study Questions:

1. Primary prevention study: Will intensive control of blood glucose slow development and subsequent progression of diabetic retinopathy?
2. Secondary prevention study: Will intensive control of blood glucose slow progression of diabetic retinopathy?

Eligibility:

1. 726 patients with type 1 diabetes mellitus (1–5 years' duration) and no diabetic retinopathy.
2. 715 patients with type 1 diabetes mellitus (1–15 years' duration) and mild-to-moderate diabetic retinopathy.

Study Groups: Intensive control of blood glucose (multiple daily insulin injections or insulin pump) versus conventional management.

Outcome Variables: Development of diabetic retinopathy or progression of retinopathy by 3 steps using modified Airlie House classification scale; neuropathy, nephropathy, and cardiovascular outcomes were also assessed.

Results: Intensive control reduced risk of developing retinopathy by 76% and slowed progression of retinopathy by 54%; intensive control also reduced risk of clinical neuropathy by 60% and albuminuria by 54%.

The effect of intensive treatment of diabetes on the development and progression of long-term complications in insulin-dependent diabetes mellitus. Diabetes Control and Complications Trial Research Group. *N Engl J Med.* 1993;329:977–986.

Intensive blood-glucose control with sulphonylureas or insulin compared with conventional treatment and risk of complications in patients with type 2 diabetes (UKPDS 33). United Kingdom Prospective Diabetes Study Group. *Lancet.* 1998;352:837–853.

Klein R, Klein BE, Moss SE, et al. Association of ocular disease and mortality in a diabetic population. *Arch Ophthalmol.* 1999;117:1487–1495.

Klein R, Klein BE, Moss SE, et al. The Wisconsin Epidemiologic Study of Diabetic Retinopathy: XVII. The 14-year incidence and progression of diabetic retinpathy and associated risk factors in type 1 diabetes. *Ophthalmology.* 1998;105:1801–1815.

Progression of retinopathy with intensive versus conventional treatment in the Diabetes Control and Complications Trial. Diabetes Control and Complications Trial Research Group. *Ophthalmology.* 1995;102:647–661.

Tight blood pressure control and risk of macrovascular and microvascular complications in type 2 diabetes: UKPDS 38. United Kingdom Prospective Diabetes Study Group. *Br Med J.* 1998;317:703–713.

Laser treatment of PDR

The development of neovascularization heralds an important change in the progression of diabetic retinopathy. Complications from PDR can result in severe visual loss if left untreated. More importantly, prompt treatment often can significantly reduce the probability of developing these adverse outcomes.

CLINICAL TRIAL 5-3

United Kingdom Prospective Diabetes Study (UKPDS)

Study Questions:

1. Will intensive control of blood glucose, in patients with type 2 diabetes, reduce the risk of microvascular complications of diabetes, including the risk of retinopathy progression?
2. Will intensive control of blood pressure, in patients with type 2 diabetes and elevated blood pressure, reduce the risk of microvascular complications of diabetes, including the risk of retinopathy progression?

Eligibility:

1. 4209 patients with newly diagnosed type 2 diabetes.
2. 1148 hypertensive patients with newly diagnosed type 2 diabetes.

Randomization:

1. Patients were randomly assigned to conventional policy starting with diet (1138 patients) or to intensive policy starting with a sulphonylurea chlorpropamide (788 patients), glibenclamide (615 patients), or glipizide (170 patients) or with insulin (1156 patients). If overweight and in the intensive group, patients were assigned to start treatment with metformin (342 patients).
2. Patients were randomly assigned to tight control of blood pressure (400 with ACE inhibitor and 398 with beta blocker) or to less tight control (390 patients).

Outcome Variables: Development of any of three aggregate adverse outcomes and specific retinopathy-related outcomes (worsening of retinopathy on a modified Airlie House scale, retinal photocoagulation, vitreous hemorrhage, and worsening of visual acuity).

Results:

1. Intensive control of blood glucose slowed progression of retinopathy and reduced the risk of other microvascular complications of diabetes. Sulphonylureas did not increase the risk of cardiovascular disease.
2. Intensive control of blood pressure slowed progression of retinopathy and reduced the risk of other microvascular and macrovascular complications of diabetes. No clinically or statistically significant difference was found in the comparison of blood pressure lowering with ACE inhibitors versus beta blockers.

The mainstay of treatment for PDR involves the use of thermal laser photocoagulation in a panretinal pattern to induce regression.

Scatter laser treatment For patients with high-risk PDR, scatter panretinal photocoagulation (PRP) treatment is almost always recommended. The goal of scatter PRP is to cause regression of existing neovascular tissue and to prevent progressive neovascularization in the future. The amount of therapy necessary to achieve these endpoints is determined by the clinical response to a standard initial treatment. Full PRP, as used in the Diabetic Retinopathy Study (DRS; Clinical Trial 5-4) and ETDRS, included 1200 or more 500-μm burns, separated from each other by one-half burn width, at 0.1 second duration (Fig 5-7). Treatments may be divided into 2 or more sessions.

After the initial standard PRP, additional incremental therapy can be applied in the attempt to achieve further regression of persistent neovascularization. Green, red, or diode laser photocoagulation may be successfully applied when vitreous hemorrhage or

CLINICAL TRIAL 5-4

Diabetic Retinopathy Study (DRS)

Study Question: Is photocoagulation (argon or xenon arc) effective for treating diabetic retinopathy?

Eligibility: Proliferative diabetic retinopathy or bilateral severe nonproliferative diabetic retinopathy, with visual acuity 20/100 or better in each eye.

Randomization: 1742 participants. One eye randomly assigned to photocoagulation (argon laser or xenon arc) and one eye assigned to no photocoagulation.

Outcome Variable: Visual acuity less than 5/200 for at least 4 months.

Results: Photocoagulation (argon or xenon) reduces risk of severe visual loss compared to no treatment. Treated eyes with high-risk PDR achieved the greatest benefit.

Status: Study completed.

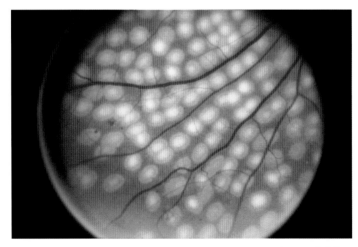

Figure 5-7 Full-scatter panretinal photocoagulation treatment used in the DRS and the ETDRS. Included are 1200 or more 500-μm burns, separated by one-half burn width. The burns in this photograph have a surrounding ring of edema, making many of the burns appear confluent. *(Photograph courtesy of Harry W. Flynn, Jr, MD.)*

cataract prevents the use of argon laser. Scatter treatment should generally be avoided in areas of prominent fibrovascular membranes, vitreoretinal traction, and tractional retinal detachment. Despite clinical regression of neovascularization, episodes of fibrovascular contracture may occur, resulting in recurrent vitreous hemorrhage and tractional or rhegmatogenous retinal detachment. Additional laser treatment may not be necessary in the absence of progressive neovascularization. Small transient vitreous hemorrhages can occasionally occur in the presence of complete PRP and can usually be observed.

Noteworthy side effects associated with scatter PRP include a decrease in night vision, color vision, and/or peripheral vision, as well as a loss of 1 or 2 lines of visual acuity in some patients. Additional side effects include glare, temporary loss of accommodation, and photopsia. Macular edema, if present prior to scatter PRP, may be aggravated by scatter therapy. Many of these side effects can be reduced by using multiple treatment sessions, applying macular focal laser prior to PRP, and using more peripheral laser placement. Great care must be taken to avoid foveal photocoagulation, especially when contact lenses that reverse the image are used.

Early photocoagulation for diabetic retinopathy. ETDRS report 9. Early Treatment Diabetic Retinopathy Study Research Group. *Ophthalmology.* 1991;98 (5 suppl):766–785.

Fong DS, Segal PP, Myers F, et al. Subretinal fibrosis in diabetic macular edema. ETDRS report 23. Early Treatment Diabetic Retinopathy Study Research Group. *Arch Ophthalmol.* 1997;115:873–877.

Current clinical threshold parameters for scatter laser treatment stem from the results of the Diabetic Retinopathy Study.

Diabetic Retinopathy Study The DRS was a randomized, prospective clinical trial evaluating PRP treatment to 1 eye of patients with clear media and advanced NPDR or PDR in both eyes (see Clinical Trial 5-4). The primary outcome measurement in the DRS was severe visual loss (SVL), defined as a visual acuity of less than 5/200 on two consecutive follow-up examinations 4 months apart. The DRS demonstrated a 50% or greater reduction in the rates of SVL in eyes treated with PRP compared to untreated control eyes during a follow-up of over 5 years (Fig 5-8).

High-risk PDR was defined as any one of following:

- mild neovascularization of the disc (NVD) with vitreous hemorrhage (Fig 5-9)
- moderate to severe NVD with or without vitreous hemorrhage (≥Standard 10A, showing ¼ to ⅓ disc area of NVD)
- moderate (½ disc area) neovascularization elsewhere (NVE) with vitreous hemorrhage (Fig 5-10)

High-risk PDR was also defined by any combination of 3 of the 4 retinopathy risk factors:

- presence of vitreous or preretinal hemorrhage
- presence of new vessels
- location of new vessels on or near the optic disc
- moderate to severe extent of new vessels

The DRS recommended prompt treatment of eyes with high-risk PDR because this group had the highest risk of SVL. The complications of argon laser PRP in the DRS were generally mild but included a decrease in visual acuity by 1 or more lines in 11% and visual field loss in 5%.

Four risk factors for severe visual loss in diabetic retinopathy. DRS report 3. Diabetic Retinopathy Study Research Group. *Arch Ophthalmol.* 1979:97:654–655.

Photocoagulation treatment of proliferative diabetic retinopathy: clinical application of Diabetic Retinopathy Study (DRS) findings. DRS report 8. Diabetic Retinopathy Study Research Group. *Ophthalmology.* 1981:88:583–600.

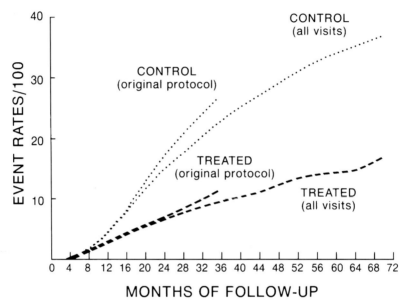

Figure 5-8 The cumulative rate of severe visual loss during the period of follow-up in the Diabetic Retinopathy Study. *(From the Diabetic Retinopathy Study Research Group. Photocoagulation treatment of proliferative diabetic retinopathy: clinical application of Diabetic Retinopathy Study (DRS) findings: DRS report 8. Ophthalmology. 1981;88:583–600.)*

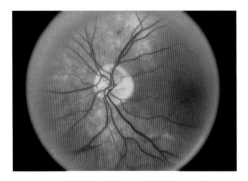

Figure 5-9 NVD with small vitreous hemorrhage. Even without vitreous hemorrhage, this amount of NVD is the lower limit of moderate NVD and is considered high-risk PDR. *(Standard photograph 10A, courtesy of the DRS.)*

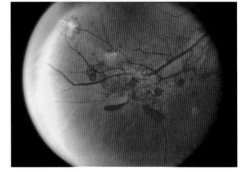

Figure 5-10 Moderate neovascularization elsewhere (NVE) with preretinal hemorrhage. *(Standard photograph 7, courtesy of the DRS.)*

Neovascularization of the iris or anterior chamber angle Small isolated tufts of neovascularization at the pupillary border are relatively common in patients with diabetes. Eyes with small isolated tufts can be carefully followed without initial treatment. Patients with contiguous neovascularization of the pupil and midstromal iris or involving the anterior chamber angle generally require prompt PRP whether or not high-risk PDR is present.

Surgical management of PDR

The 2 main sequelae of advanced PDR include vitreous hemorrhage and tractional retinal detachment. For both conditions, surgical intervention is the mainstay of contemporary management.

Vitreous hemorrhage In the 1970s, after Machemer introduced vitrectomy surgery, the indications for surgical intervention in patients with PDR included nonclearing vitreous hemorrhage for more than a year. The Diabetic Retinopathy Vitrectomy Study (DRVS; Clinical Trial 5-5) was carried out in order to determine whether there was a role for earlier vitrectomy in patients with vitreous hemorrhage secondary to PDR.

Diabetic Retinopathy Vitrectomy Study The DRVS was a randomized, prospective clinical trial investigating the role of vitrectomy in managing eyes with severe PDR (see Clinical Trial 5-5). Two outcome measurements in the DRVS were the percentages of eyes with 10/20 or 10/50 visual acuity on DRVS standardized visual acuity charts at the 2- and 4-year follow-up examinations.

The DRVS evaluated the benefit of early (1–6 months after onset of vitreous hemorrhage) versus late (at 1 year) vitrectomy for eyes with severe vitreous hemorrhage and visual loss (≤5/200). Patients with type 1 diabetes with severe vitreous hemorrhage clearly demonstrated the benefit of early vitrectomy, but no such advantage was found in mixed or type 2 patients (Table 5-1). The DRVS also showed an advantage for early vitrectomy compared with conventional management in eyes with very severe PDR.

CLINICAL TRIAL 5-5

Diabetic Retinopathy Vitrectomy Study (DRVS)

Study Questions: Is early vitrectomy preferable to deferral of vitrectomy in eyes with

1. Severe vitreous hemorrhage from proliferative diabetic retinopathy?
2. Very severe proliferative diabetic retinopathy?

Eligibility: Recent severe vitreous hemorrhage from proliferative retinopathy (616 eyes); advanced active very severe proliferative diabetic retinopathy (370 eyes, 240 with prior scatter photocoagulation).

Randomization: Early vitrectomy versus conventional management.

Outcome Variable: Visual acuity 20/40 or better.

Results: Visual acuity 20/40 or better was more frequent in early-vitrectomy groups; benefit of early vitrectomy was seen only in eyes with most severe proliferative diabetic retinopathy.

Table 5-1 DRVS Final Visual Acuity Results ≥10/20 for Eyes With Severe Vitreous Hemorrhage

Diabetes	Early Vitrectomy	Late Vitrectomy
Type 1	35.6%	11.7%
Mixed	18.6%	17.4%
Type 2	15.9%	18.1%

Advances in vitreoretinal surgery, including the development of the endolaser, have changed some of the recommendations of the DRVS. Patients with preexisting, well-placed, complete PRP treatment in the face of vitreous hemorrhage can undergo a longer period of observation. If PRP has not been performed, early intervention is usually recommended in patients with vitreous hemorrhage secondary to PDR regardless of the class of diabetes.

Early vitrectomy for severe proliferative diabetic retinopathy in eyes with useful vision: results of a randomized trial. DRVS report 3. Diabetic Retinopathy Vitrectomy Study Research Group. *Ophthalmology.* 1988;95:1307–1320.

Early vitrectomy for severe vitreous hemorrhage in diabetic retinopathy: two-year results of a randomized trial. DRVS report 2. Diabetic Retinopathy Vitrectomy Study Research Group. *Arch Ophthalmol.* 1985;103:1644–1652.

Tractional retinal detachment Complications from PDR are exacerbated by traction of the vitreous on elevated fibrovascular proliferative tissue. Partial posterior vitreous detachment frequently develops in eyes with fibrovascular proliferation, resulting in traction on the new vessels and vitreous or preretinal hemorrhage. Tractional complications such as vitreous hemorrhage, retinal detachment, or macular heterotopia may ensue, as well as progressive fibrovascular proliferation. Contraction of the fibrovascular proliferation and vitreous may result in retinal breaks and subsequent rhegmatogenous retinal detachment. The presence of chronic retinal detachment in eyes with PDR contributes to retinal ischemia and may account for the increased risk of iris neovascularization in such eyes.

Greater discussion of the surgical management of tractional retinal detachments secondary to PDR can be found in Chapter 16.

Davis MD. *Proliferative diabetic retinopathy.* In: Ryan SJ, ed. *Retina.* 3rd. St Louis: Mosby; 2001:1309– 1349.

Diabetic Macular Edema

Retinal edema threatening or involving the macula is an important visual consequence of abnormal retinal vascular permeability in diabetic retinopathy (Fig 5-11). The diagnosis of diabetic macular edema (DME) is best made by slit-lamp biomicroscopy of the posterior pole using a contact lens. Important observations include

- location of retinal thickening relative to the fovea
- presence and location of exudates
- presence of cystoid macular edema

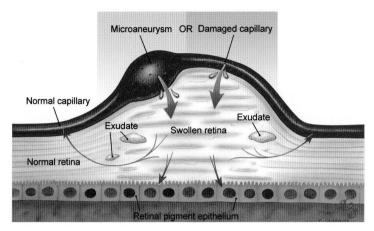

Figure 5-11 Artist's conception of the mechanism of diabetic macular edema, demonstrating development of thickening from a break in the blood–retinal barrier. *(Reproduced with permission from Ginsburg LH, Aiello LM. Diabetic retinopathy: classification, progression, and management. Focal Points: Clinical Modules for Ophthalmologists. San Francisco: American Academy of Ophthalmology; 1993, module 7. Illustration by Christine Gralapp.)*

Fluorescein angiography is useful in demonstrating the breakdown of the blood–retinal barrier by showing retinal capillary leakage. However, angiography should *not* be used to evaluate for the presence of macular edema, as this should be primarily a slit-lamp biomicroscopic diagnosis. Simple leakage on the angiogram may not always be associated with retinal thickening in the macular area.

DME may manifest as focal or diffuse retinal thickening with or without exudates. Although an overlap of categories often occurs, 2 general categories of macular edema— focal and diffuse—have been described. *Focal macular edema* is characterized by areas of focal fluorescein leakage from specific capillary lesions. It may be associated with rings of hard exudate derived from plasma lipoproteins that appear to emanate from micro-aneurysms. Resorption of fluid components results in precipitation of lipid residues, usually in the outer and inner plexiform layers but occasionally beneath the sensory retina itself. These residues are the white to yellow deposits described as *hard exudates. Diffuse macular edema* is characterized by widespread retinal capillary abnormalities associated with diffuse leakage from extensive breakdown of the blood–retinal barrier and, often, with cystoid macular edema.

Laser treatment of DME

Many of the current treatment paradigms for the management of diabetic macular edema are derived from the ETDRS, a randomized, prospective clinical trial evaluating photo-coagulation of patients with diabetes with less than high-risk PDR in both eyes. The primary outcome measurement in the ETDRS was moderate visual loss (MVL), comparing baseline with follow-up visual acuities. MVL was defined as a doubling of the visual angle (eg, a drop from 20/20 to 20/40 or from 20/50 to 20/100), a drop of 15 or more letters on ETDRS visual acuity charts, or a drop of 3 or more lines of Snellen equivalent.

The ETDRS defined clinically significant macular edema (CSME) and recommended treatment with focal laser photocoagulation for the following:

- retinal edema located at or within 500 μm of the center of the macula (Fig 5-12)
- hard exudates at or within 500 μm of the center if associated with thickening of adjacent retina (Fig 5-13)
- a zone of thickening larger than 1 disc area if located within 1 disc diameter of the center of the macula (Fig 5-14)

Results of laser treatment of DME

The ETDRS demonstrated that eyes with CSME benefited from focal argon laser photocoagulation treatment when compared to untreated eyes in a control group. Treatment for CSME reduced the risk of moderate visual loss, increased the chance of visual improvement, and was associated with only minor losses of visual field (Fig 5-15). Eyes without CSME showed no significant difference between treated eyes and control eyes during the first 2 years. In clinical practice, therefore, treatment of such eyes can be delayed until progression of edema threatens the center of the macula.

For patients with CSME who are asymptomatic and have normal visual acuity, the decision of when to begin treatment is sometimes difficult. This decision may be influenced by the proximity of exudates to the fovea, the status and course of the fellow eye, anticipated cataract surgery, or the presence of high-risk PDR. It is preferable to initiate photocoagulation for DME before scatter photocoagulation for high-risk PDR. Likewise, it is preferable to treat DME prior to cataract surgery because of potential progression of retinopathy after surgery. The ETDRS also demonstrated that subretinal fibrosis occurred less often in laser-treated eyes than in untreated control eyes. Subretinal fibrosis was associated with the presence and severity of retinal hard exudates in the macula. Table 5-2 lists the side effects of photocoagulation for macular edema.

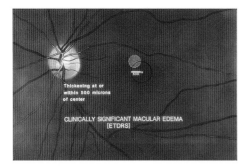

Figure 5-12 CSME: Retinal edema located at or within 500 μm of the center of the macula. *(Courtesy of the ETDRS.)*

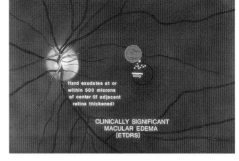

Figure 5-13 CSME: Hard exudates at or within 500 μm of the center of the macula if associated with thickening of the adjacent retina. *(Courtesy of the ETDRS.)*

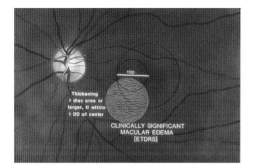

Figure 5-14 CSME: A zone of thickening larger than 1 disc area if located within 1 disc diameter of the center of the macula. *(Courtesy of the ETDRS.)*

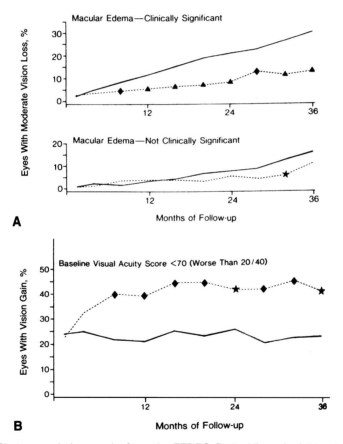

Figure 5-15 Photocoagulation results from the ETDRS. Dotted lines depict treated group; solid lines indicate control group. **A,** Visual acuity results (all eyes with macular edema). Photocoagulation for clinically significant macular edema reduces the risk of moderate visual loss by 50%. **B,** Improvement in visual acuity (more than one line), initial acuity worse than 20/40. Laser treatment for clinically significant macular edema increases the chance of visual improvement. *(Reprinted with permission from Early Treatment Diabetic Retinopathy Study Group. Photocoagulation for diabetic macular edema. ETDRS Report Number 1. Arch Ophthalmol. 1985;103:1796–1806.)*

Table 5-2 Focal Laser Photocoagulation: Side Effects and Complications

Paracentral scotomata
Transient increased edema/decreased vision
Choroidal neovascularization
Subretinal fibrosis
Photocoagulation scar expansion
Inadvertent foveolar burns

(Modified from Kim JW, AI E. Diabetic retinopathy. In: Regillo CD, Brown GC, Flynn HW Jr, eds. *Vitreoretinal Disease: The Essentials.* New York: Thieme; 1999:147.)

Early Treatment Diabetic Retinopathy Study Research Group. Focal photocoagulation treatment of diabetic macular edema. Relationship of treatment to fluorescein angiographic and other retinal characteristics at baseline: ETDRS Report 19. *Arch Ophthalmol.* 1995;113:1144–1155.

Surgical management of DME

In patients with refractory CSME, intravitreal administration of corticosteroids has been shown to be useful. Currently, several drug delivery modalities are in clinical trials that are investigating their efficacy in treating DME.

Kaiser PK, Riemann CD, Sears JE, et al. Macular traction detachment and diabetic macular edema associated with posterior hyaloidal traction. *Am J Ophthalmol.* 2001;131:44–49
Martidis A, Duker JS, Greenberg PB, et al. Intravitreal triamcinolone for refractory diabetic macular edema. *Ophthalmology.* 2002;109:920–927.

Pars plana vitrectomy and detachment of the posterior hyaloid may also be useful for treating DME, particularly when there is evidence of posterior hyaloidal traction and diffuse DME.

Diabetic Macular Ischemia

Retinal capillary nonperfusion is a feature commonly associated with progressive NPDR. Fluorescein angiography can show the extent of capillary nonperfusion. The foveal avascular zone may become irregular and enlarged because of nonperfusion of the marginal capillaries. Microaneurysms tend to cluster at the margins of zones of capillary nonperfusion. Closure of retinal arterioles may result in larger areas of nonperfusion and progressive ischemia. Evidence of enlargement of the foveal avascular zone greater than 1000 μm in diameter generally means visual loss.

Current Indications for Pars Plana Vitrectomy in Patients With Diabetes

The following are the 5 most common and traditional indications for pars plana vitrectomy in patients with diabetes:

- dense, nonclearing vitreous hemorrhage
- tractional retinal detachment involving or threatening the macula
- combined tractional and rhegmatogenous retinal detachment
- diffuse diabetic macular edema associated with posterior hyaloidal traction
- significant recurrent vitreous hemorrhage despite maximal PRP

To evaluate the presence or absence of retinal detachment in patients with dense, non-clearing vitreous hemorrhage, echography is required. If retinal detachment is present, an early vitrectomy is usually suggested. Patients with bilateral severe vitreous hemorrhage generally should undergo vitrectomy in one eye when they are medically stable.

The DRVS data indicate that, for patients with type 1 diabetes with dense vitreous hemorrhage and severe visual loss in one eye, early surgery (1–6 months after visual loss) is preferable to waiting 1 year or more. The DRVS showed no difference in outcomes of 10/20 or better between the early and late vitrectomy groups among type 2 patients with severe vitreous hemorrhage. This lack of difference may be attributable to a higher frequency in type 2 patients of diabetic maculopathy, which causes visual reduction to the 20/200 range. Because endolaser treatment was not yet available for use during the DRVS and microsurgical techniques have improved since the conclusion of the study in 1988, the outcomes of pars plana vitrectomy may now be better than those reported in the DRVS publications.

Tractional retinal detachment not involving the macula may remain stable for many years. When the macula becomes involved, immediate vitrectomy is generally recommended. Combined tractional and rhegmatogenous retinal detachment may progress rapidly, and early surgery should be considered in selected patients with bullous retinal detachment.

Additional reported indications for vitrectomy in patients with diabetes include the following:

- severe progressive fibrovascular proliferation
- anterior hyaloidal fibrovascular proliferation
- red blood cell–induced (erythroclastic) glaucoma
- anterior segment neovascularization with media opacities preventing photocoagulation
- dense premacular (subhyaloid) hemorrhage

For further discussion of vitrectomy, see Chapter 16.

Smiddy WE, Flynn HW Jr. Vitrectomy in the management of diabetic retinopathy. *Surv Ophthalmol.* 1999;43:491–507.

Photocoagulation for Diabetic Retinopathy

Based on the findings of the DRS, ETDRS, and other clinical studies, photocoagulation is generally recommended for eyes with CSME and high-risk PDR (see also Chapter 15). However, some clinical features are associated with poorer visual acuity outcomes after photocoagulation:

- diffuse macular edema with center involved
- diffuse fluorescein leakage
- macular ischemia (extensive perifoveal capillary nonperfusion)
- hard exudate deposits in the fovea
- marked cystoid macular edema

In general, the ophthalmologist views the patient's fluorescein angiogram to guide treatment for CSME. For focal leakage, direct laser therapy using green or yellow wavelengths is applied to all leaking microaneurysms between 500 and 3000 μm from the center of the macula. Parameters for focal treatment include

- 50- to 100-μm spot size
- 0.1 second or less duration
- attempt to whiten or darken microaneurysms

For diffuse leakage or zones of capillary nonperfusion adjacent to the macula, a light-intensity grid pattern using green or yellow is applied to all areas of diffuse leakage more than 500 μm from the center of the macula and 500 μm from the temporal margin of the optic disc. Parameters for local treatment in a grid pattern include:

- 50- to 100-μm spot size
- 0.1 second or less duration
- spots spaced at least 1 burn width apart

Multiple treatment sessions spread out over many months are frequently necessary for resolution of diabetic macular edema.

Early Treatment Diabetic Retinopathy Study Research Group. Treatment techniques and clinical guidelines for photocoagulation of diabetic macular edema. ETDRS report 2. *Ophthalmology.* 1987;94:761–774.

Folk JC, Pulido JS. *Laser Photocoagulation of the Retina and Choroid.* Ophthalmology Monograph 11. San Francisco: American Academy of Ophthalmology; 1997.

Cataract Surgery in Patients With Diabetes

Various studies suggest that diabetic retinopathy may progress following cataract surgery. Patients about to undergo cataract surgery who have CSME, severe NPDR, or PDR should be considered for photocoagulation prior to cataract removal if the ocular media are sufficiently clear to allow treatment. If the density of the cataract precludes adequate evaluation of the retina or treatment, prompt postoperative retinal evaluation and treatment can be considered. Patients with diabetes enrolled in the ETDRS who underwent cataract surgery usually had improved visual acuity postoperatively.

In general, all patients with preexisting diabetic retinopathy should be reevaluated following cataract surgery. The need for an adequate pupillary size in order to facilitate postoperative evaluation and treatment of the retina is a factor the cataract surgeon should consider at the time of cataract surgery. BCSC Section 11, *Lens and Cataract,* discusses the special considerations that the cataract surgeon must take into account in patients with diabetes.

Jaffe GJ, Burton TC, Kuhn E, et al. Progression of nonproliferative diabetic retinopathy and visual outcome after extracapsular cataract extraction and intraocular lens implantation. *Am J Ophthalmol.* 1992;114:448–456.

Suggested Timetables for Detailed Ophthalmic Examination of Patients With Diabetes

Patients with type 1 diabetes rarely have retinopathy during the first 5 years after diagnosis. By contrast, a significant percentage of patients with type 2 diabetes have established retinopathy at the time of initial diagnosis; these patients should have an ophthalmic examination upon diagnosis. Female patients are particularly at risk for progression of diabetic retinopathy during pregnancy. An examination is generally recommended for pregnant patients in the first trimester and thereafter at the discretion of the ophthalmologist (Table 5-3). Depending on the severity of the retinopathy and the threat to visual function from progression, the ophthalmologist may prefer to follow selected patients more often because of the anticipated need for treatment (Table 5-4).

Preferred Practice Patterns Committee, Retina Panel. *Diabetic Retinopathy.* San Francisco: American Academy of Ophthalmology; November 2003.

Sickle Cell Retinopathy

The sickle cell hemoglobinopathies of greatest ocular importance are those in which mutant hemoglobins S and/or C are inherited as alleles of normal hemoglobin A. These disorders result from a mutant gene that defines the sequence of amino acids in the

---

Table 5-3 Timetable Based on Age of Patient or Pregnancy

Age of Onset of DM/Pregnancy	Recommended Time of First Eye Examination	Routine Minimum Follow-up
0–30	Within 5 years of diagnosis	Annually
31 and older	Upon diagnosis	Annually
Pregnancy	Before conception or early in first trimester	Every 3 months or at discretion of ophthalmologist

(Modified from Preferred Patterns Committee, Retina Panel. *Diabetic Retinopathy.* San Francisco: American Academy of Ophthalmology; 1998.)

Table 5-4 Timetable Based on Retinopathy Findings

Retinal Abnormality	Suggested Follow-up
Normal or rare microaneurysms	Annually
Mild NPDR	Every 9 months
Moderate NPDR	Every 6 months
Severe NPDR	Every 4 months
CSME	Every 2–4 months* (careful follow-up)
PDR	Every 2–3 months* (careful follow-up)

* Consider laser surgery

(Modified from Preferred Practice Patterns Committee, Retina Panel. *Diabetic Retinopathy.* San Francisco: American Academy of Ophthalmology; 1998.)

β-polypeptide chain of adult hemoglobin. In sickle cell hemoglobin (SC), the valine is substituted for glutamic acid at the sixth position in the β-polypeptide chain due to a substitution of adenine for thymine. This seemingly small alteration causes a profound reduction of solubility when hemoglobin is deoxygenated, leading to deformation of red blood cells into a characteristic sickle shape when the partial pressure of oxygen is low.

Sickle cell hemoglobinopathies are most often seen in the black population. Sickle cell trait (Hb AS) affects 8% of African Americans; 0.4% have sickle cell disease (Hb SS), and 0.2% have hemoglobin SC disease (Table 5-5). Thalassemia, in which the α- or β-polypeptide chain is defective, rarely causes retinopathy. Although sickling and solubility tests (sickle cell preparations, or "preps") are reliable indicators of the presence of hemoglobin S and are therefore excellent for screening, they do not distinguish between heterozygous and homozygous states. Hemoglobin electrophoresis testing should be performed following a positive sickle cell prep. This process is described in Part III, Genetics, of BCSC Section 2, *Fundamentals and Principles of Ophthalmology,* along with detailed explanations of allelic gene defects.

Sickle cell ocular abnormalities are caused by intravascular sickling, hemolysis, hemostasis, and thrombosis. The initial event in the pathogenesis of sickle cell retinopathy is peripheral arteriolar occlusion and capillary nonperfusion, which may progress to retinal neovascularization, usually at the border between perfused and nonperfused retina.

The incidence of significant visual loss from sickle cell retinopathy is variable but appears to be relatively low in natural history studies. Serious ocular complications of proliferative sickle cell retinopathy (PSR)—including retinal neovascularization, vitreous hemorrhage, and tractional retinal detachment—are more characteristic of SC and SThal (sickle cell thalassemia) than of SS disease, although SS disease results in more systemic complications.

Clarkson JG. The ocular manifestations of sickle-cell disease: a prevalence and natural history study. *Trans Am Ophthalmol Soc.* 1992;90:481–504.

Harlan JB, Fekrat S, Lutty GA, et al. Hemoglobinopathies. In: Ryan SJ, ed. *Retina.* 3rd ed. St Louis: Mosby; 2001:1454–1471.

Table 5-5 Incidence of Sickle Cell Hemoglobinopathies in North America

Hemoglobinopathy	Incidence in Population	Incidence of Proliferative Retinopathy in Subgroups
Any sickle hemoglobin	10%	—
Sickle cell trait (AS)	8%	Uncommon
Hemoglobin C trait (AC)	2%	Uncommon
Sickle cell homozygote (SS)	0.4%	3%[*]
Sickle cell hemoglobin C (SC)	0.2%	33%[*]
Sickle cell thalassemia (SThal)	0.03%	14%[*]
Homozygous C (CC)	0.016%	Unknown

[*] Approximate

(Modified from Fekrat S, Goldberg MF. Sickle retinopathy. In: Regillo CD, Brown GC, Flynn HW Jr, eds. *Vitreoretinal Disease: The Essentials.* New York: Thieme; 1999:333.)

Nonproliferative Sickle Cell Retinopathy

The retinal changes seen in sickle cell hemoglobinopathies follow arteriolar and capillary occlusion. Anastomosis and remodeling occur in the periphery, as do the hemorrhagic sequelae of occlusion (Fig 5-16):

- salmon patch hemorrhages
- refractile (iridescent) deposits or spots
- black sunburst lesions

Clinical and histopathologic studies have shown that *salmon patch hemorrhages* represent areas of intraretinal hemorrhages occurring after a peripheral retinal arteriolar occlusion. *Refractile spots* are old, resorbed hemorrhages with hemosiderin deposition within the retina just beneath the inner limiting membrane. *Black sunburst lesions* are localized areas of retinal pigment epithelial hypertrophy, hyperplasia, and pigment migration into the retina. These lesions often have a spiculated appearance and are usually seen in a perivascular location in the periphery. The presence of hemosiderin deposition in the lesion suggests that retinal hemorrhage with extension into the subretinal space plays a role in the pathogenesis of the black sunburst lesions.

Occlusion of parafoveal capillaries and arterioles is one cause of decreased visual acuity in sickle cell retinopathy. Patients with sickle cell hemoglobinopathies may also develop spontaneous occlusion of the central retinal artery. Vascular occlusions do not inevitably lead to infarction in sickle cell retinopathy.

Fekrat S, Goldberg MF. Sickle retinopathy. In: Regillo CD, Brown GC, Flynn HW Jr, eds. *Vitreoretinal Disease: The Essentials.* New York: Thieme; 1999:333–345.

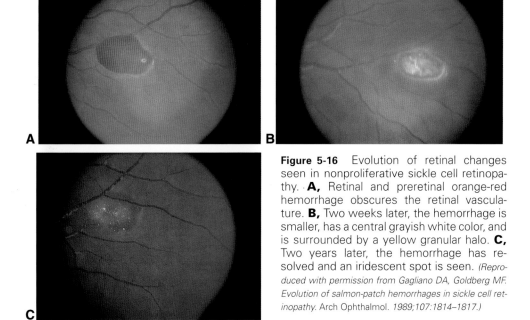

Figure 5-16 Evolution of retinal changes seen in nonproliferative sickle cell retinopathy. **A,** Retinal and preretinal orange-red hemorrhage obscures the retinal vasculature. **B,** Two weeks later, the hemorrhage is smaller, has a central grayish white color, and is surrounded by a yellow granular halo. **C,** Two years later, the hemorrhage has resolved and an iridescent spot is seen. *(Reproduced with permission from Gagliano DA, Goldberg MF. Evolution of salmon-patch hemorrhages in sickle cell retinopathy. Arch Ophthalmol. 1989;107:1814–1817.)*

Proliferative Sickle Cell Retinopathy

Proliferative sickle cell retinopathy (PSR) has been classified into the following pathogenetic sequence (Fig 5-17):

1. Peripheral arteriolar occlusions (stage 1) lead to
2. peripheral arteriovenular anastomoses (stage 2), which appear to be dilated, preexisting capillary channels. Sequential fluorescein angiograms show dynamic remodeling of the peripheral retinal vasculature.
3. Preretinal *sea fan neovascularization* (stage 3) may occur at the posterior border of areas of nonperfusion and lead to
4. vitreous hemorrhage (stage 4) and
5. tractional retinal detachment (stage 5).

Sea fan neovascularization also frequently undergoes spontaneous infarction.

> Goldberg MF. Classification and pathogenesis of proliferative sickle retinopathy. *Am J Ophthalmol.* 1971;71:649–665.

Proliferative sickle cell retinopathy (PSR) is one of many retinal vascular diseases in which fibrovascular proliferation occurs in response to retinal ischemia. Whereas the neovascularization in proliferative diabetic retinopathy (PDR) generally begins postequatorially, it is located more peripherally in PSR. Another way in which PSR differs from PDR is in the frequent occurrence of autoinfarction of the peripheral neovascularization, resulting in a white sea fan (Fig 5-18).

Other Ocular Abnormalities in Sickle Cell Hemoglobinopathies

Another clinical finding seen in many patients with SS or SC disease is segmentation of the conjunctival blood vessels. Numerous comma-shaped capillaries appear to be separated from other vessels, most often in the inferior fornix (the *comma sign*). Similarly,

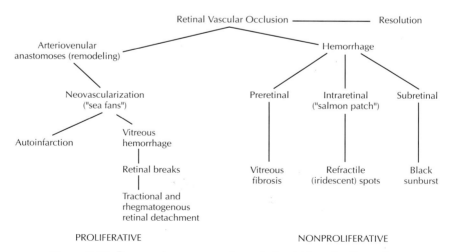

Figure 5-17 Proposed sequence of events in sickle cell retinopathy.

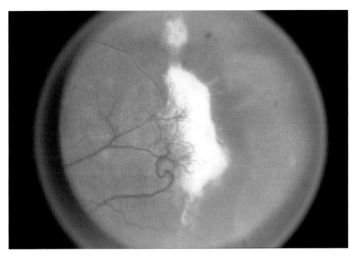

Figure 5-18 Peripheral neovascularization ("sea fan") with autoinfarction, as illustrated in the white atrophic vessels. *(Photograph courtesy of Harry W. Flynn, Jr, MD.)*

small vessels on the surface of the optic disc can exhibit intravascular occlusions, manifested as dark red spots (the *disc sign* of sickling). Angioid streaks have been reported clinically in up to 6% of cases of SS disease and in sickle cell trait. The pathogenetic nature of this association is uncertain.

Management

All black patients presenting with a traumatic hyphema should be screened for a sickling hemoglobinopathy (including trait) because of the increased risk of complications in the presence of rigid sickled erythrocytes. Intraocular pressure (IOP) control may be difficult, and ischemic optic neuropathy may result from short intervals of modest increase in IOP. In the presence of a significant hyphema with increased IOP, some authors have recommended early anterior chamber washout. In addition, the physician must be cautious in the use of carbonic anhydrase inhibitors, which may worsen sickling through the production of systemic acidosis.

McLeod DS, Merges C, Fukushima A, et al. Histopathologic features of neovascularization in sickle cell retinopathy. *Am J Ophthalmol.* 1997;124:455–472.

Wax MB, Ridley ME, Magargal LE. Reversal of retinal and optic disc ischemia in a patient with sickle cell trait and glaucoma secondary to traumatic hyphema. *Ophthalmology.* 1982;89:845–851.

Photocoagulation

Therapeutic approaches to PSR have included diathermy, cryopexy, and photocoagulation. Although recommended in the past, the use of photocoagulation to close feeder vessels to the neovascular frond is not currently recommended because of complications, including retinal and choroidal hemorrhages, breaks in Bruch's membrane, choroidal neovascularization with extension into the vitreous, retinal breaks, and retinal detachment. Peripheral scatter photocoagulation, applying lower-intensity light burns to the involved ischemic peripheral retina, may cause effective regression of active neovascular fronds and may decrease the risk of vitreous hemorrhage.

Farber MD, Jampol LM, Fox P, et al. A randomized clinical trial of scatter photocoagulation of proliferative sickle cell retinopathy. *Arch Ophthalmol.* 1991;109:363–367.

Jacobson MS, Gagliano DA, Cohen SB, et al. A randomized clinical trial of feeder vessel photocoagulation of sickle cell retinopathy: a long-term follow-up. *Ophthalmology.* 1991;98:581–585.

Vitreoretinal surgery in PSR

Surgery may be indicated for nonclearing vitreous hemorrhage and/or for rhegmatogenous, tractional, or combined retinal detachment. Retinal detachment usually begins in the ischemic peripheral retina. The tears may be at the base of sea fans and are often seen following photocoagulation treatment. Anterior segment ischemia or necrosis has been reported in association with 360° scleral buckling procedures, particularly when extensive diathermy or cryopexy has been applied. For this reason, extra precautions should be taken in treating patients with retinal detachment associated with PSR. Recommended techniques for scleral buckling procedures include

- use of local anesthesia without adjunctive epinephrine
- nonremoval of extraocular muscles
- judicious use of cryopexy
- adequate patient hydration
- use of supplementary nasal oxygen

Likewise, precautions for vitrectomy include elimination of epinephrine from the irrigating solution, cautious use of expansile gases, and avoidance of encircling scleral buckles unless necessary. Exchange transfusion is no longer favored prior to vitreoretinal surgery.

Pulido JS, Flynn HW Jr, Clarkson JG, et al. Pars plana vitrectomy in the management of complications of proliferative sickle retinopathy. *Arch Ophthalmol.* 1988;106:1553–1557.

Ryan SJ, Goldberg MF. Anterior segment ischemia following scleral buckling in sickle cell hemoglobinopathy. *Am J Ophthalmol.* 1971;72:35–50.

Peripheral Retinal Neovascularization

A number of entities besides the sickling disorders can cause peripheral neovascularization; see Table 5-6 for a differential diagnosis.

Retinopathy of Prematurity

Previously called *retrolental fibroplasia,* retinopathy of prematurity (ROP) is a proliferative retinopathy of premature and low-birth-weight infants. It is estimated that ROP causes some degree of visual loss in approximately 1300 children born each year in the United States and severe visual impairment in 250–500 of those children. Approximately 300 children per million live births have at least 1 blind eye from ROP. For an in-depth discussion of ROP, see BCSC Section 6, *Pediatric Ophthalmology and Strabismus.*

Table 5-6 Differential Diagnosis of Peripheral Retinal Neovascularization

Vascular diseases with ischemia
Proliferative diabetic retinopathy
Branch retinal vein occlusion
Branch retinal arteriolar occlusion
Carotid cavernous fistula
Sickling hemoglobinopathies (eg, SC, SS)
Other hemoglobinopathies (eg, AC, AS)
Eales disease
Retinal embolization (eg, talc)
Retinopathy of prematurity (ROP)
Familial exudative vitreoretinopathy (FEVR)
Hyperviscosity syndromes (eg, chronic myelogenous leukemia)
Aortic arch syndromes/ocular ischemic syndromes
Idiopathic retinal vasculitis, aneurysms, and neuroretinitis (IRVAN)

Inflammatory diseases with possible ischemia
Sarcoidosis
Retinal vasculitis (eg, systemic lupus erythematosus)
Uveitis, including pars planitis
Birdshot retinochoroidopathy
Toxoplasmosis
Multiple sclerosis

Miscellaneous
Incontinentia pigmenti
Long-standing retinal detachment
Choroidal melanoma
Retinitis pigmentosa
Retinoschisis

(Modified from Jampol LM, Ebroon DA, Goldbaum MH. Peripheral proliferative retinopathies: an update on angiogenesis, etiologies, and management. *Surv Ophthalmol.* 1994;38:519–540.)

Flynn JT, Bancalari E, Snyder ES, et al. A cohort study of transcutaneous oxygen tension and the incidence and severity of retinopathy of prematurity. *N Engl J Med.* 1992;326:1050–1054.
McNamara JA, Connolly BP. Retinopathy of prematurity. In: Regillo CD, Brown GC, Flynn HW Jr, eds. *Vitreoretinal Disease: The Essentials.* New York: Thieme; 1999:177–192.

The Joint Statement of the American Academy of Pediatrics, Section on Ophthalmology; the American Association for Pediatric Ophthalmology and Strabismus; and the American Academy of Ophthalmology recommends at least 2 dilated funduscopic examinations using binocular indirect ophthalmoscopy for all infants with a birth weight of less than 1500 g or with a gestational age of 28 weeks or less, as well as for selected infants between 1500 and 2000 g with an unstable clinical course who are believed to be at high risk by their attending pediatrician or neonatologist. One examination is sufficient only if it demonstrates unequivocally that the retina is fully vascularized bilaterally. The first examination should generally be performed between 4 and 6 weeks of postnatal age or, alternatively, within the 31st to 33rd week of postconceptional or postmenstrual age, whichever is later. Examinations are then generally performed every 1–2 weeks (see the following examination schedules) until the retina is fully vascularized. Signs of ROP are seen in 66% of infants with a birth weight of less than 1251 g and in 82% of those with a birth weight of less than 1000 g.

Infants with the following findings should be examined at least weekly:

- ROP less than threshold in zone I
- ROP in zone II, including:
  - stage 3 ROP without plus disease
  - stage 2 ROP with plus disease; and
  - stage 3 ROP with plus disease not yet extensive enough to justify ablative therapy

Infants with the following findings should be examined at 1- to 2-week intervals:

- less severe ROP in zone II
- no ROP, but incomplete retinal vascularization in zone I

Infants with incomplete retinal vascularization in zone II but no ROP should be examined at 2–3 week intervals. Infants found to have threshold disease should receive retinal ablative therapy (either cryotherapy or laser photocoagulation) within 72 hours of diagnosis.

> The American Academy of Pediatrics Policy Statement. Screening examination of premature infants for retinopathy of prematurity. September 2001;108 (3):809–811.
>
> Palmer EA, Flynn JT, Hardy RJ, et al. Incidence and early course of retinopathy of prematurity. The Cryotherapy for Retinopathy of Prematurity Cooperative Group. *Ophthalmology*. 1991;98:1628–1640.

Pathogenesis and Staging

Normal retinal vascularization proceeds from the optic disc to the periphery and is complete in the nasal quadrants at approximately 36 weeks of gestation and on the temporal side at 40 weeks. A vanguard of mesenchymal cells initially grows outward in the nerve fiber layer from the region of the optic disc starting at month 4–5 of gestation. These mesenchymal cells give rise to retinal capillary endothelial cells, which then form the capillary system. Some capillaries enlarge to form arterioles and venules, and some drop out as remodeling occurs (Fig 5-19). Current understanding of ROP is incomplete, but it has been suggested that the centrifugally progressing mesenchymal vascular precursor tissue is susceptible to capillary endothelial cell cytotoxicity until it has been remodeled into more mature vessels.

Exposure to excessive concentrations of oxygen during this period can lead to an injury that results in arrest of vascular development, obliteration of newly formed capillaries, and formation of a major arteriovenous shunt in the eye. These events leave a variable amount of neurosensory retina without inner retinal blood supply. Although an important contributing factor, oxygen is no longer considered the sole factor in the pathogenesis of ROP. Other factors such as low birth weight and a short gestational period also increase the risk of developing the disease.

Factors such as intercurrent illnesses, blood transfusions, and pCO_2, although statistically associated with the outcome in a univariate sense, failed to maintain a significant association when considered in a multivariate analysis. ROP has been reported in full-term infants (possibly familial exudative vitreoretinopathy?), in stillborn infants who had

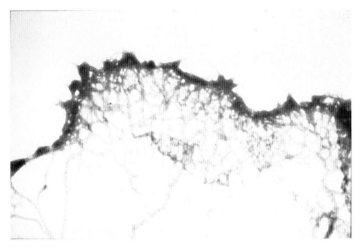

Figure 5-19 Trypsin digest preparation of the peripheral retina from the eye of a premature infant. The more posterior vascularized and peripheral avascular retina are well differentiated. Some of the retinal capillaries have remodeled to form arterioles and venules. *(Photograph courtesy of W. Richard Green, MD.)*

not received supplemental oxygen, in anencephalic infants, and in infants with congenital heart disease and significant right-to-left shunting whose pAO$_2$ never exceeded 50–60 mm Hg.

Clinically, vascularized retina in the premature infant without ROP normally blends almost imperceptibly into the anterior, gray, nonvascularized retina. With ROP, however, the juncture between the two becomes more distinct.

Classification and terminology

The international classification of ROP has been devised to standardize the specific staging and analysis of the natural history and therapy (Table 5-7). In *stage 1* ROP, the shunt is essentially flat, whereas in *stage 2,* the mesenchymal ridge is elevated (Fig 5-20). *Stage 3* ROP is distinguished by actual neovascularization (extraretinal neovascularization), with blood vessels growing through the ILM of the retina (Fig 5-21).

The international classification also defined ROP according to location of the disease (see Table 5-7). There are 3 zones: I, II, and III. *Zone I* encompasses the area included in a circle twice the radius of the optic disc-to-foveola distance. *Zone II* encompasses that area included in a circle centered on the optic disc with a radius of the distance from the optic disc to the nasal ora serrata, and *zone III* includes the remainder of the fundus outside zones I and II. An eye is classified according to the highest zone in which retinal vessels are located. Eyes with ROP in zone III typically have a good visual prognosis. The more posterior the zone at the time of discovery of the disease, the more worrisome the prognosis.

The Committee for the Classification of Retinopathy of Prematurity. An international classification of retinopathy of prematurity. *Arch Ophthalmol.* 1984;102:1130–1134.

Table 5-7 Acute ROP (International Committee on Classification of Acute ROP)

Location

Zone I: posterior retina within a 60° circle centered on the optic nerve
Zone II: from the posterior circle (zone 1) to the nasal ora serrata anteriorly
Zone III: remaining temporal peripheral retina

Extent: number of clock hours involved

Severity

Stage 1: presence of a demarcation line between vascularized and nonvascularized retina
Stage 2: presence of demarcation line that has height, width, and volume (ridge)
Stage 3: a ridge with extraretinal fibrovascular proliferation (may be mild, moderate, or
    severe, as judged by the amount of proliferative tissue present)
Stage 4: subtotal retinal detachment
    A. extrafoveal
    B. retinal detachment including fovea

Stage 5: total retinal detachment with funnel:	*Anterior*	*Posterior*
	Open	Open
	Narrow	Narrow
	Open	Narrow
	Narrow	Open

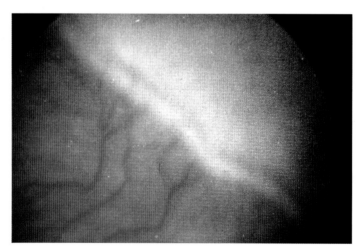

Figure 5-20 Stage 2 ROP. An elevated ridge of mesenchymal tissue is present at the border of the vascular and avascular retina. *(Photograph courtesy of William S. Tasman, MD.)*

The International Committee for the Classification of the Late Stages of Retinopathy of Prematurity. An international classification of retinopathy of prematurity. II. The classification of retinal detachment. *Arch Ophthalmol.* 1987;105:906–912.

In eyes with stage 3 ROP, the neovascularization shunts the blood from the arterial to the venous side. The more peripheral the shunt and the smaller its size and extent on the retina, the better the outlook for spontaneous regression with minimal scarring. An active shunt will be associated with dilation and increased tortuosity of the retinal vessels posteriorly. Increased and abnormal terminal arborization of retinal vessels as they approach the shunt or ridge is a notable finding in active disease. In addition, microvascular abnormalities (eg, microaneurysms, areas of capillary nonperfusion, and dilated vessels) may be visible behind the shunt.

In the vasoproliferative phase, new vessels varying greatly in size and extent arise from retinal vessels just posterior to the shunt. These new vessels adhere to the posterior hyaloid face of the vitreous and can induce contracture of the overlying vitreous gel, which in turn can lead to tractional retinal detachment (stage 4). *Stage 4,* or subtotal retinal detachment, is further divided in stages 4A and 4B (Fig 5-22). In *stage 4A,* the detachment is extrafoveal, whereas in *stage 4B,* the foveal retina is detached. In stage 5 ROP, the retina is totally detached (Fig 5-23). Vitreous hemorrhage can occur in stages 3–5, and exudative retinal detachment can also occur.

Plus disease, another term of importance emphasized in the international classification of ROP, is determined by the presence of retinal vascular dilation and tortuosity in the posterior pole (Fig 5-24). It is indicative of an actively progressing phase of the disease. If plus disease is accompanied by vascularization ending in zone I or very posterior zone II, the risk of very rapid progressive disease ("rush" disease) is significant.

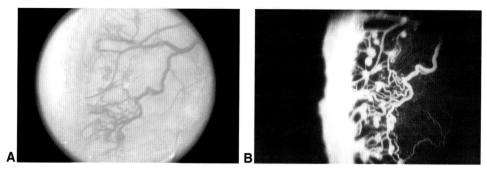

Figure 5-21 Stage 3 ROP. **A,** Arborization of retinal vessels as they approach the ridge of neovascularization. Note the orange-red color of the ridge, as compared to the more white appearance of the ridge in Stage 2 ROP (see Fig 5-20). **B,** Intravenous fluorescein angiogram corresponding to **A** at 32.6 seconds after injection shows marked hyperfluorescence as a result of leakage of dye from the extraretinal neovascularization in the ridge. *(Photographs courtesy of Gary C. Brown, MD.)*

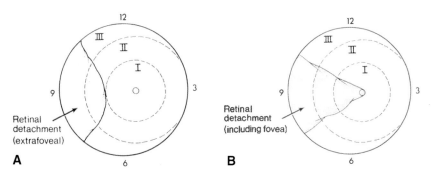

Figure 5-22 **A,** Stage 4A ROP. **B,** Stage 4B ROP. The roman numerals in each schematic indicate the zones, as per the international classification. *(Illustration courtesy of J. Arch McNamara, MD.)*

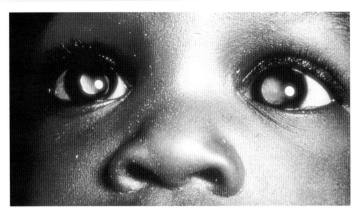

Figure 5-23 Stage 5 ROP. Bilateral total retinal detachments are present, with the retinal tissue drawn up behind the clear lens as a retrolental mass in each eye. *(Photograph courtesy of Gary C. Brown, MD.)*

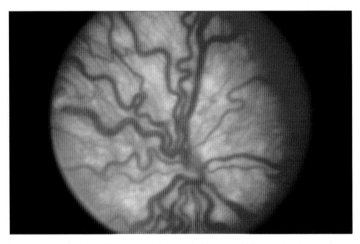

Figure 5-24 Pronounced "plus" disease in an ROP eye. The retinal arteries and veins are dilated, and the arteries in particular are tortuous. *(Photograph courtesy of Gary C. Brown, MD.)*

An important term in ROP classification is *threshold disease.* Threshold disease is characterized by more than 5 contiguous clock-hours of extraretinal neovascularization or 8 cumulative clock-hours of extraretinal neovascularization in association with plus disease and location of the retinal vessels within zone I or II (Fig 5-25).

Natural course

The systemic or local tissue factors that influence regression or progression of ROP are not known. The initial clinical sign of regression is the development of a clear zone of retina beyond the shunt, followed by the development of straight vessels crossing the shunt with an arteriovenous feeder extending into the avascular retina.

ROP is a transient disease in the majority of infants, with spontaneous regression occurring in 85% of eyes. Approximately 7% of infants with a birth weight of less than

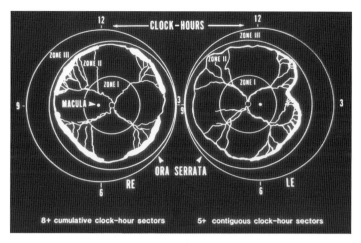

Figure 5-25 Examples of threshold disease, as characterized in the Multicenter Trial of Cryotherapy for Retinopathy of Prematurity. *(Reprinted by permission of American Medical Association from Cryotherapy for Retinopathy of Prematurity Cooperative Group. Multicenter trial of cryotherapy for retinopathy of prematurity: preliminary results. Arch Ophthalmol. 1988;106:474.)*

1251 g eventually develop threshold ROP. Those eyes that demonstrate progression undergo a gradual transition from the active to the cicatricial stage of ROP, which is associated with variable degrees of fibrosis, contracture of the proliferative tissue, and vitreous and retinal traction, macular distortion, and/or retinal detachment.

Cryotherapy for Retinopathy of Prematurity Cooperative Group. Multicenter trial of cryotherapy for retinopathy of prematurity: preliminary results. *Arch Ophthalmol.* 1988;106:471–479.

Flynn JT, Bancalari E, Bachynski BN, et al. Retinopathy of prematurity: diagnosis, severity, and natural history. *Ophthalmology.* 1987;94:620–629.

Foos RY. Chronic retinopathy of prematurity. *Ophthalmology.* 1985;92:563–574.

Associated conditions

Certain problems are more likely to occur in eyes with regressed ROP, including the following:

- myopia with astigmatism
- anisometropia
- strabismus
- amblyopia
- cataract
- glaucoma
- retinal detachment

Angle-closure glaucoma has been reported to occur during the second to fifth decades, with a mean age of 32 years in affected cases. Exudative retinopathy can also occur as a late sequela. It is important to remember that the sequelae of advanced ROP can cause problems throughout the patient's life, and long-term follow-up is crucial.

Brown MM, Brown GC, Duker JS, et al. Exudative retinopathy of adults: a late sequela of retinopathy of prematurity. *Int Ophthalmol.* 1995;18:281–285.

Michael AJ, Pesin SR, Katz LJ, et al. Management of late-onset angle-closure glaucoma associated with retinopathy of prematurity. *Ophthalmology.* 1991;98:1093–1098.

Treatment

Optimal preventive therapy for ROP is the prevention of extremely low birth weight (<1000 g). A clinical trial, the Supplemental Therapeutic Oxygen for Prethreshold ROP (STOP-ROP) trial was designed to test whether supplemental oxygen would decrease the progression to threshold ROP in infants who had prethreshold ROP. The STOP-ROP trial demonstrated that use of supplemental oxygen at pulse oximetry saturations of 96% to 99% did not cause further progression of prethreshold ROP but also did not significantly reduce the number of infants requiring peripheral ablative surgery. A subgroup analysis suggested a benefit of supplemental oxygen among infants who have prethreshold ROP without plus disease, but this finding requires additional study. Supplemental oxygen increased both the risk of adverse pulmonary events, including pneumonia and/or exacerbations of chronic lung disease, and the need for oxygen, diuretics, and hospitalization at 3 months of corrected age.

In another study, the Light-ROP study, exposure to ambient light was found to have no effect on the incidence or severity of ROP.

Reynolds JD, Hardy RJ, Kennedy KA, et al. Lack of efficacy of light reduction in preventing retinopathy of prematurity. Light Reduction in Retinopathy of Prematurity (Light-ROP) Cooperative Group. *N Engl J Med.* 1998;338:1572–1576.

The Stop-ROP Multicenter Study Group. Supplemental therapeutic oxygen for prethreshold retinopathy of prematurity (STOP-ROP), a randomized, controlled trial. I: Primary outcomes. *Pediatrics.* 2000;105:295–310.

Vitamin E and other antioxidants were investigated for their potential efficacy in decreasing the incidence of ROP; however, interest in testing the use of antioxidant therapy in a multicenter trial diminished due to concerns about side effects of vitamin E and because of the demonstrated efficacy of surgical intervention in patients with threshold ROP.

Cryotherapy to the avascular anterior retina in ROP eyes with threshold disease has been demonstrated to reduce by approximately half the incidence of an unfavorable outcome such as macular dragging, retinal detachment, or retrolental cicatrix formation (Figs 5-26, 5-27). These sequelae are reduced from 47% to 25% at 1 year of follow-up, and the visual results in such cases have been shown to parallel the anatomic results. At 10 years, eyes that received cryotherapy were still much less likely than control eyes to be blind. Cryotherapy should be performed in conjunction with pediatric consultation because 5% of treated patients can develop respiratory or cardiorespiratory arrest.

Brown GC, Tasman WS, Naidoff M, et al. Systemic complications associated with retinal cryoablation for retinopathy of prematurity. *Ophthalmology.* 1990;97:855–858.

Cryotherapy for Retinopathy of Prematurity Cooperative Group. Multicenter trial of cryotherapy for retinopathy of prematurity: ophthalmological outcomes at 10 years. *Arch Ophthalmol.* 2001;119:1110–1118.

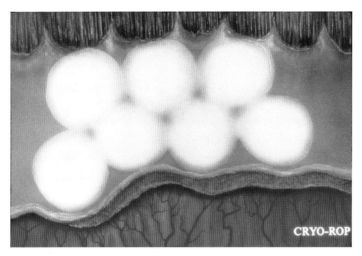

Figure 5-26 Cryotherapy to the anterior avascular retina in an eye with threshold ROP. *(Reprinted by permission of American Medical Association from Cryotherapy for Retinopathy of Prematurity Cooperative Group. Multicenter trial of cryotherapy for retinopathy of prematurity: preliminary results. Arch Ophthalmol. 1988;106:474.)*

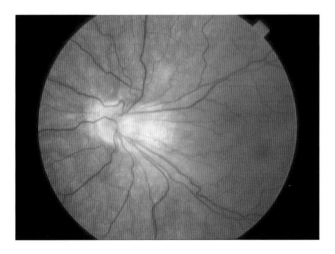

Figure 5-27 Temporal dragging of the retina in an eye with chronic changes of ROP. *(Photograph courtesy of Gary C. Brown, MD.)*

In the Early Treatment for Retinopathy of Prematurity Randomized Trial, a multicenter, prospective, randomized trial, infants with bilateral high-risk prethreshold ROP had 1 eye randomized to early treatment with ablation of the avascular retina, whereas the fellow eye was managed conventionally (that is, observation until the eye either reached threshold disease and was treated or the ROP regressed without progressing to threshold). High risk was determined using a model based on the Multicenter Trial of Cryotherapy for Retinopathy of Prematurity natural history cohort; this model used demographic characteristics of the infants and clinical features of ROP to classify eyes with prethreshold ROP as high risk or low risk. In infants with high-risk prethreshold ROP, earlier treatment was associated with a reduction in unfavorable grating visual acuity outcomes (from 19.5% to 14.5%; p = 0.01) and a reduction in unfavorable structural outcomes (from 15.6% to 9.1%; p < 0.001) at 9 months. Further analyses supported retinal ablative therapy for eyes with type 1 ROP, defined as zone I, any stage ROP with plus disease; zone I, stage 3 ROP without plus disease; or zone II, stage 2 or 3 ROP with plus disease. Analyses supported a wait-and-watch approach to type 2 ROP, defined as zone I, stage 1 or 2 ROP without plus disease or zone II, stage 3 ROP without plus disease; these eyes should be considered for treatment only if they progress to type 1 or threshold ROP.

> Early Treatment for Retinopathy of Prematurity Cooperative Group. Revised indications for the treatment of retinopathy of prematurity: results of the Early Treatment for Retinopathy of Prematurity Randomized Trial. *Arch Ophthalmol.* 2003;121:1684–1694.
>
> Good WV, Hardy RJ. The multicenter study of early treatment for retinopathy of prematurity (ETROP). ETROP Multicenter Study Group. *Ophthalmology.* 2001;108:1013–1014.
>
> Quinn GE, Young TL. Retinopathy of prematurity. *Focal Points: Clinical Modules for Ophthalmologists.* San Francisco: American Academy of Ophthalmology; 2001, module 11.

Most ophthalmologists who treat threshold or prethreshold ROP are now using laser therapy rather than retinal cryoablation. The treatment is applied in a full-scatter fashion to the avascular anterior retina with the indirect ophthalmoscope (Figs 5-28, 5-29, 5-30). Laser therapy is believed to be less traumatic systemically than cryoablation; it also appears to improve the chances for a better visual outcome. Largely because of its superior clinical efficacy, laser therapy also appears to be a substantially more cost-effective modality than cryotherapy.

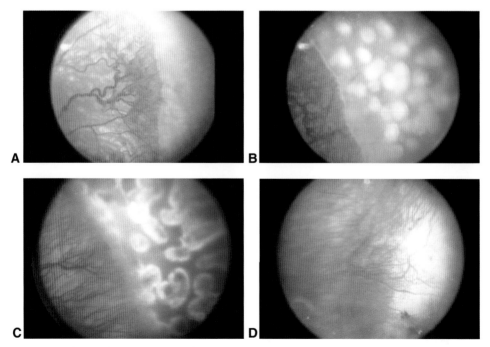

Figure 5-28 Laser photocoagulation for threshold ROP. **A,** Threshold eye prior to laser therapy. **B,** Immediately after laser therapy. **C,** 1 week after laser therapy. **D,** 3 months after laser therapy. *(Photographs courtesy of Gary C. Brown, MD.)*

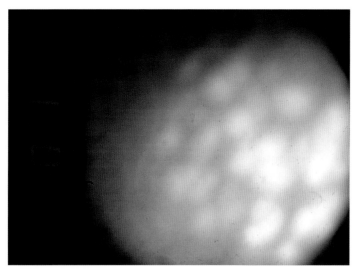

Figure 5-29 Dense laser pattern in avascular retina with plus disease and flat neovascularization. *(Photograph courtesy of Philip J. Ferrone, MD.)*

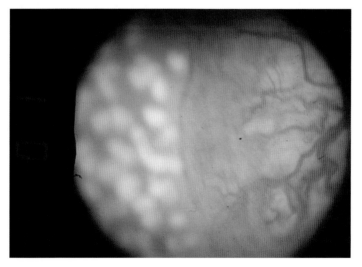

Figure 5-30 Flat neovascularization with florid plus disease. *(Photograph courtesy of Philip J. Ferrone, MD.)*

Brown GC, Brown MM, Sharma S, et al. Cost-effectiveness of treatment for threshold retinopathy of prematurity. *Pediatrics.* 1999;104:e47.

Connolly BP, McNamara JA, Sharma S, et al. A comparison of laser photocoagulation with trans-scleral cryotherapy in the treatment of threshold retinopathy of prematurity. *Ophthalmology.* 1998;105:1628–1631.

Laser ROP Study Group. Laser therapy for retinopathy of prematurity. *Arch Ophthalmol.* 1994;112:154–156.

McNamara JA, Tasman W, Brown GC, et al. Laser photocoagulation for stage 3+ retinopathy of prematurity. *Ophthalmology.* 1991;98:576–580.

Vander JF, Handa J, McNamara JA. Early treatment of posterior retinopathy of prematurity: a controlled trial. *Ophthalmology.* 1997;104:1731–1736.

Attempts have been made to treat eyes with progressive, active-phase ROP using scleral buckling or a lens-sparing vitrectomy in eyes with stage 4 ROP. For eyes with stage 5 disease, vitrectomy surgery combined with scissors dissection of the fibrovascular membranes and adherent vitreous has been anatomically successful in fully or partially reattaching the retina in approximately 30% of eyes. Nevertheless, with a median follow-up of 5 years, only 25% of retinas in eyes with initial partial or total reattachment after surgery remained fully attached. Among the patients whose retinas were initially reattached, only 10% will eventually have ambulatory vision. Eyes with surgical intervention in stage 4A rather than in 4B or 5 have a more favorable course. Although several authors have reported anatomic success in reattaching the retina in eyes with stage 4B or stage 5 ROP-related retinal detachments, visual outcome is rarely better than 20/400. More recently, it has been reported that lens-sparing vitrectomy for tractional 4A ROP-related retinal detachments may reduce the progression to stage 4B and 5 ROP, with the potential for improved visual outcome.

Capone A Jr, Trese MT. Lens-sparing vitreous surgery for tractional stage 4A retinopathy of prematurity retinal detachments. *Ophthalmology.* 2001:2068–2070.

Noorily SW, Small K, de Juan E Jr, et al. Scleral buckling surgery for stage 4B retinopathy of prematurity. *Ophthalmology.* 1992;99:263–268.

Quinn GE, Dobson V, Barr CC, et al. Visual acuity of eyes after vitrectomy for retinopathy of prematurity: follow-up at 5½ years. The Cryotherapy for Retinopathy of Prematurity Cooperative Group. *Ophthalmology.* 1996;103:595–600.

Trese MT. Scleral buckling for retinopathy of prematurity. *Ophthalmology.* 1994;101:23–26.

Trese MT, Droste PJ. Long-term postoperative results of a consecutive series of stages 4 and 5 retinopathy of prematurity. *Ophthalmology.* 1998;105:992–997.

Venous Occlusive Disease

Branch Retinal Vein Occlusion

The ophthalmoscopic findings of acute branch retinal vein occlusion (BRVO) include superficial hemorrhages, retinal edema, and often cotton-wool spots (nerve fiber layer infarcts) in a sector of retina drained by the affected vein (Fig 5-31). Branch retinal vein occlusions most commonly occur at an arteriovenous crossing, and the degree of macular involvement determines the level of visual impairment. When the occlusion does not occur at an arteriovenous crossing, the possibility of an underlying inflammatory condition should be considered. The mean age for patients at the time of occurrence is in their sixties.

The obstructed vein is dilated and tortuous, and, with time, the corresponding artery may become narrowed and sheathed. The quadrant most commonly affected is the superotemporal (63%); nasal occlusions are rarely detected clinically. A variant of BRVO based on congenital variation in central vein anatomy may involve either the superior half or inferior half of the retina (hemispheric or hemicentral retinal vein occlusion, Fig 5-32).

The Eye Disease Case-Control Study identified the following abnormalities as risk factors for the development of BRVO:

- history of systemic arterial hypertension
- cardiovascular disease
- increased body mass index at 20 years of age
- history of glaucoma

Diabetes mellitus was not a major independent risk factor.

Histologic studies suggest that common adventitia binds the artery and the vein together at the arteriovenous crossing and that thickening of the arterial wall compresses the vein, resulting in turbulence of flow, endothelial cell damage, and thrombotic occlusion. The thrombus may extend histologically to the capillary bed. Secondary arterial narrowing often develops in the area of occlusion.

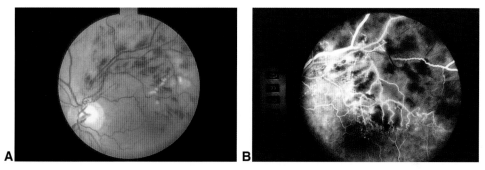

Figure 5-31 **A,** Superotemporal branch retinal vein occlusion. **B,** Fluorescein angiogram corresponding to **A** reveals pronounced retinal capillary nonperfusion in the distribution of the retina drained by the obstructed vein. *(Photograph courtesy of Gary C. Brown, MD.)*

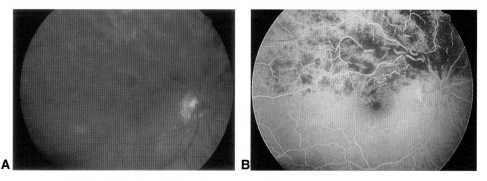

Figure 5-32 **A,** Hemispheric retinal vein occlusion. Photograph shows superior involvement with intraretinal hemorrhage. **B,** Fluorescein angiography shows blockage of underlying details in areas of hemorrhage: ischemia is probably minimal. Note that the foveal avascular zone is intact.

Frangieh GT, Green WR, Barraquer-Somers E, et al. Histopathologic study of nine branch retinal vein occlusions. *Arch Ophthalmol*. 1982;100:1132–1140.

Risk factors for branch retinal vein occlusion. The Eye Disease Case-Control Study Group. *Am J Ophthalmol*. 1993;116:286–296.

Visual prognosis in BRVO is most closely related to the extent of capillary damage and retinal ischemia. Fluorescein angiography is used to assess the extent and location of retinal capillary nonperfusion, as shown in Figure 5-31. The integrity of the parafoveal capillaries is an important prognostic factor for visual recovery. Vision may be reduced in acute cases from macular edema, retinal hemorrhage, or perifoveal retinal capillary occlusion. The hemorrhage resolves over time, and capillary compensation and collateral formation may permit restitution of flow with resolution of the edema and improvement in visual function. In other eyes, however, progressive capillary closure may occur.

Extensive retinal ischemia (greater than 5 disc diameters) results in neovascularization from the retina or optic nerve in approximately 40% of eyes, and 60% of such eyes will develop preretinal bleeding if laser photocoagulation is not performed. Overall, approximately 50%–60% of patients with all types of BRVO will maintain visual acuity of 20/40 or better after 1 year.

Argon laser scatter photocoagulation for prevention of neovascularization and vitreous hemorrhage in branch vein occlusion: a randomized clinical trial. Branch Vein Occlusion Study Group. *Arch Ophthalmol*. 1986;104:34–41.

Fekrat S, Finkelstein D. Venous occlusive disease. In: Regillo CD, Brown GC, Flynn HW Jr, eds. *Vitreoretinal Disease: The Essentials*. New York: Thieme; 1999:117–132.

Findings in eyes with permanent visual loss from BRVO include the following:

- macular ischemia
- cystoid macular edema
- macular edema with hard lipid exudates
- pigmentary macular disturbance
- subretinal fibrosis
- epiretinal membrane formation

Less commonly, vision is lost from vitreous hemorrhage or tractional and/or rhegmatogenous retinal detachment, which typically develops following a break in the retina adjacent to, or underlying, an area of retinal neovascularization.

Photocoagulation

Photocoagulation therapy in BRVO is considered for the 2 major complications: (1) chronic macular edema in eyes with intact perifoveal retinal capillary perfusion and (2) posterior segment neovascularization. For eyes with macular edema, it is suggested that therapy be delayed for at least 3 months to permit the maximum spontaneous resolution of the edema and intraretinal blood. Despite the persistence of macular edema, some eyes will not be candidates for treatment because of permanent structural alterations caused by central retinal capillary shutdown. Neovascularization of the iris is seen in approximately 1% of eyes with BRVO. Scatter panretinal laser photocoagulation can be considered in such instances to prevent the development of neovascular glaucoma.

Photocoagulation for macular edema accompanying BRVO is usually given to eyes with vision falling in the 20/40–20/200 range if the perifoveal retinal capillaries are intact. It is typically administered with the argon laser and is focused on edematous retina within the arcades drained by the obstructed vein (Fig 5-33). Areas of capillary leakage as identified by recent fluorescein angiography are treated with a light grid pattern using 100-µm and 200-µm spots. Leaking microvascular abnormalities may be treated directly, but prominent collateral vessels should be avoided.

The Branch Vein Occlusion Study

The Branch Vein Occlusion Study (BVOS) demonstrated that argon laser photocoagulation improved the visual outcome to a significant degree in eyes with BRVO in which the foveal vascularity was intact but macular edema had reduced vision to 20/40–20/200. Patients with distinct areas of macular capillary nonperfusion were excluded. Treated eyes were more likely to gain 2 lines of visual acuity (65%) compared with untreated eyes (37%). Furthermore, treated eyes were more likely to have 20/40 or better vision at 3-years' follow-up (60% compared with 34% untreated), with a mean visual acuity improvement of 1.3 ETDRS lines versus 0.2 line in untreated patients. Overall, mean visual acuity in the treated group was in the 20/40–20/50 range; in the untreated group, it was 20/70.

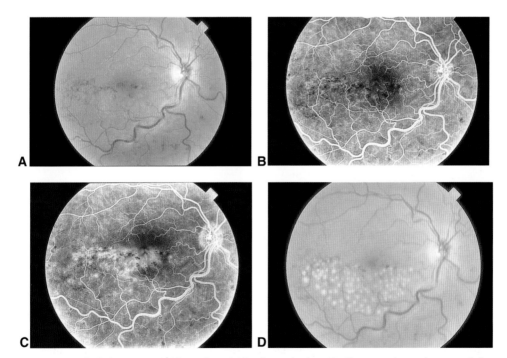

Figure 5-33 A, Inferotemporal branch retinal vein occlusion. **B,** Fluorescein angiogram of *A* at 49 seconds after injection reveals that the perifoveolar retinal capillary bed is essentially intact. **C,** At 393 seconds after injection, intraretinal leakage of dye is present. **D,** Laser photocoagulation given in a full-scatter grid using 100-µm spot size burns with the argon green laser. *(Photographs courtesy of Gary C. Brown, MD.)*

Argon laser photocoagulation for macular edema in branch vein occlusion. The Branch Vein Occlusion Study Group. *Am J Ophthalmol.* 1984;98:271–282.

Panretinal photocoagulation to the area of retinal capillary nonperfusion is also effective in causing regression of the new vessels in eyes with retinal or disc neovascularization (Fig 5-34). The BVOS has shown that scatter argon laser photocoagulation reduces from 22% to 12% the risk of developing neovascularization in eyes that had recently sustained a BRVO involving a retinal area of at least 5 disc diameters. Although patients with large areas of nonperfusion, such as that shown in Figure 5-31, were found to be at significant risk for development of neovascularization, the BVOS concluded that ischemia alone was not an indication for treatment provided that follow-up could be maintained. Rather, it recommended that patients should be observed for the development of neovascularization, which is an indication for photocoagulation.

The BVOS also showed that scatter argon laser photocoagulation reduced the risk of vitreous hemorrhage from 60% to 30% in eyes with a recent BRVO in which neovascularization was already detectable. Clinically, it is important to distinguish collateral vessels from neovascularization of the disc or retina. Complete laser therapy may not be possible in the presence of vitreous hemorrhage, and in such cases, peripheral retinal cryoablation or staged photocoagulation may be useful.

Vitrectomy surgery and/or a scleral buckling procedure may be indicated for eyes that develop nonresorbing vitreous hemorrhage or retinal detachment (see also Chapters 11 and 16).

Finkelstein D, Clarkson JG, Hillis A. Branch and central vein occlusions. *Focal Points: Clinical Modules for Ophthalmologists.* San Francisco: American Academy of Ophthalmology; 1997, module 9.

Pars plana vitrectomy

Pars plana vitrectomy with arteriovenous sheathotomy has been reported in small, uncontrolled series of patients with decreased vision due to BRVO and macular edema unresponsive to laser treatment or not eligible for laser treatment according to BVOS criteria (eg, macular ischemia, persistent and extensive macular hemorrhage). This treat-

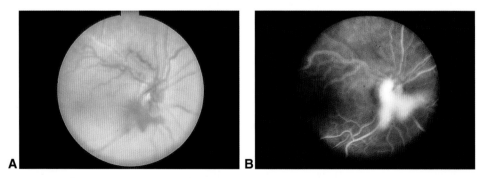

Figure 5-34 A, Neovascularization of the disc (NVD) occurring secondary to a superotemporal BRVO. **B,** Fluorescein angiogram corresponding to **A** at 18 seconds after injection reveals marked hyperfluorescence of the new vessels originating on the optic disc. *(Photographs courtesy of Gary C. Brown, MD.)*

ment modality has not yet been investigated in a prospective, randomized controlled clinical trial.

Opremcak EM, Bruce RA. Surgical decompression of branch retinal vein occlusion via arteriovenous crossing sheathotomy: a prospective review of 15 cases. *Retina.* 1999;19:1–5.

Shah GK, Sharma S, Fineman MS, et al. Arteriovenous adventitial sheathotomy for the treatment of macular edema associated with branch retinal vein occlusion. *Am J Ophthalmol.* 2000;129:104–106.

Intravitreal triamcinolone

A prospective, randomized controlled clinical trial to investigate the safety and efficacy of intravitreal triamcinolone in patients with macular edema associated with BRVO and central retinal vein occlusion (CRVO), the SCORE Study, has been funded by the National Eye Institute.

Central Retinal Vein Occlusion

Long associated with a characteristic fundus appearance of dilated and tortuous retinal veins, a swollen optic disc, intraretinal hemorrhages, and retinal edema, CRVO is now classified by 2 ends of the spectrum of disease:

- *nonischemic,* a milder form sometimes referred to as *partial, perfused,* or *venous stasis retinopathy*
- *ischemic,* a form characterized by at least 10 disc areas, as demonstrated by fluorescein angiography, of retinal capillary nonperfusion on a posterior pole view; also known as *nonperfused, complete,* or *hemorrhagic*

An intermediate, or indeterminate, form also exists, but more than 80% of these eyes progress to the ischemic form.

Baseline and early natural history report. The Central Vein Occlusion Study. Central Vein Occlusion Study Group. *Arch Ophthalmol.* 1993;111:1087–1095.

Histologic studies suggest that most forms of CRVO have a common mechanism: thrombosis of the central retinal vein at and posterior to the level of the lamina cribrosa. In some instances, an atherosclerotic central retinal artery may impinge on the central retinal vein, causing turbulence, endothelial damage, and thrombus formation.

Nonischemic CRVO is characterized by mild dilation and tortuosity of all branches of the central retinal vein, with dot-and-flame hemorrhages in all quadrants of the retina (Fig 5-35). Macular edema with decreased visual acuity and mild optic disc swelling may or may not be present. Fluorescein angiography usually demonstrates prolongation of the retinal circulation time with breakdown of capillary permeability but minimal areas of nonperfusion. Anterior segment neovascularization is rare in nonischemic CRVO. In some eyes, the presence of mild vitreous cells may indicate a combined inflammatory and occlusive mechanism (papillophlebitis).

Ischemic CRVO is usually associated with more extensive 4-quadrant hemorrhage and retinal edema (Fig 5-36). Marked venous dilation is present, and variable numbers of cotton-wool spots are frequently found. Fluorescein angiography typically shows widespread capillary nonperfusion, as well as prolonged intraretinal circulation. The visual

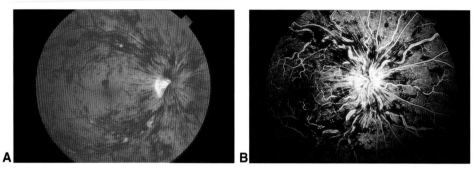

Figure 5-35 **A,** Nonischemic, or perfused, CRVO in an eye with 20/40 vision. Dilated retinal veins and retinal hemorrhages are present, as well as occasional cotton-wool spots, but a foveolar reflex is still present. **B,** Fluorescein angiogram corresponding to **A** at 33 seconds after injection reveals perfusion of the retinal capillary bed. *(Photographs courtesy of Gary C. Brown, MD.)*

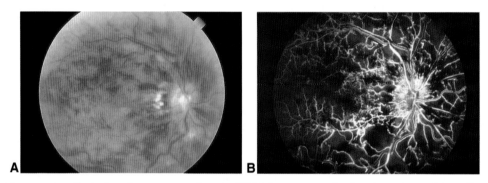

Figure 5-36 **A,** Ischemic, or nonperfused, CRVO in an eye with hand motions vision. The veins are dilated and retinal hemorrhages are present. In contrast to the nonischemic variant, marked retinal edema casts a yellow hue to the background fundus appearance and obscures the foveolar reflex. **B,** Fluorescein angiogram corresponding to **A** at 18 seconds after injection reveals widespread retinal capillary nonperfusion, which causes the midsize and larger retinal vessels to stand out in relief from the gray, nonperfused areas. *(Photographs courtesy of Gary C. Brown, MD.)*

prognosis is generally poor in ischemic CRVO, with approximately 10% of eyes achieving vision better than 20/400. In addition, the incidence of iris neovascularization is high (up to 60%) in very ischemic eyes, usually occurring at a mean of 3–5 months after the onset of symptoms.

> Zegarra H, Gutman FA, Conforto J. The natural course of central retinal vein occlusion. *Ophthalmology.* 1979;86:1931–1942.

Patients may have premonitory symptoms of transient obscuration of vision prior to overt retinal manifestations. Both types of CRVO are similar with regard to patient age at onset (although nonischemic generally occurs at a slightly younger age), associated local and systemic findings, and laboratory studies. Although CRVO can occur and lead to severe visual loss at younger ages, 90% of patients are older than 50 years at the time of onset. Systemic associations noted in the Eye Disease Case-Control Study include:

- systemic arterial hypertension
- diabetes mellitus
- open-angle glaucoma

Increased intraorbital pressure is a rare but potentially important cause of central vein occlusion.

Fekrat S, Finkelstein D. Venous occlusive disease. In: Regillo CD, Brown GC, Flynn HW Jr, eds. *Vitreoretinal Disease: The Essentials.* New York: Thieme; 1999:117–132.

Gutman FA. Evaluation of a patient with central retinal vein occlusion. *Ophthalmology.* 1983;90:481–483.

Risk factors for central retinal vein occlusion. The Eye Disease Case-Control Study Group. *Arch Ophthalmol.* 1996;114:545–554.

It is common for patients presenting with CRVO to have elevated IOP or frank open-angle glaucoma either in the affected eye only or in both eyes. CRVO can also be followed by a transient shallowing of the anterior chamber that, in some instances, leads to angle-closure glaucoma.

Oral contraceptives and diuretics have been implicated in CRVO. Unusual diseases that affect the blood vessel wall or cause alteration in clotting mechanisms and blood viscosity may be associated with a CRVO-like picture. Examples include blood dyscrasias (polycythemia vera), dysproteinemias, and causes of vasculitis (eg, sarcoidosis, systemic lupus erythematosus), and such hypercoagulable conditions as hyperhomocysteinemia, protein S deficiency, and protein C deficiency.

It is particularly important to recognize that hyperviscosity retinopathy can mimic a typical CRVO. However, the retinal findings in hyperviscosity retinopathy are generally bilateral and usually related to dysproteinemia such as Waldenström macroglobulinemia or multiple myeloma. In many cases, the hyperviscosity can be reversed by plasmapheresis. Diagnostic testing includes serum protein electrophoresis and measurements of whole blood viscosity.

Evaluation and management

The ocular evaluation of CRVO requires measurement of IOP to help detect glaucoma. Gonioscopy should be performed in both eyes to determine a predilection toward angle-closure glaucoma, evidence of previous angle-closure glaucoma, or signs of iris neovascularization. Any elevation of IOP in the affected or fellow eye should be treated (see also BCSC Section 10, *Glaucoma*).

The examiner should attempt to determine whether the vein occlusion is of the nonischemic or ischemic type. Fluorescein angiography demonstrates diffuse leakage in the former type and widespread capillary nonperfusion in the latter. The presence of a relative afferent pupillary defect (Marcus Gunn pupil) may be a useful indicator that a CRVO is of the ischemic type. The retinopathy associated with carotid occlusive disease may simulate CRVO and should be differentiated by determination of retinal artery pressure and carotid evaluation.

Kearns TP. Differential diagnosis of central retinal vein obstruction. *Ophthalmology.* 1983;90:475–480.

Management considerations for patients with CRVO include treatment of any associated medical conditions, such as hypertension, diabetes, and elevated cholesterol. When tests for common risk factors for CRVO are negative, consider ordering selected tests in young patients with CRVO to rule out thrombophilias, especially in patients with bilateral CRVO, a history of previous thrombosis, or a family history of thrombosis. Grid pattern photocoagulation for macular edema in CRVO was evaluated prospectively by the Central Vein Occlusion Study Group (CVOS). The initial median visual acuity was 20/160 in treated eyes and 20/125 in control eyes. Final median acuity was 20/200 in treated eyes and 20/160 in control eyes. Thus, even though grid laser treatment in the macula reduced angiographic evidence of macular edema, it yielded no benefit in improving visual acuity. However, there was a trend in the CVOS that grid laser treatment might be beneficial in improving visual acuity for eyes with macular edema in younger patients.

Evaluation of grid pattern photocoagulation for macular edema in central vein occlusion. The Central Vein Occlusion Study Group M report. *Ophthalmology.* 1995;102:1425–1433.

Lahey JM, Tunc M, Kearney J, et al. Laboratory evaluation of hypercoagulable states in patients with central retinal vein occlusion who are less than 56 years of age. *Ophthalmology.* 2002;109:126–131.

Patients with CRVO should be warned of the importance of reporting worsening vision, because some eyes with initially perfused CRVO progress to an ischemic pattern. Corticosteroids and therapies to reduce platelet adhesiveness (aspirin/dipyridamole) have been suggested, but their efficacy and risk remain unproven. Systemic anticoagulation is not typically recommended. Case reports and small case series have reported that intravitreal triamcinolone acetonide may be associated with decreased macular edema and improved visual acuity in some patients with CRVO; however, this treatment modality has not yet been evaluated in a prospective, randomized, controlled clinical trial. Surgical decompression of CRVO via radial optic neurotomy (which involves sectioning the posterior scleral ring) and retinal vein cannulation with an infusion of tissue plasminogen activator (tPA) have been reported in uncontrolled series; the efficacy and risk of these procedures are unproven.

Opremcak EM, Bruce RA, Lomeo MD, et al. Radial optic neurotomy for central retinal vein occlusion: a retrospective pilot study of 11 consecutive cases. *Retina.* 2001;21:408–415.

Iris neovascularization

The CVOS found that the most important risk factor predictive of iris neovascularization in central venous occlusive disease is poor visual acuity. Other risk factors the study found to be associated with the development of iris neovascularization include increasing amounts of retinal capillary nonperfusion and intraretinal blood. A decreased electroretinographic bright-flash, dark-adapted b:a–wave amplitude ratio may also help to distinguish between the ischemic and nonischemic forms of CRVO but has not been shown to add to these risk factors predictive of iris neovascularization.

The CVOS reported that scatter panretinal laser photocoagulation (PRP)—when used before any iris neovascularization has occurred—failed to result in a statistically significant difference in the incidence of iris neovascularization, even though these study participants assigned to scatter PRP had a greater average amount of retinal capillary nonperfusion than did control participants. Because 20% of participants who had received scatter PRP before any iris neovascularization developed still developed the condition, careful follow-up of cases at high risk of developing iris neovascularization is necessary, even when laser is given prophylactically. The CVOS thus recommended waiting for early iris neovascularization to develop before performing PRP; however, it also suggested that prophylactic PRP should be considered for ischemic eyes when close follow-up is not possible or seems unlikely.

Natural history and clinical management of central retinal vein occlusion. The Central Vein Occlusion Study Group. *Arch Ophthalmol.* 1997;115:486–491.

A randomized clinical trial of early panretinal photocoagulation for ischemic central vein occlusion. The Central Vein Occlusion Study Group N report. *Ophthalmology.* 1995;102:1434–1444.

Retinopathy of Carotid Occlusive Disease

Under chronic circumstances, ipsilateral carotid occlusive disease, originally called *venous stasis retinopathy,* can cause a retinopathy similar in appearance to a partial occlusion of the central retinal vein. Hemorrhages in carotid occlusive disease are commonly splotchy, round, and more often located in the midperipheral retina. Typically, the retinal veins are dilated with both CRVO and carotid artery occlusive disease, but most often they are tortuous only in CRVO. A helpful method to differentiate between the two entities is to measure the retinal artery pressure by ophthalmodynamometry. CRVO will have normal artery pressure, whereas carotid occlusive disease will have a low artery pressure.

Arterial Occlusive Disease

The blood supply to the inner layers of the retina comes entirely from the central retinal artery, unless a cilioretinal artery is present (15%–30% of eyes). Retinal ischemia will result from disease affecting the afferent vessels anywhere from the common carotid artery to the intraretinal arterioles. The signs and symptoms of arterial obstruction depend on the vessel involved: whereas occlusion of a peripheral extramacular arteriole may be asymptomatic, ophthalmic artery disease can cause total blindness.

Precapillary Retinal Arteriole Obstruction

Acute obstruction of a precapillary retinal arteriole leads to the formation of a nerve fiber layer (NFL) infarct, or cotton-wool spot, thus inhibiting axoplasmic transport in the NFL. Cotton-wool spots are typically ¼ disc area or less in size and usually fade in 5–7 weeks, although those seen in association with diabetic retinopathy often remain longer (Fig 5-37). A subtle retinal depression caused by inner retinal ischemic atrophy may develop in the area of prior ischemia. The effect on visual function, including loss of visual acuity and field defects, is related to the size and location of the occluded area.

Diabetic retinopathy, the most common cause of cotton-wool spots, was discussed earlier in this chapter. Although the clinical findings are similar, many other diverse causes of precapillary arteriolar closure have been identified.

These other causes include

- systemic arterial hypertension
- cardiac embolic disease
- carotid artery obstructive disease
- sickle cell retinopathy
- radiation retinopathy
- vasculitis
- collagen-vascular disease
- leukemia
- acquired immunodeficiency syndrome (AIDS)

The observation of even 1 cotton-wool spot in the fundus of a patient without diabetes should alert the clinician to initiate a workup for an underlying systemic etiology.

Brown GC, Brown MM, Hiller T, et al. Cotton-wool spots. *Retina.* 1985;5:206–214.
Jampol LM. Arteriolar occlusive diseases of the macula. *Ophthalmology.* 1983;90:534–539.

Branch Retinal Artery Occlusion

Although an acute branch retinal artery occlusion (BRAO) may initially not be apparent ophthalmoscopically, within hours to days it leads to an edematous opacification of the retina caused by infarction in the distribution of the affected vessel (Fig 5-38). With time, the occluded vessel recanalizes, perfusion returns, and the edema resolves; however, a permanent field defect remains. Beyond the posterior pole, occlusion may be clinically silent.

Occlusion at any site is a result of embolization or thrombosis of the affected vessel. Three main varieties of emboli are recognized:

- cholesterol emboli (Hollenhorst plaques) arising in the carotid arteries (Fig 5-39)
- platelet-fibrin emboli associated with large-vessel arteriosclerosis
- calcific emboli arising from diseased cardiac valves

Rare causes of emboli include cardiac myxoma, fat emboli from long-bone fractures, septic emboli from infective endocarditis, and talc emboli in intravenous drug users.

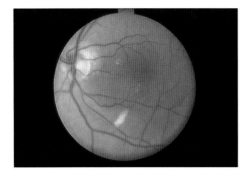

Figure 5-37 Cotton-wool spot. *(Photograph courtesy of Gary C. Brown, MD.)*

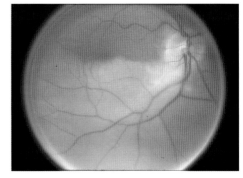

Figure 5-38 Inferotemporal branch retinal artery obstruction. The visual acuity was 20/30 but returned to 20/20 over several weeks. *(Photograph courtesy of Gary C. Brown, MD.)*

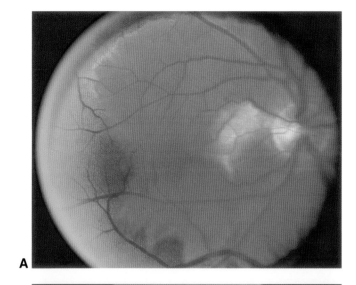

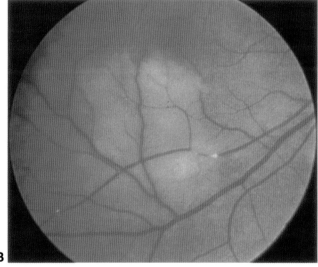

Figure 5-39 BRAO. **A,** Branch artery occlusion that could be mistaken for cilioretinal artery occlusion with swollen whitened retina in distribution of the artery. **B,** Note Hollenhorst plaques and zone of intraretinal infarction and edema below the macula.

Rarely, migraine in patients less than 30 years of age causes ocular arterial occlusions. Other associations include:

- trauma
- coagulation disorders
- sickle cell disease
- oral contraceptive use
- mitral valve prolapse
- inflammatory and/or infectious etiologies such as toxoplasmic retinochoroiditis and syphilis
- connective tissue disorders, including giant cell arteritis

Management is directed toward determining systemic etiologic factors. No specific ocular therapy has been proven consistently effective to improve the visual prognosis. Pressure on the globe may dislodge an embolus from a large central vessel toward a more peripheral location.

Arruga J, Sanders MD. Ophthalmologic findings in 70 patients with evidence of retinal embolism. *Ophthalmology.* 1982;89:1336–1347.

Brown GC, Magargal LE, Shields JA, et al. Retinal arterial obstruction in children and young adults. *Ophthalmology.* 1981;88:18–25.

Central Retinal Artery Occlusion

Sudden, severe, and painless loss of vision in one eye is characteristic of central retinal artery occlusion (CRAO). The retina becomes opaque and edematous, particularly in the posterior pole where the nerve fiber and ganglion cell layers are thickest (Fig 5-40). The orange reflex from the intact choroidal vasculature beneath the foveola thus stands out in contrast to the surrounding opaque neural retina, producing the *cherry-red spot.*

With time, the central retinal artery reopens or recanalizes and the retinal edema clears; however, the effect on visual acuity is usually devastating because the retina has been infarcted. In one study, 66% of eyes had final vision worse than 20/400, and 18% of eyes had vision of 20/40 or better. Most cases of 20/40 or better vision occur in the presence of a patent cilioretinal artery, which preserves the central macula (Fig 5-41). Loss of vision to the level of no light perception is often associated with choroidal vascular insufficiency (ophthalmic artery occlusion) in addition to occlusion of the central retinal artery (Fig 5-42).

Studies in nonhuman primates have suggested that irreversible damage to the sensory retina occurs after 90 minutes of complete CRAO. Nevertheless, clinical return of vision can be seen in some instances even if the obstruction has persisted for many hours.

CRAO is often caused by atherosclerosis-related thrombosis occurring at the level of the lamina cribrosa. Embolization may be important in some cases, as are hemorrhage under an atherosclerotic plaque, thrombosis, spasm, and dissecting aneurysm within the central retinal artery. Overall, emboli are seen in the retinal arterial system in approximately 20% of eyes with CRAO.

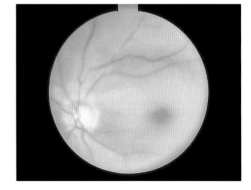

Figure 5-40 CRAO with superficial retinal opacification and a cherry-red spot in the foveola. The visual acuity was hand motions. *(Photograph courtesy of Gary C. Brown, MD.)*

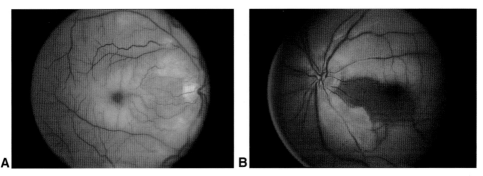

Figure 5-41 A, An acute embolic CRAO produces sudden vision loss in a 68-year-old man. Visual acuity was 20/400. A prominent cherry-red spot was present. **B,** Acute CRAO with cilioretinal artery sparing is seen in this fundus photograph. Diffuse ischemic retinal whitening of the inner retina is observed. The inferior macula is spared as a result of the cilioretinal artery. *(Used with permission from Quillen DA, Blodi BA, eds.* Clinical Retina. *Chicago: AMA Press; 2002:121. Copyright © 2002, American Medical Association. All rights reserved.)*

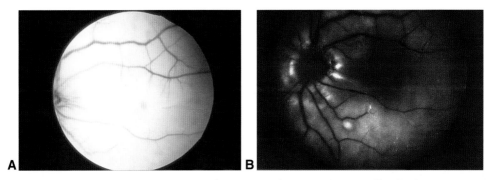

Figure 5-42 A, Acute ophthalmic artery obstruction. Severe retinal opacification is present and a cherry-red spot is absent. The visual acuity was no light perception. **B,** Fluorescein angiogram corresponding to **A** at 27 seconds after injection reveals hypofluorescence of the retinal vessels, the choroid, and the optic disc. *(Photographs courtesy of Gary C. Brown, MD.)*

Embolic phenomena within the carotid distribution may include transient ischemic attacks (TIA) to the retinal circulation, the most frequent cause of amaurosis fugax. Bright cholesterol emboli, or Hollenhorst plaques, seen typically at retinal arterial bifurcations suggest a carotid atheromatous origin and, when accompanied by relevant symptoms and findings, may be an indication for carotid artery treatment. Systemic etiologic considerations, as outlined for BRAO, are important and require evaluation. It should be noted that the leading cause of death in patients with retinal arterial obstruction is cardiovascular disease.

Brown GC, Magargal LE. Central retinal artery obstruction and visual acuity. *Ophthalmology.* 1982;89:14–19.

Hayreh SS, Kolder HE, Weingeist TA. Central retinal artery occlusion and retinal tolerance time. *Ophthalmology.* 1980;87:75–78.

Giant cell arteritis accounts for approximately 1%–2% of cases of CRAO. For this reason, an erythrocyte sedimentation rate (ESR) should be obtained in cases of CRAO in which emboli are not readily visible. Testing the C-reactive protein level is also recommended. Unlike the ESR, which has a rather wide range of "normal" values, the range of "normal" serum C-reactive protein levels is smaller and does not vary by age. Obtaining both ESR and C-reactive protein levels improves the sensitivity and specificity of giant cell arteritis diagnosis. If giant cell arteritis is suspected as a cause, corticosteroid therapy should be promptly instituted because the second eye can become involved by CRAO within hours to days after the first, and a temporal artery biopsy should be obtained. See BCSC Section 1, *Update on General Medicine,* for further discussion of giant cell arteritis.

Management

If therapy for CRAO is to be instituted, it should theoretically be undertaken without delay. Unfortunately, the efficacy of treatment is questionable. Steps include reduction in IOP by ocular massage, anterior chamber paracentesis, or retrobulbar anesthesia. Other treatments advocated in the past include inhalation therapy with 95% oxygen–5% carbon dioxide mixture, and the use of oral acetazolamide and aspirin.

> Atebara NH, Brown GC, Cater J. Efficacy of anterior chamber paracentesis and Carbogen in treating acute nonarteritic central retinal artery occlusion. *Ophthalmology.* 1995;102: 2029–2034.
>
> Brown GC. Arterial occlusive disease. In: Regillo CD, Brown GC, Flynn HW Jr, eds. *Vitreoretinal Disease: The Essentials.* New York: Thieme; 1999:97–115.

Experimental data have shown that ischemic retinal damage may arise not only from the presence of retinal nonperfusion but also from a cascade of events that injure cells after the tissue becomes reperfused. In the future it may be possible to minimize damage with drugs that block this cascade of oxidative and membrane damage.

Iris neovascularization will develop in approximately 18% of eyes with acute CRAO at 1–12 weeks after the event, with a mean time of approximately 4–5 weeks. Full-scatter PRP is effective in eradicating the new iris vessels in about two thirds of cases.

Ocular Ischemic Syndrome

Ocular ischemic syndrome is the name given to the ocular symptoms and signs attributable to chronic, severe carotid artery obstruction, although chronic ophthalmic artery obstruction can cause a similar clinical picture. Atherosclerosis is the most common etiology, but possible causes include Eisenmenger syndrome, giant cell arteritis, and other inflammatory conditions. Most patients are older than 55 years of age. Typically, a 90% or greater ipsilateral obstruction is necessary to cause the ocular ischemic syndrome. Both eyes are involved in about 20% of cases.

Symptoms include visual loss usually occurring over a period of weeks to months, aching pain localized to the orbital area of the affected eye, and prolonged recovery following exposure to a bright light. Anterior segment signs include iris neovascularization in two thirds of eyes, and an anterior chamber cellular response is seen in about one fifth of eyes. Despite the fact that iris neovascularization is very prevalent, only half of the eyes with it show an increase in IOP; most likely, the low or normal IOP found in the other half is caused by impaired ciliary body perfusion. Posterior segment signs include narrowed retinal arteries, dilated (but generally not tortuous) retinal veins, retinal hemorrhages, microaneurysms, and neovascularization of the optic disc and/or retina (Fig 5-43).

Fluorescein angiography reveals delayed choroidal filling in 60% of eyes, delayed arteriovenous transit time in 95% of eyes, and prominent vascular staining (particularly of the arteries) in 85% of eyes. Electroretinography often discloses diminished amplitude of the a- and b-waves as a result of outer and inner layer retinal ischemia, respectively.

Approximately one half of patients with ocular ischemic syndrome also have ischemic cardiovascular disease, one fourth have had a previous cerebrovascular accident, and one fifth have peripheral atherosclerotic vascular disease so severe that a previous surgical procedure was necessary. The stroke rate is increased over that in the general population, and the 5-year mortality is approximately 40%. As with retinal arterial obstruction, the majority of deaths occur secondary to the complications of cardiovascular disease.

The natural history of vision in eyes with the ocular ischemic syndrome is uncertain, but when rubeosis iridis is present, more than 90% of those eyes are legally blind within a year after the disease is discovered. Full-scatter PRP is effective in eradicating rubeosis in about 35% of eyes.

The most definitive treatment for the ocular ischemic syndrome appears to be carotid endarterectomy, although visual results are generally anecdotal. Unfortunately, the procedure is ineffective when there is a 100% obstruction, which is often the case in ocular ischemic syndrome patients. Extracranial to intracranial bypass surgery has been attempted in such cases but has been shown to be ineffective in preventing visual loss or stroke.

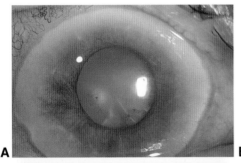

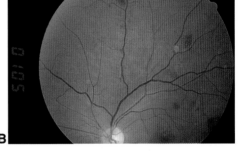

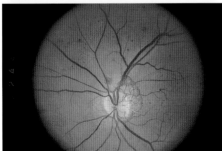

Figure 5-43 A, Ocular ischemic syndrome is caused by insufficient blood flow to the eye. Many patients present with iris neovascularization. Patients with anterior chamber angle involvement may develop neovascular glaucoma. **B,** Funduscopic examination usually reveals intraretinal hemorrhages. The retinal arteries are narrowed, and the veins may be slightly dilated. **C,** Optic disc neovascularization develops in approximately one third of patients. *(Used with permission from Quillen DA, Blodi BA, eds.* Clinical Retina. *Chicago: AMA Press; 2002:143. Copyright © 2002, American Medical Association. All rights reserved.)*

In eyes with iris neovascularization and low or normal IOP as a result of impaired ciliary body perfusion and decreased aqueous formation, endarterectomy may improve the ciliary body perfusion, which, in turn, can lead to increased aqueous formation and a severe rise in IOP.

Brown GC. Arterial occlusive disease. In: Regillo CD, Brown GC, Flynn HW Jr, eds. *Vitreoretinal Disease: The Essentials.* New York: Thieme; 1999:97–115.

Brown GC. Ocular ischemic syndrome. In: Ryan SJ, ed. *Retina.* 3rd ed. St Louis: Mosby; 2001:1516–1529.

Data from the North American Symptomatic Carotid Endarterectomy Trial Collaborators are applicable to some patients with the ocular ischemic syndrome. The study demonstrated that symptomatic patients [those with a history of amaurosis fugax, a hemispheric transient ischemic attack (TIA), or a nondisabling stroke] with a 70%–99% carotid artery stenosis have a 2-year stroke rate of 9% in the endarterectomy group versus a 26% rate in a control group treated with antiplatelet agents. A similar study performed by the European Carotid Surgery Trialists' Collaborative Group found no benefit to endarterectomy compared to antiplatelet agents in a symptomatic group with a 0%–29% carotid stenosis. In patients with a symptomatic 50%–69% stenosis, the 5-year stroke rate is approximately 16% with endarterectomy and 22% among those treated medically. Thus, the treatment benefit effect for this subgroup is only moderate.

Barnett HJ, Taylor DW, Eliasziw M, et al. Benefit of carotid endarterectomy in patients with symptomatic moderate or severe stenosis. North American Symptomatic Carotid Endarterectomy Trial Collaborators. *N Engl J Med.* 1998;339:1415–1425.

Beneficial effect of carotid endarterectomy in symptomatic patients with high-grade carotid stenosis. North American Symptomatic Carotid Endarterectomy Trial Collaborators. *N Engl J Med.* 1991;325:445–453.

MRC European Carotid Surgery Trial: interim results for symptomatic patients with severe (70–99%) or with mild (0–29%) carotid stenosis. European Carotid Surgery Trialists' Collaborative Group. *Lancet.* 1991;337:1235–1243.

Vasculitis

Vasculitis from any cause can lead to similar pathologic sequelae and may accompany primary inflammatory disease elsewhere in the eye. The early clinical manifestations are generally nonspecific, with perivascular infiltrates and sheathing of the retinal vessels (vascular wall thickening with vessel involution; Fig 5-44). Distinct involvement of exclusively retinal arteries or veins is less common than diffuse changes. Causes of retinal vasculitis include

- giant cell arteritis
- polyarteritis
- systemic lupus erythematosus
- Behçet syndrome
- inflammatory bowel diseases
- multiple sclerosis
- pars planitis

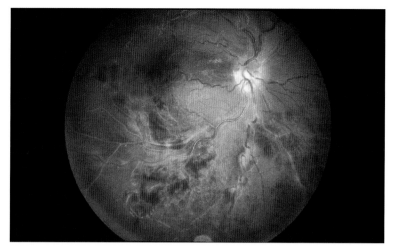

Figure 5-44 Retinal vasculitis in an eye of a patient with Crohn disease. Retinal hemorrhages and edema are present, as is prominent sheathing of the retinal vessels. *(Photograph courtesy of Gary C. Brown, MD.)*

- sarcoidosis
- syphilis
- toxoplasmosis
- viral retinitides
- Lyme disease
- cat-scratch disease

The masquerade syndromes should also be considered. See BCSC Section 9, *Intraocular Inflammation and Uveitis,* for further discussion of most of these conditions and Section 5, *Neuro-Ophthalmology,* for discussion of multiple sclerosis.

Primary idiopathic retinal vasculitis has been termed *Eales disease.* This disease, which occurs primarily in males, is an obliterative periphlebitis that usually involves the peripheral retina of both eyes and often results in retinal neovascularization with vitreous hemorrhage. An associated tuberculin hypersensitivity may be present.

A clinical picture indistinguishable from past retinal vasculitis may result from chronic embolism or thrombosis without inflammation. Evaluation includes a search for possible causes: cardiac valvular disease, cardiac arrhythmias, ulcerated atheromatous disease of the carotid vessels, and hemoglobinopathies.

Idiopathic retinal vasculitis, aneurysms, and neuroretinitis (IRVAN) describes a syndrome characterized by the presence of retinal vasculitis, multiple macroaneurysms, neuroretinitis, and peripheral capillary nonperfusion. Systemic investigations are generally noncontributory and oral prednisone has demonstrated little benefit. Capillary nonperfusion is frequently sufficiently severe to warrant panretinal laser photocoagulation.

Chang TS, Aylward GW, Davis JL, et al. Idiopathic retinal vasculitis, aneurysms, and neuro-retinitis. Retinal Vasculitis Study. *Ophthalmology.* 1995;102:1089–1097.

Gieser SC, Murphy RP. Eales' disease. In: Tasman W, Jaeger EA, eds. *Duane's Clinical Ophthalmology.* Philadelphia: Lippincott; 1991: vol 3, ch 16, pp 1–5.

Mandava N, Yannuzzi LA. Miscellaneous retinal vascular conditions. In: Regillo CD, Brown GC, Flynn HW Jr, eds. *Vitreoretinal Disease: The Essentials.* New York: Thieme; 1999: 193–211.

Cystoid Macular Edema

Cystoid macular edema (CME) is characterized by intraretinal edema contained in honeycomb-like cystoid spaces. Fluorescein angiography shows the source of edema to be abnormal perifoveal retinal capillary permeability, seen as multiple small focal fluorescein leaks and late pooling of the dye in cystoid spaces. Optical coherence tomography findings of CME include diffuse retinal thickening with cystic areas of low reflectivity (reduced reflectivity) more prominently evident in the outer plexiform layers. This finding correlates with histopathology studies reported in the literature. On occasions, a nonreflective cavity can be appreciated underneath the neurosensory retina, which is consistent with subretinal fluid accumulation. Because of Henle's fiber layer, this pooling classically forms a flower-petal pattern (Fig 5-45). Severe cases may be associated with vitritis (vitreous cells) and optic nerve head swelling.

Gass JD, Norton EW. Follow-up study of cystoid macular edema following cataract extraction. *Trans Am Acad Ophthalmol Otolaryngol.* 1969;73:665–682.

Abnormal permeability of the perifoveal retinal capillaries may occur in a wide variety of conditions, including diabetic retinopathy, central and branch retinal vein occlusion, any type of uveitis (particularly pars planitis), and retinitis pigmentosa. These capillary changes may also follow any type of ocular surgery, such as cataract extraction, retinal detachment surgery, vitrectomy, glaucoma procedures, photocoagulation, and cryopexy. Subretinal disease (choroidal neovascularization) must also be considered when CME is detected; see Chapter 4.

Rare causes of cystic macular change of different pathogenesis (such as juvenile retinoschisis, Goldmann-Favre disease, some cases of retinitis pigmentosa, and nicotinic acid maculopathy) are distinguishable by the clinical setting, family history, and the lack of late fluorescein leakage into the cystlike spaces.

The term *Irvine-Gass syndrome* is used for CME following cataract surgery, which is a common and important setting. The incidence may be as high as 60% of patients who have undergone intracapsular lens extraction and may be lower when the posterior capsule remains intact. Intraocular lens implantation at the time of extracapsular surgery does not appear to increase the incidence of CME. The peak incidence occurs 6–10 weeks postoperatively, with spontaneous resolution occurring clinically in approximately 95% of uncomplicated cases, usually within 6 months. Most such cases of CME are mild and asymptomatic; it is relevant to distinguish between symptomatic, or *clinical,* CME and edema apparent only on fluorescein angiography (*angiographic* CME). More severe CME may result in permanent visual loss. The incidence of CME increases with significant postoperative uveitis and with surgical complications such as vitreous loss or iris prolapse. Increased incidence may be related to IOL complications and photic effects as well. See also BCSC Section 11, *Lens and Cataract.*

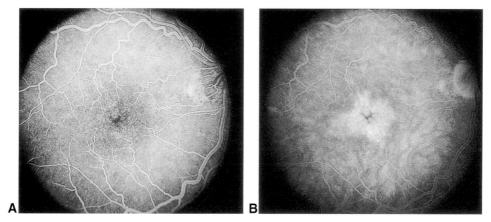

Figure 5-45 CME. Fluorescein angiogram demonstrates hyperfluorescent dilated capillaries in early frames **(A)** with late intraretinal accumulation of fluorescein in a petaloid pattern **(B).** Disc staining is also commonly associated.

Berkow JW, Flower RW, Orth DH, et al. *Fluorescein and Indocyanine Green Angiography: Technique and Interpretation.* 2nd ed. Ophthalmology Monograph 5. San Francisco: American Academy of Ophthalmology; 1997:117–118.

Although the source of edema has been demonstrated, the precise cause of CME is unknown. Inflammation is undoubtedly important, as evidenced by clinical and pathologic association with varying degrees of iritis, cyclitis, vitritis, and retinal phlebitis. Other important clinical associations include systemic vascular disease such as hypertension or diabetes and age greater than 60 years.

The effect on therapy for CME is difficult to evaluate because of the high rate of spontaneous resolution, but it is reasonable to treat eyes with any clinical evidence of intraocular inflammation. Pharmacologic therapy may be considered for prophylaxis as well as for established edema. For prophylaxis of CME, several studies have demonstrated that topical and systemic indomethacin is effective in reducing the incidence of angiographic CME. Topical, periocular, and systemic corticosteroids have been used, as well as prostaglandin inhibitors and carbonic anhydrase inhibitors, which are believed to enhance fluid transport across the RPE. Corticosteroids may be beneficial for established CME, but the recurrence rate is high following cessation of steroid therapy. Improvement of visual acuity in eyes with chronic aphakic or pseudophakic CME has been demonstrated in a multicenter clinical trial using topical 0.5% ketorolac tromethamine (Acular).

CME may be associated with vitreous adhesions to the iris or a corneoscleral wound, presumably on the basis of persistent uveitis and perhaps vitreoretinal traction. Interruption of the vitreous strands by vitrectomy surgery or use of the Nd:YAG laser may be helpful.

Cox SN, Hay E, Bird AC. Treatment of chronic macular edema with acetazolamide. *Arch Ophthalmol.* 1988;106:1190–1195.

Flach AJ, Jampol LM, Weinberg D, et al. Improvement in visual acuity in chronic aphakic and pseudophakic cystoid macular edema after treatment with topical 0.5% ketorolac tromethamine. *Am J Ophthalmol.* 1991;112:514–519.

Fung WE. Surgical therapy for chronic aphakic cystoid macular edema. *Ophthalmology.* 1982;89:898–901.

Harbour JW, Smiddy WE, Rubsamen PE, et al. Pars plana vitrectomy for chronic pseudo-phakic cystoid macular edema. *Am J Ophthalmol.* 1995;120:302–307.

Heier JS, Topping TM, Baumann W, et al. Ketorolac versus prednisolone versus combination therapy in the treatment of acute pseudophakic cystoid macular edema. *Ophthalmology.* 2000;107:2034–2039.

Weisz JM, Bressler NM, Bressler SB, et al. Ketorolac treatment of pseudophakic cystoid macular edema identified more than 24 months after cataract extraction. *Ophthalmology.* 1999;106:1656–1659.

Coats Disease

Coats disease (retinal telangiectasia) is defined by the presence of vascular anomalies, including telangiectatic vessels, venous dilation, microaneurysms, and fusiform capillary dilation, frequently associated with exudative retinal detachment and a degree of capillary nonperfusion as defined by clinical examination and fluorescein angiography. Despite the presence of retinal capillary nonperfusion, posterior segment neovascularization is distinctly unusual. The abnormal vessels are incompetent, resulting in the accumulation of serum and other blood components in and under the retina. Any portion or all of the capillary system may be involved. Variation in the clinical findings is wide, ranging from mild retinal vascular abnormalities and minimal exudation to extensive areas of retinal telangiectasia associated with massive leakage and exudative retinal detachment, as may be detected in children (Coats reaction; Fig 5-46).

This retinal condition is not hereditary and is not associated with systemic vascular abnormalities. However, entities such as retinitis pigmentosa and others may occasionally be associated with retinal telangiectasia. Usually only 1 eye is involved, and there is a marked male predominance (85%). Gradual progression with increasing exudation occurs over time. The severity and rate of progression appear greater in patients under the age of 4 years, in whom massive exudative retinal detachment may simulate retinoblastoma. Coats disease should be included in the differential diagnosis of leukocoria in this age group. BCSC Section 4, *Ophthalmic Pathology and Intraocular Tumors,* discusses retinoblastoma in depth.

Patients with peripheral areas of telangiectasia or other vascular anomalies typically present with lipid deposition in an otherwise angiographically normal macula, as hard exudate tends to accumulate in the macula. Similar findings when seen initially in adults probably represent late decompensation of preexisting vascular anomalies. Occasionally, a disciform scar in the macula is the initial finding. Differential diagnosis may include

- dominant (familial) exudative vitreoretinopathy
- facioscapulohumeral muscular dystrophy
- retinopathy of prematurity

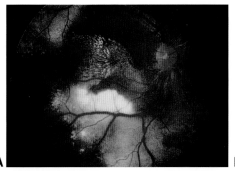

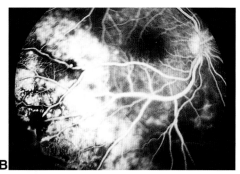

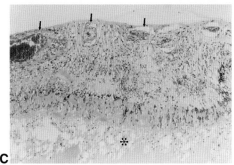

Figure 5-46 "Light bulb" aneurysms in Coats disease. **A,** Retinal telangiectasia, "light bulb" aneurysms, beading of vessel walls, capillary dilatation, and massive retinal edema sourrounded by subretinal exudate in an 8-year-old boy with Coats disease. **B,** Fluorescein angiogram showing retinal vascular telangiectasis, areas of capillary dilatation and nonperfusion, beading of vessels, and "light bulb" aneurysms typical of Coats disease. **C,** Histopathology of Coats disease demonstrating retina with gliosis and focal loss of the normal lamellar architecture. Telangiectatic blood vessels *(arrows)* are present in the inner aspect of the retina, causing massive intraretinal and subretinal exudation and focal areas of hemorrhage. The retina is detached by subretinal exudate containing numerous foamy lipid-laden macrophages *(asterisk)*. (Hematoxylin and eosin, ×100.) *(Used with permission from Scott IU, Flynn HW Jr, Rosa RH Jr. Other retinal vascular diseases: hypertensive retinopathy, venous and arterial occlusive disease, retinal artery macroaneurysms, sickle cell retinopathy, Coats' disease, juxtafoveal telangiectasis, and Eales disease. In: Parrish RK, ed.* The University of Miami Bascom Palmer Eye Institute Atlas of Ophthalmology. *Philadelphia: Current Medicine; 2000:300.)*

For milder cases, diabetic retinopathy, BRVO, juxtafoveal retinal telangiectasis, and radiation retinopathy may be considered.

Treatment of Coats disease generally consists of photocoagulation, cryotherapy, and, in severe cases, retinal reattachment surgery. Photocoagulation and cryotherapy are effective in obliterating the vascular anomalies and in halting progression. Multiple treatments may be necessary, and long-term follow-up is important to detect recurrences.

Horn G, Rabb MF, Lewicky AO. Retinal telangiectasis of the macula: a review and differential diagnosis. *Int Ophthalmol Clin.* 1981;21:139–155.

Ridley ME, Shields JA, Brown GC, et al. Coats' disease: evaluation of management. *Ophthalmology.* 1982;89:1381–1387.

Parafoveal (Juxtafoveal) Retinal Telangiectasis

Clinically apparent retinal telangiectasis and ectasia of the capillary bed, confined to the juxtafoveolar region of one or both eyes, may result in visual loss from capillary incompetence and exudation (Fig 5-47). Histopathologic evidence suggests that this is not a true telangiectasia but rather consists of structural abnormalities similar to diabetic

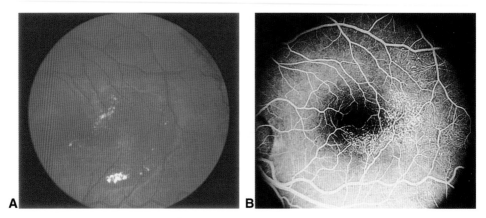

Figure 5-47 Parafoveal telangiectasis, type 1. Note retinal exudate and typical capillary anomalies, primarily in temporal macula.

microangiopathy, with deposits of excess basement membrane within the retinal capillaries. The entity has been subdivided into 3 groups:

- *Group 1:* Unilateral parafoveal telangiectasis, congenital or acquired
- *Group 2:* Bilateral parafoveal telangiectasis (Fig 5-48)
- *Group 3:* Bilateral perifoveal telangiectasis with retinal capillary obliteration

Group 1, which typically occurs in males, resembles a localized variant of Coats disease with a circinate type of exudate. Patients in group 2, either males or females, usually have bilateral thickening of the retina, most pronounced in the temporal fovea. RPE hyperplasia is often present, and choroidal neovascularization may subsequently develop. Visual loss ranges from mild to severe. More than one third of patients with this variant will have an abnormal glucose tolerance test. Cases in group 3 show progressive loss from the obliteration of the perifoveal capillaries.

Photocoagulation treatment may be indicated for group 1 cases and can be successful in resolving exudation. Group 2 and group 3 eyes typically do not respond to photocoagulation. The differential diagnosis includes, but is not limited to, branch vein or venule obstruction, diabetes, radiation retinopathy, and carotid artery disease.

Gass JD, Blodi BA. Idiopathic juxtafoveolar retinal telangiectasis: update of classification and follow-up study. *Ophthalmology.* 1993;100:1536–1546.

Park DW, Schatz H, McDonald HR, et al. Grid laser photocoagulation for macular edema in bilateral juxtafoveal telangiectasis. *Ophthalmology.* 1997;104:1838–1846.

Arterial Macroaneurysms

Retinal arterial macroaneurysms are acquired retinal vascular abnormalities (Fig 5-49). Large macroaneurysms can actually traverse the full thickness of the retina. Visual loss may occur from sub-ILM hemorrhage, intraretinal or subretinal hemorrhage, retinal edema involving the macula, or vitreous hemorrhage. Other retinal findings may include arteriolar emboli, capillary telangiectasia, and vascular occlusions (arteriolar or venous).

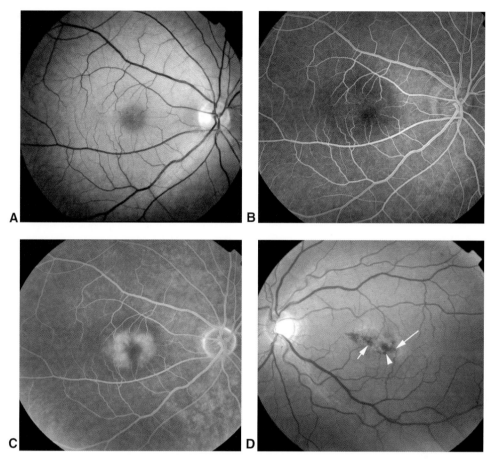

Figure 5-48 **A,** Red-free photograph showing bilateral parafoveal telangiectasis. The patient has telangiectasis in the temporal juxtafoveal macula, early right-angle vein formation, and fine crystals in the inner retina. **B,** Early-phase fluorescein photograph showing telangiectasis. **C,** In the late-phase fluorescein photograph, there is hyperfluorescence from inner retinal leakage of fluorescein. **D,** Arrowheads point to pigment hyperplasia typically seen in this condition. *(Photographs courtesy of Richard Spaide, MD.)*

Arterial macroaneurysms are frequently multiple, although only 10% of cases are bilateral. They are associated with systemic arterial hypertension in about two thirds of cases. Sclerosis and spontaneous closure often accompany macroaneurysm-related hemorrhage; only rarely does bleeding occur more than once.

Laser photocoagulation treatment may be considered if increasing edema in the macula impinges on central visual function. The surface of the leaking abnormality may be treated lightly with large spot size (200–500 μm) burns; treatment to the retina immediately adjacent to the aneurysm may also be considered. Caution should be used when treating abnormalities along arterial vessels that supply the central macula, because one of the complications of therapy is thrombosis and retinal arterial obstruction distal to the macroaneurysm.

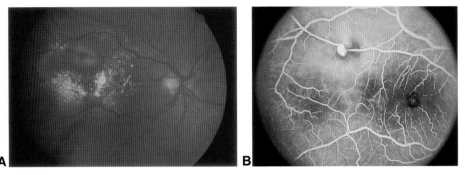

Figure 5-49 A, Arterial macroaneurysm associated with leakage, manifested as exudate encroaching into the fovea. **B,** Fluorescein angiogram demonstrates arterial macroaneurysm, as well as relative hypofluorescence from blocking effect of exudate.

Brown DM, Sobol WM, Folk JC, et al. Retinal arteriolar macroaneurysms: long-term visual outcome. *Br J Ophthalmol.* 1994;78:534–538.

Chew EY, Murphy RP. Acquired retinal macroaneurysms. In: Ryan SJ, ed. *Retina.* 3rd ed. St Louis: Mosby; 2001:1500–1504.

Rabb MF, Gagliano DA, Teske MP. Retinal arterial macroaneurysms. *Surv Ophthalmol.* 1988;33:73–96.

Phakomatoses

Conventionally, a number of syndromes referred to as *phakomatoses* ("mother spot") are grouped loosely by the common features of ocular and systemic involvement of a congenital nature. Most, but not all, are hereditary. With the exception of Sturge-Weber syndrome, the phakomatoses involve the neuroretina and its circulation. For further discussion of the phakomatoses, see BCSC Section 5, *Neuro-Ophthalmology,* and Section 6, *Pediatric Ophthalmology and Strabismus.*

von Hippel–Lindau Disease (Retinal Angiomatosis)

Capillary hemangiomas develop in the retina and optic nerve head in retinal angiomatosis. The early lesions are small and easily overlooked clinically but may be seen in fluorescein angiography. A fully developed lesion is a spherical orange-red tumor fed by a dilated, tortuous retinal artery and drained by an engorged vein (Fig 5-50). Multiple angiomas may be found in the same eye, and bilateral involvement occurs in 50% of patients. Angiomas affecting the optic nerve head and peripapillary retina may be more difficult to recognize because of the absence of visible afferent and efferent dilated vessels. Lesions in such locations are predominantly subretinal or epiretinal (exophytic or endophytic).

An angiomatous variant has been described, with the lesion located peripherally and not associated with large feeding and draining vessels nor with systemic manifestations. Angiomatous variants have also been reported with the late sequelae of ROP.

Leakage of plasma constituents from an angioma may lead to serous detachment of the retina and/or accumulation of exudate in the macula, resulting in reduction in visual

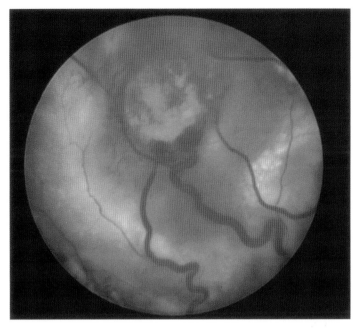

Figure 5-50 Patient with von Hippel disease, showing peripheral angioma with surrounding exudate and retinal detachment. Note dilation of feeder arteriole and draining venule.

acuity (Fig 5-51). Occasionally, vitreous hemorrhage or tractional detachment may occur. Neovascularization of the optic disc, retina, and/or iris may develop following retinal detachment.

Retinal angiomatosis has both a hereditary and a sporadic form. The mode of transmission is autosomal dominant, often with incomplete penetrance and variable expression. The retinal and/or optic disc lesions have also been referred to as *von Hippel lesions*. When retinal angiomatosis is associated with central nervous system (CNS) and visceral involvement, the eponym *von Hippel–Lindau disease* is used. For a more extensive discussion of von Hippel–Lindau disease, see BCSC Section 6, *Pediatric Ophthalmology and Strabismus*.

Central nervous system tumors (hemangioblastomas of the cerebellum, medulla, pons, and spinal cord) occur in 20% of patients. The visceral lesions include cysts of the kidney, pancreas, liver, epididymis, and ovary. Renal cell carcinoma, meningiomas, and pheochromocytomas have also been associated. When an ocular lesion is discovered, a systemic workup should also be considered for possible renal cell carcinoma and pheochromocytoma, as well as for CNS lesions. The leading causes of death in patients with von Hippel–Lindau disease are cerebellar hemangioblastoma and renal cell carcinoma.

Gass JD, Braunstein R. Sessile and exophytic capillary angiomas of the juxtapapillary retina and optic nerve head. *Arch Ophthalmol*. 1980;98:1790–1797.

Hardwig P, Robertson DM. von Hippel–Lindau disease: a familial, often lethal, multisystem phakomatosis. *Ophthalmology*. 1984;91:263–270.

Shields JA, Decker WL, Sanborn GE, et al. Presumed acquired retinal hemangiomas. *Ophthalmology*. 1983;90:1292–1300.

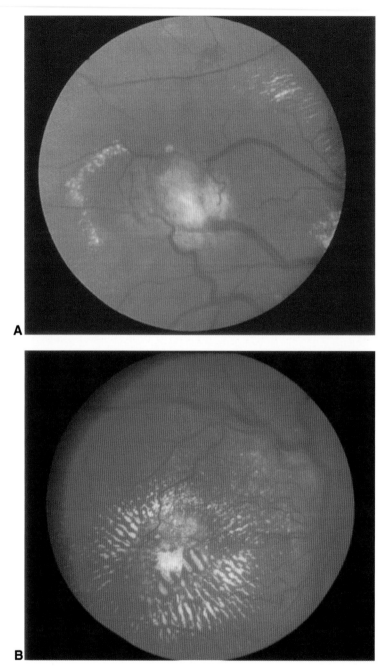

Figure 5-51 **A,** Patient with von Hippel disease, showing peripheral angiomatous lesion with surrounding zones of intraretinal exudate. **B,** Exudative maculopathy associated with peripheral angioma.

Many retinal angiomas are believed to enlarge over time, with an increase in the exudative component. Ocular management therefore generally includes treatment of all identified retinal angiomas and careful follow-up to detect recurrence or the development of new lesions. Photocoagulation and cryotherapy have been used to treat the angiomatous lesions directly. Shrinkage of the angioma, attenuation of the afferent vessels, and resorption of the subretinal fluid will occur with successful treatment. Therefore, consideration may be given to treating smaller retinal angiomas. Early diagnosis increases the likelihood for successful treatment. Treatment is hazardous and may be associated with a temporary, marked increase in the amount of exudation, which may occasionally result in the development of a total retinal detachment. Rarely, retinal capillary angiomas may involute spontaneously. A case report described involution of a retinal capillary hemangioma with reduction in subretinal fluid and improvement in visual acuity following photodynamic therapy.

Atebara NH. Retinal capillary hemangioma treated with verteporfin photodynamic therapy. *Am J Ophthalmol.* 2002;134:788–790.

Shields JA, Shields CL. Tumors of the retina and optic disc. In: Regillo CD, Brown GC, Flynn HW Jr, eds. *Vitreoretinal Disease: The Essentials.* New York: Thieme; 1999:439–453.

Congenital Retinal Arteriovenous Malformations (Racemose Angioma, Wyburn-Mason Syndrome)

Congenital retinal arteriovenous communications are rare developmental anomalies. No intervening capillary bed exists in racemose angioma. The abnormalities may range from a single arteriovenous communication to a complex anastomotic system.

Lesions are typically unilateral, nonhereditary, and located in the retina or optic nerve. They do not show leakage on fluorescein angiography. The retinal lesions may be associated in some cases with similar ipsilateral vascular malformations in the brain, face, and orbit (Wyburn-Mason syndrome). Associated central nervous vascular malformations tend to be located deeply and follow the optic tract. Many of the retinal malformations remain asymptomatic. If the lesions are large, however, they may be associated with subretinal fluid and exudate.

Retinal Cavernous Hemangioma

Although most cases of cavernous hemangioma are sporadic and restricted to the retina or optic nerve head, they may occur in a familial (autosomal dominant) pattern and may be associated with intracranial and skin hemangiomas. For this reason, cavernous hemangioma may be considered one of the phakomatoses.

Retinal cavernous hemangioma is characterized by the formation of grapelike clusters of thin-walled saccular angiomatous lesions in the inner retina or on the optic nerve head (Fig 5-52). The blood flow in these lesions is derived from the retinal circulation and is relatively stagnant, producing a characteristic fluorescein picture. These dilated saccular lesions fill slowly during angiography, and plasma-erythrocyte layering occurs as a result of the sluggish blood flow. Fluorescein leakage is characteristically absent, correlating with the absence of subretinal fluid and exudate in retinal cavernous

Figure 5-52 **A,** Large retinal cavernous hemangioma in inferior retina of right eye. Color photograph shows the dilated and tortuous vein with grapelike saccular clusters of angiomatous lesions that could be mistaken for retinal neovascularization. These lesions are usually stable and require no treatment. **B,** Fluorescein angiogram (late transit at 43.3 seconds) shows poor blood flow and uneven filling of the vascular lesion. **C,** Even by 60.8 seconds the vascular tree is not completely filled. Late phases typically show accumulation of dye in the saccular lesions with no sign of leakage.

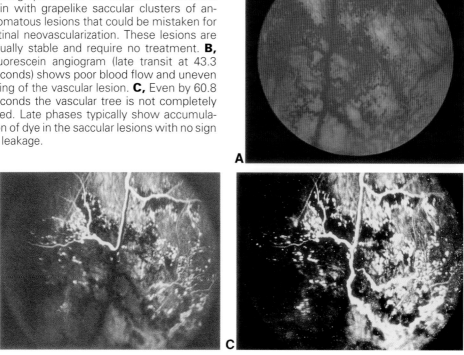

hemangioma and serving to differentiate it from retinal telangiectasis, von Hippel retinal angiomatosis, and racemose aneurysm of the retina.

Rarely, the hemangiomas may bleed into the vitreous, but they usually remain asymptomatic. Vitreous traction is thought to be the cause of hemorrhage in these cases. Treatment of retinal cavernous hemangiomas is usually not indicated unless recurrent vitreous hemorrhage develops, in which case photocoagulation or cryotherapy may be effective.

The authors wish to acknowledge the contributions of Robert Equi, MD, to this chapter.

CHAPTER 6

Choroidal Disease

Certain noninflammatory choroidal diseases that are most appropriately discussed in the context of associated involvement of the retina are covered in this chapter. Inflammatory disorders of the retina and choroid are discussed in Chapter 7. See also BCSC Section 9, *Intraocular Inflammation and Uveitis*. Intraocular tumors, such as melanoma, are covered in BCSC Section 4, *Ophthalmic Pathology and Intraocular Tumors*.

Bilateral Diffuse Uveal Melanocytic Proliferation

A rare paraneoplastic disorder affecting the choroid, bilateral diffuse uveal melanocytic proliferation (BDUMP) causes diffuse thickening of the choroid, reddish or brownish patches, cataracts, and serous retinal detachment. As the name suggests, usually a bilateral proliferation of benign melanocytes is associated with or often heralds a systemic cancer. These proliferations can look like large nevi (Fig 6-1). Some BDUMP lesions appear to be areas of depigmentation of the RPE that have associated hyperfluorescence during fluorescein angiography. These spots look reddish. The more common tumors associated with BDUMP are cancer of the ovaries, uterus, and lung, but they may also occur with cancer of the colon, pancreas, gall bladder, and esophagus.

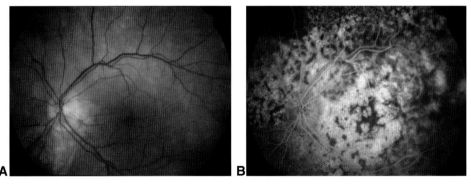

Figure 6-1 Bilateral diffuse uveal melanocytic proliferation (BDUMP). **A,** Note the large nevuslike regions of increased pigmentation and thickening of the choroid. **B,** Fluorescein angiography demonstrates decreased fluorescence in the region of the melanocytic proliferation in the superonasal portion of the photograph. There is a leopard spot pattern to the fluorescence in the posterior pole, secondary to chronic subretinal fluid. *(Photographs courtesy of Mark Johnson, MD).*

Gass JD, Gieser RG, Wilkinson CP, et al. Bilateral diffuse uveal melanocytic proliferation in patients with occult carcinoma. *Arch Ophthalmol.* 1990;108:527–533.

Choroidal Perfusion Abnormalities

Although the bulk of blood flow into the eye goes to the choroid, perfusion abnormalities in the choroid are sometimes difficult to diagnose. Retinal vascular occlusion is readily visible by ophthalmoscopy and is straightforwardly confirmed by fluorescein angiography. Choroidal vascular occlusion may produce changes that vary from clinically evident to quite subtle. In addition, it is not uncommon for choroidal vascular abnormalities to be associated with retinal vascular abnormalities such as cotton-wool spots and intraretinal hemorrhages. Most of the entities that cause choroidal vascular abnormalities affect the circulation from the arterioles to the choriocapillaris. On rare occasions, choroidal blood flow abnormalities may be related to venous outflow problems. Diagnosis of choroidal blood flow abnormalities often requires angiography with both fluorescein and indocyanine green (Fig 6-2).

One of the most commonly seen groups of diseases that lead to choroidal vascular compromise are those that acutely cause severely elevated blood pressure, such as malignant hypertension or eclampsia. In addition to retinal abnormalities, patients with these diseases commonly develop serous detachment of the retina associated with areas of yellow placoid discoloration of the RPE (Fig 6-3). The perfusion abnormalities may range from focal infarction of the choriocapillaris to fibrinoid necrosis of larger arterioles. Although the choroid has a rich circulation, the blood flow occurs in a segmental fashion such that there is very little collateral flow after a focal occlusion. Resolution of smaller infarcts produces small patches of atrophy and pigmentary abnormalities called Elschnig spots. Linear aggregations of these spots are called Siegrist streaks.

Inflammatory conditions, chiefly various types of arteritis, may affect the choroidal circulation as well. Giant cell arteritis may cause occlusion of one or more short posterior ciliary arteries, leading to broad areas of choroidal nonperfusion (Fig 6-4). Patients with this condition may have concurrent central retinal artery occlusion that dominates the clinical picture. Wegener's granulomatosis is a disorder characterized by necrotizing granulomatous lesions of the upper and lower respiratory tracts, glomerulonephritis, and generalized focal necrotizing vasculitis. Ocular manifestations occur in 30%–50% of patients and may include retinal vascular occlusion, choroidal vascular occlusion, or both (Fig 6-5).

An embolic phenomenon, particularly microemboli, may occur in a variety of diseases. In these entities, the choroidal circulation appears to be more affected than is the retinal circulation. Because of the rapid deceleration of the blood flow and the larger volumetric flow within the choroid, platelet emboli may be more likely to become lodged there. Thrombotic thrombocytopenic purpura causes a classic pentad of findings: microangiopathic hemolytic anemia, thrombocytopenia, fever, and neurologic and renal dysfunction. Patients with this condition may also have multifocal yellow placoid areas and associated serous detachment of the retina. A similar fundus picture may occur in patients with disseminated intravascular coagulation, where consumption of coagulation

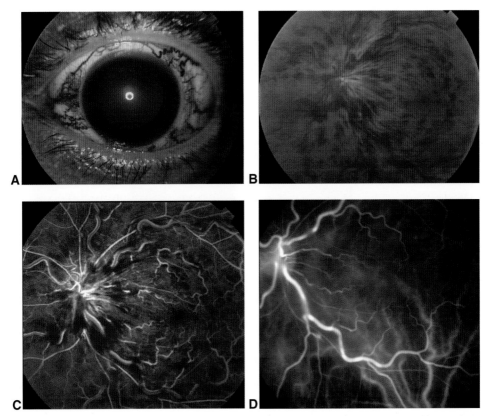

Figure 6-2 A, The left eye of this patient was proptotic and had dilated episcleral vessels. **B,** Color fundus photograph of the left eye shows a swollen optic nerve head, dilated and tortuous veins, and intraretinal hemorrhages. **C,** Fluorescein angiography of the left eye shows swelling of the optic nerve, blocking of the background fluorescence from retinal hemorrhages and a global delay in venous filling. Note how some venous segments show laminar filling whereas others do not. **D,** Indocyanine green (ICG) angiography shows hypovascularity with dilation of the remaining choroidal veins. *(From Chung JE, Spaide RF, Warren FA. Dural arteriovenous malformation and superior ophthalmic vein occlusion. Retina. 2004;24:491–492.)*

proteins, involvement of cellular elements, and release of fibrin degradation products lead to hemorrhage from multiple sites and ischemia from microthrombi.

On rare occasion choroidal ischemia may result from iatrogenic reasons. Thermal laser photocoagulation and, rarely, photodynamic therapy has caused choroidal vascular occlusion with resultant segmental ischemia. Ocular compression related to cataract surgery has also caused choroidal ischemia in some patients.

Gaudric A, Coscas G, Bird AC. Choroidal ischemia. *Am J Ophthalmol.* 1982;94:489–498.

Iida T, Spaide RF, Kantor J. Retinal and choroidal arterial occlusion in Wegener's granulomatosis. *Am J Ophthalmol* 2002;133:151–152.

Kinyoun JL, Kalina RE. Visual loss from choroidal ischemia. *Am J Ophthalmol.* 1986;101:650–656.

Melton RC, Spaide, RF: Visual problems as a presenting sign for thrombotic thrombocytopenic purpura. *Retina.* 1996;16:78–80.

Spaide RF, Goldbaum M, Wong DWK, et al. Serous detachment of the retina. *Retina.* 2003;23:820–846.

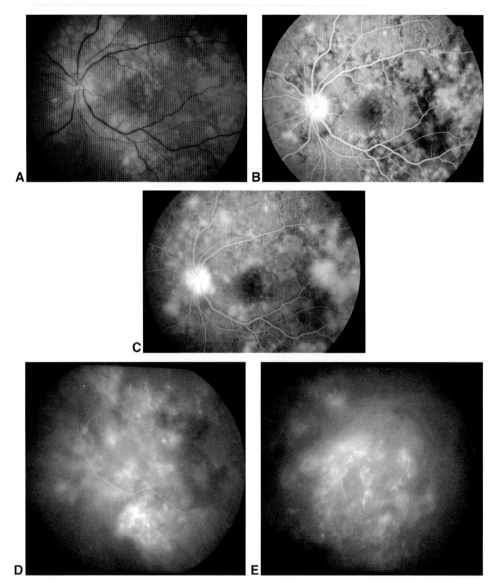

Figure 6-3 Preeclampsia with HELLP syndrome (hemolysis, elevated liver enzymes, and low platelet count). **A,** This patient had a serous detachment of the retina and multiple yellowish placoid areas at the level of the RPE and inner choroid. **B,** The early fluorescein angiographic frames showed reticular patterns of decreased choroidal perfusion bordering areas of hyper-fluorescence. Early leakage from the level of the RPE is evident and becomes more apparent in the later phases of the fluorescein angiogram **(C).** There is also staining of and leakage from the optic nerve. **D,** The ICG angiogram shows profound choroidal vascular filling defects alternating with areas of abnormal vessel leakage and staining, a finding rarely seen in ICG angiography. **E,** In the late phase, numerous arterioles show staining of their walls, indicative of severe vascular damage. *(From Spaide RF, Goldbaum M, Wong DWK, et al. Serous detachment of the retina. Retina. 2003;23:820–846.)*

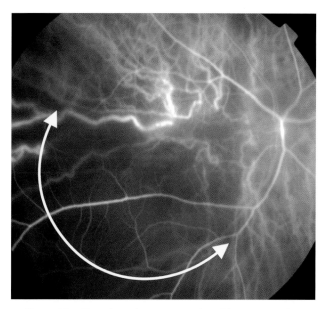

Figure 6-4 Giant cell arteritis. One day after severe visual loss secondary to arteritic anterior ischemic optic neuropathy, this patient underwent ICG angiography, which showed a segmental area of choroidal nonperfusion *(arrow)*. *(Photograph courtesy of Richard Spaide, MD.)*

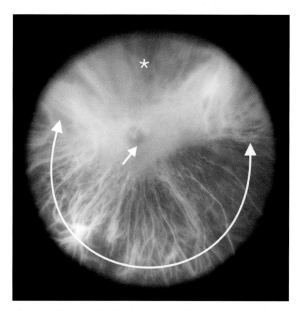

Figure 6-5 Wegener's granulomatosis. Early phase of wide-angle ICG angiography of the left eye revealed a widespread filling defect of the arterioles and choriocapillaris in the inferior fundus *(arcuate arrow)* and in a segmental area of the superior fundus *(*)*. Occlusion of the infratemporal retinal artery is also seen *(small arrow)*. *(From Iida T, Spaide RF, Kantor J. Retinal and choroidal arterial occlusion in Wegener's granulomatosis. Am J Ophthalmol. 2002;133:151–152. Copyright © 2002, with permission from Elsevier.)*

Choroidal Hemangioma

Isolated choroidal hemangiomas are reddish orange but well-circumscribed tumors of varying thickness that may be discovered during routine examination or discovered because of induced hyperopia or visual blurring related to induced hyperopia from the tumor or from the serous detachment induced by the tumor. Circumscribed hemangiomas transilluminate readily and have distinctive echographic and angiographic characteristics (Fig 6-6). Large choroidal vessels are visible early during indocyanine green angiography, and the tumefactions show a characteristic washed-out pattern in later phases of the angiogram. They are not usually associated with Sturge-Weber syndrome.

In contrast, the hemangioma seen with Sturge-Weber syndrome (encephalofacial cavernous hemangiomatosis) is diffuse and may be discovered through diagnosis or treatment of associated developmental glaucoma or amblyopia in children. The areas involved with the hemangioma have a typical "tomato catsup" appearance, where the underlying choroidal markings are not visible. The choroidal hemangiomas in Sturge-Weber may sometimes be overlooked because of their diffuse nature and because the hemangioma may blend imperceptibly into adjacent normal choroid. Also typical is the relatively constant finding of an ipsilateral facial nevus flammeus (port-wine stain) in patients with this syndrome.

Overlying retinal alteration, which presumably depends on the degree of choroidal exudation and RPE dysfunction, ranges from cystic change alone to frank neurosensory detachment. Retinal vascular leakage in the form of hard exudate is not commonly seen. Hemangiomas have been treated with a variety of modalities, including laser photocoagulation, cryopexy, external beam and plaque radiation, and photodynamic therapy. Each of these has had therapeutic success, with photodynamic therapy with verteporfin especially showing potential.

Barbazetto I, Schmidt-Erfurth U. Photodynamic therapy of choroidal hemangioma: two case reports. *Graefes Arch Clin Exp Ophthalmol.* 2000;283:214–221.

Madreperla SA, Hungerford JL, Plowman PN, et al. Choroidal hemangiomas: visual and anatomic results of treatment by photocoagulation or radiation therapy. *Ophthalmology.* 1997;104:1773–1779.

Uveal Effusion Syndrome

Net water movement across the vitreous cavity and posterior eye wall can be altered by abnormal uveoscleral aqueous outflow. This alteration may be caused by abnormal scleral composition or thickness, as in nanophthalmos, scleritis, idiopathic uveal effusion syndrome, and other states. Hyperopia frequently accompanies such settings, and glaucoma is also common. Choroidal and ciliary body thickening, RPE alterations, and exudative retinal detachment may occur transiently or permanently. Fluorescein angiography usually shows a leopard spot pattern of hypofluorescent spots and most, if not almost all, correctly diagnosed patients show no leakage (Fig 6-7)

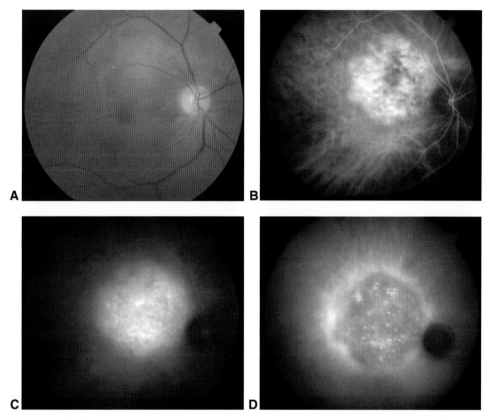

Figure 6-6 Choroidal hemangioma. **A,** The typical reddish orange elevation of a circumscribed choroidal hemangioma. **B,** Soon after ICG injection, the hypervascular nature of the hemangioma is revealed. **C,** There is hyperfluorescence of the tumefaction in the midphases of the angiogram, from a combination of dye within and leakage from the vessels of the hemangioma. **D,** In the late phase of the angiogram, the dye washes out of the lesion, leaving visible hyperfluorescent areas from leakage outside of the tumefaction. *(From Spaide RF, Goldbaum M, Wong DWK, et al. Serous detachment of the retina.* Retina. *2003;23:820–846.)*

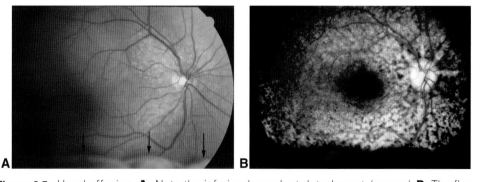

Figure 6-7 Uveal effusion. **A,** Note the inferior dependent detachment *(arrows).* **B,** The fluorescein angiogram shows a leopard spot pattern of hypofluorescent spots but no leaks. *(From Spaide RF, Goldbaum M, Wong DWK, et al. Serous detachment of the retina.* Retina. *2003;23:820–846.*

Posterior pole manifestations in the uveal effusion syndrome may be accompanied by ocular findings such as ciliochoroidal detachment and abnormal episcleral vessels. Visual function may fluctuate with the natural course of the disease. Although encouraging anatomic results can be obtained with scleral surgical approaches such as scleral windows, the visual results may be less rewarding because of chronic, irreversible changes. A high index of suspicion should be maintained for uveal effusion syndrome when examining a young patient with hyperopia who has been diagnosed with either central serous chorioretinopathy or a retinal detachment without an obvious retinal defect.

Brockhurst RJ. Nanophthalmos with uveal effusion: a new clinical entity. *Arch Ophthalmol.* 1975;93:1989–1999.

Johnson MW, Gass JD. Surgical management of the idiopathic uveal effusion syndrome. *Ophthalmology.* 1990;97:778–785.

CHAPTER 7

Focal and Diffuse Chorioretinal Inflammation

A variety of inflammatory disorders present with yellow-white lesions of the retina and choroid. The following descriptions highlight the clinical features, epidemiology, and potential treatments of various focal and diffuse chorioretinal inflammatory disorders. BCSC Section 9, *Intraocular Inflammation and Uveitis*, also discusses and illustrates many of the entities covered in this chapter.

Gass JD. *Stereoscopic Atlas of Macular Diseases: Diagnosis and Treatment.* 4th ed. St Louis: Mosby; 1997:601–736.

Guyer DR, Yannuzzi LA, Chang S, et al, eds. *Retina–Vitreous–Macula.* Philadelphia: Saunders; 1999:535–828.

Regillo CD, Brown GC, Flynn HW Jr, eds. *Vitreoretinal Disease: The Essentials.* New York: Thieme; 1999.

Noninfectious Chorioretinopathies

White Dot Syndromes

The term *white dot syndromes* has been generally used to describe the following diseases:

- acute posterior multifocal placoid pigment epitheliopathy (APMPPE)
- multiple evanescent white dot syndrome (MEWDS)
- serpiginous choroidopathy
- birdshot retinochoroidopathy
- multifocal choroiditis and panuveitis syndrome (MCP)
- punctate inner choroidopathy (PIC)

See Table 7-1. Other noninfectious chorioretinal inflammatory disorders are discussed later in this chapter.

Acute posterior multifocal placoid pigment epitheliopathy

APMPPE is an acute-onset bilateral inflammatory disease causing decreased vision in one eye first and often in the second eye days later. It presents with yellow, creamy, placoid lesions in the macula at the level of the RPE (Fig 7-1). APMPPE occurs in otherwise

Table 7-1 White Dot Syndromes

	Sex	Pathology	Laterality	Size	Morphology	Location	Color	A/C	VIT	FA	EOG	ERG	Prognosis	Etiology	Treatment
APMPPE	=	RPE Choroid	Bi	Large	Placoid	Posterior pole	White Scar	+	50%	Block Stain	↓	↓	80% Good	50% Viral	None
MEWDS	F>M (4:1)	RPE Retina	80% Uni	100–200 μm	Granular macula	Perifoveal	White	–	+	Early "Wreath"	↓	↓	Recover	50% Viral	None
Serpiginous	=	Choroid RPE	Bi	Large	Serpiginous	Disc Macula	Yellow Gravy	–	30%	Loss of chorio-capillaries	↓		Poor	?	None Immuno-suppressives
Birdshot	M:F (1:2)	Choroid RPE	Bi	100–300 μm	Ovoid	Posterior equator	Creamy, no pigment	30%	100%	Vessel Leak Mac/ON		↓	Chronic	S-Ag CMI	CSA
MCP	F>M (3:1)	Choroid RPE	80% Bi	50–350 μm	Punched out	Multifocal	Yellow pigment ring	52%	98%	Early Stain		↑↓	Poor	EBV?	Steroids Acyclovir?
PIC	F>M	Choroid RPE	Bi	50–100 μm	Discrete; well-circumscribed	Posterior pole	Yellow-white	–	–	Early Stain			May develop subretinal fibrosis	EBV?	Steroids?

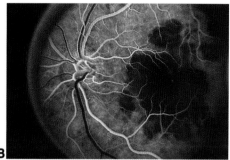

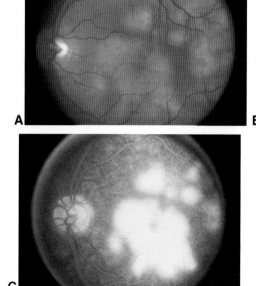

Figure 7-1 Acute posterior multifocal placoid pigment epitheliopathy (APMPPE). **A,** Multiple yellowish placoid lesions in the posterior pole. **B,** Early-phase angiogram demonstrates hypofluorescence from nonperfusion of the choriocapillaris or blocked fluorescence by the RPE lesions. **C,** Late-phase angiogram demonstrates hyperfluorescence in the areas involved. *(Photographs courtesy of J. Donald M. Gass, MD.)*

healthy young adults in the second to third decades of life, with no sex predilection. The etiology is unknown, but a viral prodrome occurs in about one third of patients.

Diagnosis is based on clinical history and ophthalmoscopic features. The fluorescein angiographic changes seen in the acute phase of the disease characteristically demonstrate blockage of fluorescence in the early frames, with even, diffuse late staining. Controversy exists concerning whether APMPPE is a result of primary disease of the pigment epithelium or is caused by obstruction of choroidal circulation with secondary pigment epithelial reaction. No evidence has shown that corticosteroids or any other medications are beneficial. Most patients start to experience improvement in the fundus appearance in 1–2 weeks. Visual acuity recovery occurs within weeks, and this disease has a generally good visual prognosis. In one series of 30 patients with over 5 years' follow-up, all but 2 of the eyes had 20/30 or better visual acuity. Despite the improvement in visual acuity, patients with APMPPE do continue to have self-reported complaints of visual dysfunction.

Several case reports have highlighted potential CNS vasculitic changes associated with APMPPE.

Comu S, Verstraeten T, Rinkoff JS, et al. Neurological manifestations of acute posterior multifocal placoid pigment epitheliopathy. *Stroke.* 1996;27:996–1001.

Gass, JDM. *Stereoscopic Atlas of Macular Diseases: Diagnosis and Treatment.* St Louis: Mosby; 1997: 668–675.

Multiple evanescent white dot syndrome

MEWDS is an acute-onset syndrome characterized by multiple small gray-white dots at the level of the deep retina/RPE in the posterior pole (Fig 7-2). Some patients also develop

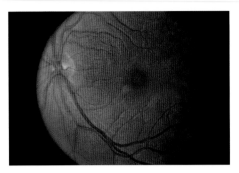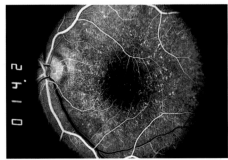

Figure 7-2 Multiple evanescent white dot syndrome (MEWDS). Note the presence of foveal granularity in addition to the white dots noted in the deep retina. *(Photographs courtesy of Tom S. Chang, MD.)*

an unusual foveal granularity that is nearly pathognomic of this condition that consists of tiny yellow-orange dots at the level of the RPE (Fig 7-2B). Vitritis may or may not be appreciated. Patients typically complain of a unilateral (80%) decrease in visual acuity. MEWDS occurs in otherwise healthy individuals with myopia in the second to fifth decades, more often in women than in men. The etiology is unknown, but a viral prodrome occurs in about 50% of patients.

Diagnosis is based on clinical history and ophthalmoscopic features. Fluorescein angiography demonstrates that each white dot comprises multiple punctate hyperfluorescent spots in a wreathlike cluster, with late staining. Indocyanine green (ICG) angiography demonstrates multiple hypofluorescent dots and hypofluorescence around the optic nerve. Enlargement of the physiologic blind spot may be seen on visual field testing, and a transient afferent pupillary defect is sometimes seen. Decreased a-wave amplitudes may be demonstrated on electroretinogram (ERG) testing. Treatment is not required because most patients start to experience improvement in the fundus appearance in 2–6 weeks, and central visual recovery usually follows. Rarely, MEWDS can be recurrent or bilateral or have persistent visual field defects.

A related entity is referred to as *idiopathic enlargement of the blind spot syndrome (IEBSS)*. This condition shares demographic features with MEWDS, with the noted absence of retinal lesions.

Jampol LM, Sieving PA, Pugh D. Multiple evanescent white dot syndrome. I. Clinical findings. *Arch Ophthalmol.* 1984;102:671–674.

Serpiginous choroidopathy (geographic choroiditis, helicoid peripapillary choroidopathy)

Serpiginous choroidopathy, a recurrent inflammatory disease of the choroid, causes a serpiginous (pseudopodial) or geographic (maplike) pattern of scars in the posterior fundus (Fig 7-3). Patients complain of decreased visual acuity and central or paracentral scotomata. Acute-onset lesions have a geographic zone of gray-yellow discoloration of the RPE, which spreads centrifugally outward from the optic disc and macula in a jigsawlike pattern. These lesions are hypofluorescent in the early phases but stain in the later phases on angiography and may appear similar to the lesions of APMPPE. Unlike APMPPE, however, serpiginous choroidopathy is a chronic and recurrent disease. As

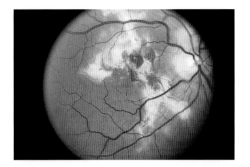
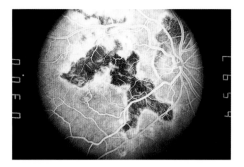

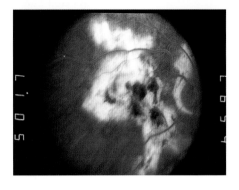

Figure 7-3 Serpiginous choroidopathy. *(Photographs courtesy of Tom S. Chang, MD.)*

active areas become atrophic over weeks to months, new lesions can occur elsewhere or contiguously with atrophic lesions. Dense scotomata corresponding to involved areas develop in all patients, and the second eye may be affected months or years later. Rarely, choroidal neovascularization may develop at the margin of an area of chorioretinal atrophy.

Treatment with immunosuppressive agents, systemic steroids, or acyclovir has been attempted, but the results of this treatment are generally poor. More potent immunosuppressive treatment with cyclosporine, azathioprine, and prednisone appears to halt disease activity in some patients. When lesions spread to involve the center of the macula, visual acuity remains at a very low level.

Hooper PL, Kaplan HJ. Triple agent immunosuppression in serpiginous choroiditis. *Ophthalmology.* 1991;98:944–952.

Tom D, Yannuzzi LA. Serpiginous choroiditis. In: Guyer DR, Yannuzzi LA, Chang S, et al, eds. *Retina–Vitreous–Macula.* Philadelphia: Saunders; 1999:553–564.

Birdshot retinochoroidopathy

Birdshot retinochoroidopathy, or *vitiliginous chorioretinitis,* occurs in patients in the fourth to sixth decades. Women are affected more often than men. Patients present with symptoms of floaters, blurred vision, and peripheral photopsia. Nyctalopia and loss of color vision may occur later. Examination reveals vitritis (100%), a variable degree of disc edema and vascular sheathing, and characteristic yellow ovoid "birdshot" chorioretinal lesions most numerous in the nasal retina (Fig 7-4). The ERG is reduced or extinguished. The fluorescein angiogram is often unremarkable, and the choroidal lesions appear more visible on ophthalmoscopy. One interesting fluorescein angiographic phe-

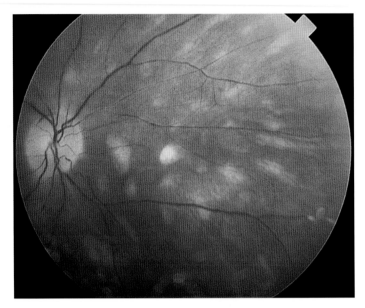

Figure 7-4 Birdshot retinochoroidopathy. *(Photograph courtesy of Tom S. Chang, MD.)*

nomenon that is seen in patients with this condition is the presence of "quench-ing,"whereby dye appears to disappear rapidly from the retinal circulation. Approximately 90% of patients are HLA-A29 positive. BCSC Section 9, *Intraocular Inflammation and Uveitis,* discusses the human leukocyte antigens in detail.

Vision loss may be caused by optic atrophy, cystoid macular edema (CME), or mac-ular choroidal neovascularization (CNV). The disease is chronic, bilateral, and prone to recurrent episodes of inflammation. In advanced cases, treatment may include periocular or systemic steroids or immunosuppressants. Visual acuity outcomes depend on the nature and extent of the disc and macular disease.

Gasch AT, Smith JA, Whitcup SM. Birdshot retinochoroidopathy. *Br J Ophthalmol.* 1999;83:241–249.

Gass JDM. *Stereoscopic Atlas of Macular Disease: Diagnosis and Treatment.* 4th ed. St. Louis: Mosby; 1997: 710–713.

Multifocal choroiditis and panuveitis syndrome

MCP is a bilateral disease that predominantly affects women between the second and sixth decades. Symptoms include decreased vision, floaters, photopsia, and visual field defects such as an enlarged blind spot. Patients present with a bilateral vitritis and mul-tifocal choroiditis (Fig 7-5). The multiple yellow choroidal lesions later evolve into cho-rioretinal scars similar to the "punched-out" lesions seen in ocular histoplasmosis (OHS) (see Chapter 4). However, unlike patients with OHS, patients with MCP have some degree of vitritis and often mild anterior segment inflammation. Topical, periocular, and sys-temic corticosteroids may help to reduce the choroidal and vitreous inflammation, whereas more potent immunosuppression may be effective for lesions threatening fixa-tion. Subfoveal CNV and CME may be late complications. In spite of treatment with corticosteroids, visual outcomes are often poor.

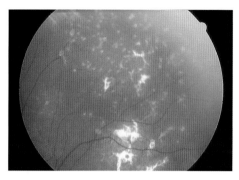 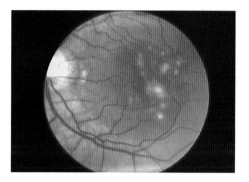

Figure 7-5 Multifocal choroiditis with subretinal fibrosis. *(Photograph courtesy of Janet L. Davis, MD.)*

Figure 7-6 Punctate inner choroidopathy.

Dreyer RF, Gass JD. Multifocal choroiditis and panuveitis: a syndrome that mimics ocular histoplasmosis. *Arch Ophthalmol.* 1984;102:1776–1784.

Michel SS, Ekong A, Baltatzis S, et al. Multifocal choroiditis and panuveitis: immunomodulatory therapy. *Ophthalmology.* 2002;109:378–383.

Punctate inner choroidopathy

PIC tends to occur in young patients with myopia. More than 90% of these patients are women. Patients present with symptoms of bilateral loss of central visual acuity, as well as prominent photopsia and scotomata. Fundus examination during the acute phase shows small (100–300 μm) round yellow lesions at the level of the RPE or inner choroid that may coalesce and form a serous retinal detachment (Fig 7-6). Scotomata usually correspond to the location of these lesions. Mild optic disc edema may be visible, but iritis and vitritis are not seen. The lesions fill and stain during the late phase of fluorescein angiography, especially if a serous detachment is present. Lesions later become atrophic yellow-white scars, which may become pigmented or enlarge over time. These scars appear very similar to those seen in OHS and multifocal choroiditis.

Oral and regional corticosteroids have been used without adverse effect in patients with PIC, but spontaneous improvement usually occurs without treatment. The prognosis for visual acuity is generally good, and the condition seems not to recur. However, one third of eyes develop CNV within a site of old scarring; some of the CNV involutes spontaneously. Photopsia may persist for years.

Watzke RC, Packer AJ, Folk JC, et al. Punctate inner choroidopathy. *Am J Ophthalmol.* 1984;98:572–584.

Other Noninfectious Choroidopathies

Acute zonal occult outer retinopathy

Acute zonal occult outer retinopathy (AZOOR), a presumed inflammatory disorder, damages broad zones of the outer retina in one eye or both eyes. AZOOR usually occurs in young women, with an acute onset in one eye. Initial symptoms include photopsia, visual field loss, and sometimes an enlarged blind spot. The fundi may appear normal on initial presentation, or mild vitritis may be seen (Fig 7-7). Angiography may show retinal and optic nerve head capillary leakage, especially in patients with evidence of vitritis. The ERG often shows decreased rod and cone amplitudes under both photopic and scotopic conditions. Visual field testing may show scotomata, which can enlarge over weeks or months.

Some patients recover from AZOOR, whereas others have persistent large visual field defects. Permanent visual field loss is often associated with late development of fundus changes. Depigmentation of large zones of RPE usually corresponds with scotomata; narrowed retinal vessels may be seen within these areas. The late fundus appearance in some patients may resemble cancer-associated retinopathy or retinitis pigmentosa. Most patients retain good vision in at least one eye. No treatment has any proven benefit.

Gass JD. Acute zonal occult outer retinopathy. Donders Lecture: The Netherlands Ophthalmological Society, Maastricht, Holland, June 19, 1992. *J Clin Neuroophthalmol.* 1993;13:79–97.

Gass JD, Agarwal A, Scott IU. Acute zonal occult outer retinopathy: a long-term follow-up study. *Am J Ophthalmol.* 2002;134:329–339.

Sarcoid panuveitis

Posterior segment manifestations of sarcoidosis are numerous and, in some cases, nonspecific. They can include intermediate uveitis with snowbank formation; vitritis with characteristic snowballs in the inferior periphery; retinal periphlebitis, specifically with formation of candlewax drippings; multifocal choroiditis; and optic nerve swelling (Fig 7-8).

See BCSC Section 9, *Intraocular Inflammation and Uveitis,* for workup and treatment of sarcoidosis.

Jabs DA, Johns CJ. Ocular involvement in chronic sarcoidosis. *Am J Ophthalmol.* 1986;102:297–301.

Moorthy RS, Rao NA. Noninfectious chorioretinal inflammatory conditions. In: Regillo CD, Brown GC, Flynn HW Jr, eds. *Vitreoretinal Disease: The Essentials.* New York: Thieme; 1999:415–438.

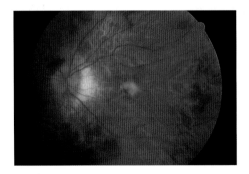 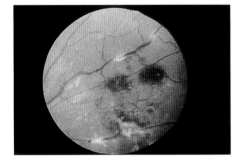

Figure 7-7 Acute zonal occult outer retinopathy. *(Photograph courtesy of J. Donald M. Gass, MD.)*

Figure 7-8 Sarcoidosis, retinal vascular sheathing.

Behçet syndrome

Behçet syndrome, a chronic recurrent systemic disease, consists of a classic triad of aphthous oral ulcers, genital ulcers, and acute iritis with hypopyon. Other systemic manifestations include arthritis, epididymitis, and intestinal ulcers. Behçet syndrome produces an occlusive vasculitis in the skin, circulatory system, and central nervous system, including the eyes. It tends to affect men more than women and is particularly common in Japan, Southeast Asia, the Middle East, and the Mediterranean region. The etiology is unknown, but it is associated with HLA-B5101.

Anterior segment involvement is more common and includes severe uveitis, often with hypopyon formation. Posterior segment involvement may include an occlusive retinal vasculitis, intraretinal hemorrhages, macular edema, focal areas of retinal necrosis, ischemic optic neuropathy, and marked vitritis. Treatment of retinal disease is with corticosteroids and, in severe cases, with immunosuppressants such as cyclosporine. Despite treatment, the visual prognosis is often poor.

James DG, Spiteri MA. Behçet's disease. *Ophthalmology*. 1982;89:1279–1284.

Michelson JB, Friedlaender MH. Behçet's disease. *Int Ophthalmol Clin*. 1990;30:271–278.

Vogt-Koyanagi-Harada syndrome

Vogt-Koyanagi-Harada syndrome (VKH) is a systemic inflammatory disorder that predominantly affects individuals with darker skin pigmentation and shows a slight female predilection. It is a bilateral granulomatous panuveitis associated with dermatologic and neurologic manifestations. Posterior segment findings are characterized by yellow-white exudates at the level of the RPE with serous retinal detachment in the posterior pole during active inflammation phases. Isolated posterior segment findings in the absence of systemic involvement is frequently referred to as *Harada's disease*. An anterior chamber reaction and significant vitritis usually occur. In the late stages of the disease, diffuse pigmentary changes in the RPE layer can lead to atrophy, giving the choroid a "sunset-glow" appearance. Punched-out atrophic lesions can sometimes be seen in the periphery. HLA-DRB*0405 has a strong association with VKH syndrome in Japanese patients.

Fluorescein angiography is helpful in the diagnosis of VKH syndrome by revealing multiple punctate hyperfluorescent dots, with leakage of dye into the subretinal space. Echography may be useful in demonstrating diffuse choroidal thickening in the acute phase. Specific systemic findings include vitiligo, alopecia, poliosis, and meningeal signs. The course is occasionally recurrent, but these episodes respond well to systemic steroids. The visual prognosis with treatment is generally good, but visual outcomes may be adversely influenced by secondary glaucoma, subfoveal CNV, complicated cataract, and phthisis bulbi.

Moorthy RS, Inomata H, Rao NA. The Vogt-Koyanagi-Harada syndrome. *Surv Ophthalmol*. 1995;39:265–292.

Rubsamen PE, Gass JD. Vogt-Koyanagi-Harada syndrome: clinical course, therapy, and long-term outcome. *Arch Ophthalmol*. 1991;109:682–687.

Pars planitis

Pars planitis is a specific idiopathic clinical entity characterized by a bilateral intermediate uveitis typically seen in young adults and children. Patients may present with complaints of decreased vision and/or floaters, usually because there are few anterior uveitic symptoms, such as red eye, pain, or photophobia. Ocular manifestions include inflammatory exudates on the inferior pars plana ("snowbanking"), aggregates of vitreous cells ("snowballs"), and diffuse vitritis. There may be associated retinal phlebitis, CME, and optic nerve head swelling. Fluorescein angiography may show diffuse peripheral venular leakage and late staining. Peripheral neovascularization may give rise to vitreous hemorrhage. Macular epiretinal membranes and retinal detachment may also occur. The disease may be chronic or self-limited, and exacerbations may respond to topical or sub-Tenon's administration of steroids. The visual prognosis is usually good but may be limited by CME, posterior subcapsular cataract, or band keratopathy. Recalcitrant uveitis can be treated with transscleral cryopexy applied to the snowbanks. Pars plana vitrectomy may be considered for serious complications of the disease, including retinal detachment, uveitis, cataracts, and severe CME.

Hooper PL. Pars planitis. *Focal Points: Clinical Modules for Ophthalmologists.* San Francisco: American Academy of Ophthalmology. 1993, module 11:9–11.

Malinowski SM, Pulido JS, Folk JC. Long-term visual outcome and complications associated with pars planitis. *Ophthalmology.* 1993;100:818–825.

Intraocular lymphoma

Intraocular lymphoma was previously referred to as *reticulum cell sarcoma, histiocytic lymphoma,* and *non-Hodgkin lymphoma of the CNS.* Intraocular lymphoma typically presents in the sixth or seventh decades of life, with bilateral iritis, vitritis, retinal vasculitis, and creamy yellow-appearing sub–retinal pigment epithelial infiltrates (Fig 7-9) and may be mistaken for uveitis. The diagnosis should be suspected if large, solid confluent RPE detachments are present. These solid RPE detachments can spontaneously involute and are thought to be distinctive for the diagnosis of intraocular lymphoma. Disc edema can be seen. The diagnosis is confirmed with pars plana vitrectomy and cytologic examination

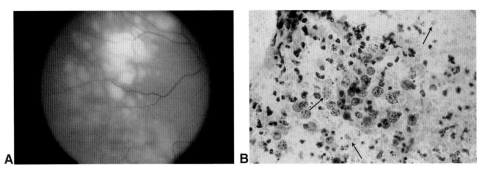

Figure 7-9 A, Sub–retinal pigment epithelial infiltrates in a patient with intraocular lymphoma. **B,** Cytologic preparation of vitreous cells in a patient with lymphoma. There are many atypical cells with large nuclei and multiple nucleoli. Cell ghosts *(arrows)* are also present. *(Photographs courtesy of David J. Wilson, MD.)*

of the specimen by an experienced cytopathologist. Cytologic examination is more important in establishing the diagnosis than are immunologic markers. This condition should be suspected in any elderly patient with chronic nonresponsive uveitis. Systemic evaluation for CNS involvement is required. Despite treatment with chemotherapy and/or radiation, the prognosis is poor, with a low 5-year survival rate. BCSC Section 4, *Ophthalmic Pathology and Intraocular Tumors,* discusses this condition in greater depth.

Gass JDM. *Stereoscopic Atlas of Macular Disease: Diagnosis and Treatment.* 4th ed. St Louis: Mosby; 1997:880–889.

Gill MK, Jampol LM. Variations in the presentation of primary introcular lymphoma: case reports and a review. *Surv Ophthalmol.* 2001;45:463–471.

Valluri S, Moorthy RS, Khan A, et al. Combination treatment of intraocular lymphoma. *Retina.* 1995;15:125–129.

Infectious Chorioretinopathies

The following is a brief description of some of the disease entities that may result in decreased vision from an infectious chorioretinopathy.

Endogenous Bacterial Endophthalmitis

Endogenous bacterial endophthalmitis typically begins as a focal or multifocal chorioretinal lesion that spreads into the vitreous (Fig 7-10). Initially, the lesions are flat or slightly elevated chorioretinal infiltrates. A wide range of bacteria can lead to endogenous bacterial endophthalmitis, including: *Streptococcus* spp, *Staphylococcus aureus, Serratia,* and *Bacillus.*

Using medical consultation, the extraocular source of infection should be determined and appropriately treated with systemic therapy. Endocarditis and infections of the gastrointestinal or urinary tract are the most commonly associated etiologies. Medical evaluation usually includes cultures of the vitreous and the extraocular sites. Treatment commonly includes intravenous antibiotics and also intravitreal antibiotics when significant vitreous involvement is present.

Binder MI, Chua J, Kaiser PK, et al. Endogenous endophthalmitis: an 18-year review of culture-positive cases at a tertiary care center. *Medicine (Baltimore).* 2003;82:97–105.

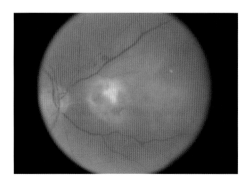

Figure 7-10 Focal endogenous bacterial endophthalmitis. *(Photograph courtesy of Janet L. Davis, MD.)*

Davis JL. Infectious chorioretinal inflammatory conditions. In: Regillo CD, Brown GC, Flynn HW Jr, eds. *Vitreoretinal Disease: The Essentials.* New York: Thieme; 1999:393–415.

Okada AA, Johnson RP, Liles WC, et al. Endogenous bacterial endophthalmitis: report of a ten-year retrospective study. *Ophthalmology.* 1994;101:832–838.

Equi RA, Green WR. Endogenous *Serratia marcescens* endophthalmitis with dark hypopyon: case report and review. *Surv Ophthalmol.* 2001;46:259–268.

Tuberculosis

Mycobacterium tuberculosis may hematogenously disseminate to the eye; the choroid is the most common initial site of intraocular tuberculosis. Tuberculous panophthalmitis was more common in the era before effective antimycobacterial therapy was available, but it was still a rare disease. Ocular involvement was usually associated with disseminated disease and tended to be severe.

An upsurge of mycobacterial infection has occurred in the era of AIDS. The patient may present with decreased vision from macular involvement or vitritis. Posterior segment examination shows choroidal tubercles, which are single or multiple polymorphic yellow-white lesions with indistinct borders. The tubercles are initially flat, one or several disc diameters in size, and exhibit variable amounts of pigmentation. Vitritis, papillitis, and an overlying serous retinal detachment may be seen with the choroidal lesions (Fig 7-11).

Treatment of ocular tuberculosis is similar to that of the pulmonary disease. A 4-drug regimen of isoniazid, rifampin, pyrazinamide, and either streptomycin or ethambutol is recommended by the Centers for Disease Control. Treatment should be coordinated with a medical specialist.

Blodi BA, Johnson MW, McLeish WM, et al. Presumed choroidal tuberculosis in a human immunodeficiency virus infected host. *Am J Ophthalmol.* 1989;108:605–607.

Recillas-Gispert C, Ortega-Larrocea G, Arellanes-Garcia L, et al. Chorioretinitis secondary to *Mycobacterium tuberculosis* in acquired immune deficiency syndrome. *Retina.* 1997;17:437–439.

Cat-scratch Disease

Cat-scratch disease is characterized by regional lymphadenopathy, fever, and malaise that appear 2 weeks after a cat scratch. Parinaud oculoglandular syndrome (conjunctival inflammation with preauricular adenopathy) may be seen in about 7% of patients with

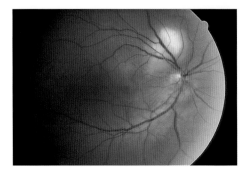

Figure 7-11 A choroidal granuloma caused by tuberculosis is located superior to the optic nerve. *(Photograph courtesy of Janet L. Davis, MD.)*

cat-scratch disease. *Bartonella henselae* has been isolated as the etiologic agent in the disease (Fig 7-12). *B henselae* has also been isolated from patients who present with fundus findings identical to Leber stellate neuroretinitis. Occasionally, branch retinal artery occlusions in the setting of retinal vasculitis with focal retinitis can be seen in patients with active cat-scratch disease. Serologic testing for *B henselae* is now available. Treatment with doxycycline (100 mg bid) or ciprofloxacin (750 mg bid) appears to be effective.

Brazis PW, Stokes HR, Ervin FR. Optic neuritis in cat scratch disease. *J Clin Neuroophthalmol.* 1986;6:172–174.

Cohen SM, Davis JL, Gass DM. Branch retinal arterial occlusions in multifocal retinitis with optic nerve edema. *Arch Ophthalmol.* 1995;113:1271–1276.

Freund KB. Leber's idiopathic stellate neuroretinitis. In: Guyer DR, Yannuzzi LA, Chang S, et al, eds. *Retina-Vitreous-Macula.* Philadelphia: Saunders; 1999:885–888.

Necrotizing Herpetic Retinitis

Necrotizing herpetic retinitis was formerly called *acute retinal necrosis (ARN)* before herpes simplex and herpes zoster viruses were identified as the causative agents. Typically, a healthy patient presents with symptoms of ocular pain and reduced vision. Iritis, episcleritis, or vitritis may be seen on the initial examination. The disease may be bilateral at onset in 20% of patients; in patients without bilateral onset, subsequent involvement of the fellow eye is very common. In immunocompromised patients, a similar disease, progressive outer retinal necrosis (PORN) syndrome, can manifest. PORN is distinguished from necrotizing herpetic retinitis by its more rapid progression and its characteristic sparing of the retinal vessels.

Large areas of retinal whitening with necrosis are seen more often in the peripheral retina (Fig 7-13). These areas coalesce and spread centripetally. Optic neuritis, arteriolitis, and vascular occlusions are associated findings. As the retinal opacification clears, large retinal breaks in the necrotic retina may occur, and the risk of retinal detachment is high.

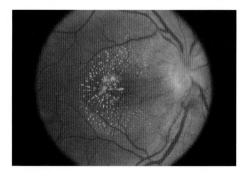

Figure 7-12 Cat-scratch disease *(Bartonella henselae). (Photograph courtesy of George Alexandrakis, MD.)*

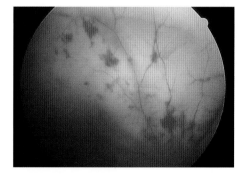

Figure 7-13 Necrotizing herpetic retinitis (acute retinal necrosis) with intraretinal hemorrhage and full-thickness opacification of the retina. *(Photograph courtesy of Janet L. Davis, MD.)*

The incidence of bilaterality and retinal detachment may be higher in AIDS patients. In immunocompetent patients, initial therapy involves IV acyclovir (800 mg 5 times daily) or oral famciclovir (Famvir; 500 mg tid). Treatment is continued until clinical evidence of retinitis resolution is observed. Oral acyclovir (800 mg 5 times a day for 3 months) may decrease the risk of infection of the second eye. In immunocompetent patients who do not respond to systemic therapy, intravitreal injections of foscarnet and ganciclovir may be of benefit. The risk of retinal detachment appears to be highest 8–12 weeks after the onset of the disease. Prophylactic use of laser photocoagulation to demarcate the borders of retinal necrosis may decrease the risk of retinal detachment.

Davis JL. Infectious chorioretinal inflammatory conditions. In: Regillo CD, Brown GC, Flynn HW Jr, eds. *Vitreoretinal Disease: The Essentials.* New York: Thieme; 1999:399–401.

Luu KK, Scott IU, Chaudhry NA, et al. Intravitreal antiviral injections as adjunctive therapy in the management of immunocompetent patients with necrotizing herpetic retinopathy. *Am J Ophthalmol.* 2000;129:811–813.

Scott IU, Luu KM, Davis JL. Intravitreal antivirals in the management of patients with acquired immunodeficiency syndrome with progressive outer retinal necrosis. *Arch Ophthalmol.* 2002;120:1219–1222.

Toxoplasmic Chorioretinitis

Toxoplasmic chorioretinitis is probably the most common cause of posterior segment infection worldwide. *Toxoplasma gondii* is an obligate, intracellular parasitic protozoon that causes a necrotizing chorioretinitis. Most cases of toxoplasmosis are now assumed to be acquired.

Unilateral decrease in visual acuity is the most common symptom of toxoplasmosis. A unifocal area of acute-onset inflammation adjacent to an old chorioretinal scar is virtually pathognomonic for toxoplasmic chorioretinitis (Fig 7-14). Focal condensation

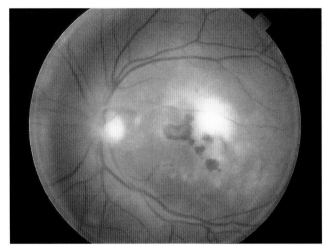

Figure 7-14 Active toxoplasmic chorioretinitis adjacent to an area of chorioretinal scarring from previous inflammation. *(Photograph courtesy of Carl D. Regillo, MD.)*

of vitreous and inflammatory cells may be seen overlying the pale yellow or gray-white raised lesion in the posterior pole. Perivasculitis and arteriolar narrowing may be seen near the inflamed area.

In immunocompromised patients (eg, HIV-positive, elderly) toxoplasmic chorioretinitis can clinically resemble necrotizing herpetic retinitis.

Neuroimaging is warranted in AIDS patients presenting with these findings because intracranial toxoplasmic lesions have been reported in up to 29% of these patients who have toxoplasmic chorioretinitis. Small extramacular lesions may be observed without treatment. Sight-threatening lesions are treated for 5–6 weeks with pyrimethamine, sulfadiazine, and folinic acid (Table 7-2). Prednisone in low doses of 30–40 mg for 2–3 weeks can be useful to reduce macular or optic nerve inflammation, but it should always be used in conjunction with antibiotics. Bactrim and clindamycin can also be employed. Folinic acid protects against the decrease in platelets and white blood cells induced by pyrimethamine. AIDS patients require chronic suppressive treatment.

Davis JL. Infectious chorioretinal inflammatory conditions. In: Regillo CD, Brown GC, Flynn HW Jr, eds. *Vitreoretinal Disease: The Essentials*. New York: Thieme; 1999:401–404.

Johnson MW, Greven CM, Jaffe GJ, et al. Atypical, severe toxoplasmic retinochoroiditis in elderly patients. *Ophthalmology*. 1997;104:48–57.

Endogenous Yeast (*Candida*) Endophthalmitis

Endogenous yeast endophthalmitis is most often caused by *Candida* spp. Affected patients frequently have a history of indwelling catheters, chronic antibiotic use, abdominal surgery, or immunosuppression. They also frequently have a history of hyperalimentation, recent abdominal surgery, and/or diabetes mellitus. The initial intraocular inflammation is usually mild to moderate, and yellow-white choroidal lesions may be single or multiple. Subretinal infiltrates may coalesce into a mushroom-shaped white nodule that projects through the retina into the vitreous (Fig 7-15).

The diagnosis is usually made through the clinical history and characteristic features in the posterior segment. Systemic and intraocular cultures help to confirm the clinical diagnosis. The ophthalmologist should usually seek infectious disease consultation to evaluate the patient for systemic disease and to assist with treatment planning. If the

Table 7-2 Standard Therapy for Ocular Toxoplasmosis: Drugs and Dosage

Pyrimethamine	75–100 mg loading dose (2 days) 25–50 mg daily until the lesion is healed (usually 4–6 weeks)
Sulfadiazine	2.0–4.0 g loading dose (2 days) 0.5–1.0 g qid until the lesion is healed (usually 4–6 weeks)
Folinic Acid	5 mg 3 times a week during pyrimethamine therapy
Prednisone	0.5–1 mg/kg daily for 3–6 weeks (starting at the third day) Taper off according to clinical response Weekly assays of white blood cells and platelets

(Modified with permission from Dodds. EM. Ocular toxoplasmosis: clinical presentations, diagnosis, and therapy. *Focal Points: Clinical Modules for Ophthalmologists*. San Francisco: American Academy of Ophthalmology; 1999, module 10.)

Figure 7-15 Endogenous yeast *(Candida)* endophthalmitis. **A,** Vitreous infiltrates in a "string of pearls" configuration. **B,** Endogenous endophthalmitis before treatment. **C,** Endogenous endophthalmitis resolved after treatment with vitrectomy and intravitreal amphotericin B. *(Photographs courtesy of Harry W. Flynn, Jr, MD.)*

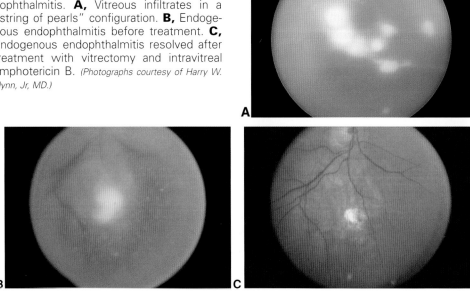

macula is not involved, visual prognosis after treatment is generally good. Focal chorioretinal lesions are often successfully treated with systemic medications. Intravenous amphotericin B does not penetrate well into the vitreous, but fluconazole does penetrate well and has fewer systemic side effects.

Intraocular cultures are best obtained by pars plana vitrectomy, as it is difficult to culture the localized vitreous clusters of fungus from a random vitreous tap. After the completion of the vitrectomy, intravitreal amphotericin B is usually injected, but successful treatment has been reported by vitrectomy alone in conjunction with systemic fluconazole.

Davis JL. Infectious chorioretinal inflammatory conditions. In: Regillo CD, Brown GC, Flynn HW Jr, eds. *Vitreoretinal Disease: The Essentials.* New York: Thieme; 1999:408–409.

Essman TF, Flynn HW Jr, Smiddy WE, et al. Treatment outcomes in a 10-year study of endogenous fungal endophthalmitis. *Ophthalmic Surg Lasers.* 1997;28:185–194.

Rao NA, Hidayat AA. Endogenous mycotic endophthalmitis: variations in clinical and histopathologic changes in candidiasis compared with aspergillosis. *Am J Ophthalmol.* 2001;132:244–251.

Endogenous Mold *(Aspergillus)* Endophthalmitis

Endogenous mold endophthalmitis is a rare but often devastating infection that occurs in immunosuppressed patients and intravenous drug users. It is reported most frequently as a cause of endogenous endophthalmitis after liver transplantation. Symptoms include the acute onset of ocular pain and visual loss. Intraocular inflammation is generally more severe than in *Candida* endophthalmitis, and the chorioretinal lesion seen with *Aspergillus* is usually larger and progresses rapidly. A characteristic large yellow infiltrate is often present in or near the macula. The inflammatory exudate may layer to form a subretinal or subhyaloidal hypopyon. Vitritis, vasculitis, and retinal necrosis are often associated.

Pars plana vitrectomy with diagnostic cultures and injection of intravitreal amphotericin B are usually recommended, especially if vitritis is present. Visual acuity outcomes are frequently poor as a result of the associated macular lesion (Fig 7-16).

Hunt KE, Glasgow BJ. *Aspergillus* endophthalmitis: an unrecognized endemic disease in orthotopic liver transplantation. *Ophthalmology.* 1996;103:757–767.

Weishaar PD, Flynn HW Jr, Murray TG, et al. Endogenous *Aspergillus* endophthalmitis: clinical features and treatment outcomes. *Ophthalmology.* 1998;105:57–65.

Diffuse Unilateral Subacute Neuroretinitis

Diffuse unilateral subacute neuroretinitis (DUSN) is a rare condition that occurs in otherwise healthy, often young, patients and is due to the presence of a subretinal nematode. Prompt diagnosis and treatment of the condition can help prevent visual loss. The clinical findings in this disease can be divided into acute and end-stage manifestations. In the acute phase, patients often present with decreased visual acuity, vitritis, papillitis, and crops of gray-white or yellow-white outer retinal lesions (Fig 7-17). The clustering

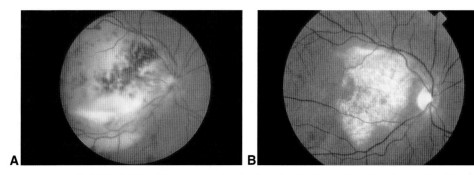

Figure 7-16 **A,** Mild vitritis, diffuse macular chorioretinal lesion with subretinal and subhyaloid hypopyon, intraretinal hemorrhage, and papillitis. **B,** Same eye 2 months after treatment shows macular scar, preserved overlying retinal vessels, temporal disc pallor. Final visual acuity was 20/400. *(Reproduced with permission from Weishaar PD, Flynn HW Jr, Murray TG, et al. Endogenous Aspergillus endophthalmitis. Ophthalmology. 1998;105:60.)*

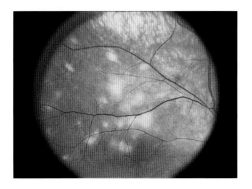

Figure 7-17 Diffuse unilateral subacute neuroretinitis (DUSN). *(Photograph courtesy of Tom S. Chang, MD.)*

of the retinal lesions is important because this often helps to localize the causative nematode. If left untreated, patients ultimately develop late sequelae, which may include optic atrophy, retinal arterial narrowing, diffuse retinal pigment epithelial changes, and an abnormal electroretinogram. The late findings of this condition are often misinterpreted as unilateral retinitis pigmentosa.

DUSN may be caused by a helminthic infection with *Toxocara canis, Baylisascaris procyonis,* or *Ancylostoma caninum.* The characteristic lesions are believed to result from a single nematode migrating within the subretinal space. If the nematode can be visualized, which occurs in less than half of cases, it should be treated with photocoagulation. After the worm is killed, visual acuity loss usually does not progress. In any unilateral presentation of "white dots," it is important that this condition be considered. Although previously thought to be endemic in some areas, that belief was likely due to under-awareness. DUSN has been diagnosed in patients in many countries and climates.

Gass JD. *Stereoscopic Atlas of Macular Diseases: Diagnosis and Treatment.* 4th ed. St Louis: Mosby; 1997:622–628.

Syphilitic Chorioretinitis

Syphilitic chorioretinitis usually occurs in the secondary stage of syphilis and is often associated with a positive rapid plasma reagin (RPR) or Venereal Disease Research Laboratory (VDRL) test, except in HIV-infected patients. It can present with a wide variety of symptoms and findings, including choroiditis, retinitis, retinal vasculitis, optic neuritis, neuroretinitis, and even exudative retinal detachment. Characteristic findings are yellow placoid chorioretinal lesions in the posterior pole (Fig 7-18). Treatment is the same as

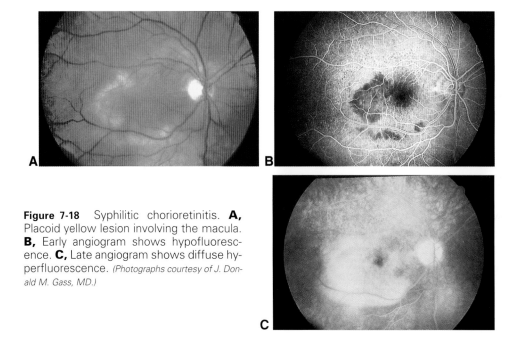

Figure 7-18 Syphilitic chorioretinitis. **A,** Placoid yellow lesion involving the macula. **B,** Early angiogram shows hypofluorescence. **C,** Late angiogram shows diffuse hyperfluorescence. *(Photographs courtesy of J. Donald M. Gass, MD.)*

for neurosyphilis, and most cases respond quickly. Corticosteroids are of limited value in decreasing posterior segment inflammation.

Gass JD, Braunstein RA, Chenoweth RG. Acute syphilitic posterior placoid chorioretinitis. *Ophthalmology.* 1990;97:1288–1297.

Tamesis RR, Foster CS. Ocular syphilis. *Ophthalmology.* 1990;97:1281–1287.

Lyme Disease

Lyme disease is caused by *Borrelia burgdorferi,* which is transmitted to humans by ticks from its usual animal reservoirs: rodents, deer, birds, cats, and dogs. The early stage of Lyme disease may present with a follicular conjunctivitis. At the early stage, systemic manifestations consist of myalgias, arthralgias, fever, headache, malaise, and a characteristic annular erythematous skin lesion with central clearing at the site of the tick bite. In later stages, as patients develop neurologic or musculoskeletal manifestations, they may exhibit keratitis, uveitis, vitritis, and optic neuritis. Chronic iridocyclitis and vitritis in patients who reside in endemic areas or who have had recent tick bites should suggest Lyme disease. Unfortunately, serologic diagnosis is plagued by high rates of false-positive and false-negative results. Diagnosis of "ocular Lyme disease" should not be made on the basis of serologic findings alone. Treatment for early disease is with tetracycline, doxycyclin, or penicillin; advanced disease may require intravenous ceftriaxone or penicillin.

Karma A, Seppala I, Mikkila H, et al. Diagnosis and clinical characteristics of ocular Lyme borreliosis. *Am J Ophthalmol.* 1995;119:127–135.

Winward KE, Smith JL, Culbertson WW, et al. Ocular Lyme borreliosis. *Am J Ophthalmol.* 1989;108:651–657.

Toxocariasis

Toxocariasis usually presents as a severe unilateral intraocular inflammatory response in a child or young adult. Although toxocariasis is the product of systemic inflammation from the nematode *Toxocara canis,* systemic manifestations such as visceral larval migrans, fever, and eosinophilia are relatively uncommon. *T canis* is a common intestinal parasite in dogs that may be acquired by humans after ingestion of soil or vegetables infected with the ova. The parasite migrates to the liver and lungs and may disseminate systemically from there.

Ocular manifestations include a severe uveitis or posterior segment granuloma, often with a fibrocellular stalk extending from the disc to a posterior granuloma (Fig 7-19). Patients usually have elevated intraocular levels of antibodies to *T canis.* Inflammation is worsened by the death of the nematode. Antihelminthic therapy is usually not effective in ocular or systemic disease. Intensive local and systemic corticosteroids are necessary to control the acute intraocular inflammation. The visual prognosis depends on the location of posterior segment inflammation or the resulting scar tissue, as well as the presence of macular traction or retinal detachment.

Bains HS, Jampol LM, Caughron MC et al. Vitritis and chorioretinitis in a patient with West Nile virus infection. *Arch Ophthalmol.* 2003;121:205–207.

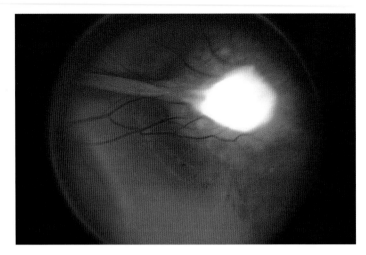

Figure 7-19 Toxocariasis (fibrotic granuloma). *(Photograph courtesy of Harry W. Flynn, Jr, MD.)*

Biglan AW, Glickman LT, Loves LA Jr. Serum and vitreous *Toxocara* antibody in nematode endophthalmitis. *Am J Ophthalmol.* 1979;88:898–901.

Ellis GS Jr, Pakalnis VA, Worley G, et al. *Toxocara canis* infestation: clinical and epidemiological associations with seropositivity in kindergarten children. *Ophthalmology.* 1986;93: 1032–1037.

Cytomegalovirus Infection

Retinitis caused by cytomegalovirus (CMV) is the most common ocular opportunistic infection in patients with AIDS. Retinal manifestations usually occur after the patient's $CD4^+$ count drops below 50. Patients often present with decreased visual acuity and floaters. CMV retinitis has a characteristic appearance that consists of opacification of the retina with areas of hemorrhage, exudate, and necrosis (Fig 7-20). There is often an

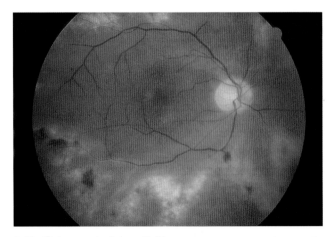

Figure 7-20 Cytomegalovirus retinitis. *(Photograph courtesy of Janet L. Davis, MD.)*

appearance of superficial granularity. Periphlebitis and even frosted branch angiitis may be seen. The degree of overlying vitreous inflammation is highly variable and may be related to the extent to which the patient is immunocompromised. Because the diagnosis is not usually made unless the lesions enlarge (over 1–2 weeks) to at least 750 µm in size, CMV retinitis, early in its course, may resemble cotton-wool spots. Serology is of limited value because exposure to CMV is common.

CMV retinitis is initially managed with either intravenous ganciclovir or foscarnet. After high-dose induction of 5 mg/kg twice daily of ganciclovir or 90 mg/kg twice daily of foscarnet for 2 weeks, patients who respond well may be switched to lower-dose daily intravenous therapy or oral ganciclovir therapy. Cidofovir is another agent approved by the FDA for treatment of CMV, and it can be administered intravenously once per week for 2 induction doses and then every 2 weeks for maintenance. Those patients whose retinitis progresses despite induction or who have disease that imminently threatens the macula may benefit from intravitreal injection with fomiversen. Ganciclovir and foscarnet can also be injected, but this mode of administration has not been FDA approved. Because ganciclovir has myelotoxic side effects and cidofovir can result in renal toxicity, those patients who cannot tolerate systemic administration of these drugs or who progress despite it may benefit from intravitreal insertion of a ganciclovir implant that delivers adequate concentrations of the drug for approximately 8 months. CMV retinitis is complicated by retinal detachment in 40%–50% of patients within the first year. Small peripheral detachments may benefit from laser demarcation, but most cases require pars plana vitrectomy with silicone oil intraocular tamponade. Highly active antiretroviral therapy (HAART) may reduce or eliminate the need for specific anti-CMV treatment. BCSC Section 9, *Intraocular Inflammation and Uveitis,* discusses CMV in greater detail in Chapter 14, Ocular Involvement in AIDS.

Graham KB, Pinnolis MK, D'Amico DJ. Retinal manifestations of the acquired immunodeficiency syndrome: diagnosis and treatment. In: Albert DM, Jakobiec FA, eds. *Principles and Practice of Ophthalmology.* 2nd ed. Philadelphia: Saunders; 2000:2119– 2134.

Holland GN. Treatment options for cytomegalovirus retinitis: a time for reassessment. *Arch Ophthalmol.* 1999;117:1549–1550.

Martin DF, Dunn JP, Davis JL, et al. Use of the ganciclovir implant for the treatment of cytomegalovirus retinitis in the era of potent antiretroviral therapy: recommendations of the International AIDS Society-USA panel. *Am J Ophthalmol.* 1999;127:329–339.

Macdonald JC, Torriani FJ, Morse LS, et al. Lack of reactivation of cytomegalovirus (CMV) retinitis after stopping CMV maintenance therapy in AIDS patients with sustained elevations in CD4 T cells in response to highly active antiretroviral therapy. *J Infect Dis.* 1998;177:1182–1187.

Nussenblatt RB, Lane HC. Human immunodeficiency virus disease: changing patterns of intraocular inflammation. *Am J Ophthalmol.* 1998;125:374–382.

Rhegmatogenous retinal detachment in patients with cytomegalovirus retinitis: the Foscarnet-Ganciclovir Cytomegalovirus Retinitis Trial. The Studies of the Ocular Complications of AIDS (SOCA) Research Group in Collaboration with the AIDS Clinical Trials Group (ACTG). *Am J Ophthalmol.* 1997;124:61–70.

The authors wish to acknowledge the contributions of Robert Equi, MD, to this chapter.

CHAPTER 8

Congenital and Stationary Retinal Disease

Color Vision (Cone System) Abnormalities

Congenital Color Deficiency

Color vision defects can be divided into 2 groups: congenital and acquired. Whereas hereditary congenital color vision defects are almost always X-linked recessive red-green abnormalities that affect 5%–8% of males and 0.5% of females, acquired defects are more often of the blue-yellow variety and affect males and females equally.

Typical male color-deficient subjects may find that pastel pinks or yellows are difficult to distinguish from greens, but relatively few subjects will confuse pure red with pure green. Patients with a blue-yellow defect tend to confuse pastel or dark blues and greens. Because congenital blue-yellow defects are exceedingly rare, the detection of a blue-yellow defect should alert the ophthalmologist to the possibility of acquired disease.

A normal individual, who requires all 3 primary colors of light (red, green, and blue) to match an arbitrary color, is classified as a *trichromat*. Abnormal subjects who require only 2 of the 3 standards to match with any color are called *dichromats*. Individuals who require 3 colors, but in abnormal proportions, are called *anomalous trichromats*. Persons with a red-green deficiency related primarily to a loss or abnormality of the red-sensitive cone pigment are said to have a *protan* defect, whereas those with loss or abnormality of the green-sensitive cone pigment have a *deutan* defect. Blue-yellow color deficiency is a *tritan* defect. Table 8-1 shows the traditional classification of color vision deficits on the basis of color matching.

The class of anomalous trichromats makes up the largest group of color-deficient persons. They are really "color weak" rather than color deficient, and the spectrum of severity of protanomaly and deuteranomaly is wide. Patients with a mild abnormality, for example, may fail some of the sensitive Ishihara test plates but have no trouble naming colors or passing the less sensitive Farnsworth Panel D-15 test (see Chapter 3). The genetic abnormality in these patients is only a slight alteration in the wavelength maxima of the absorption curve of the affected pigment.

The genes for the cone visual pigments have been isolated, and the basis for color deficiency turns out to be more complicated than the classification just described. Normal males have 1 red-pigment gene, and they may have 1 to 3 green-pigment genes in a tandem array on their single X chromosome. Unequal homologous recombination

Table 8-1 Classification and Incidence of Color Vision Defects

Color Vision	Inheritance	Incidence In Male Population (%)
Hereditary		
Trichromats		
Normal		92.0
Deuteranomalous	XR	5.0
Protanomalous	XR	1.0
Tritanomalous	AD	0.0001
Dichromats		
Deuteranopes	XR	1.0
Protanopes	XR	1.0
Tritanopes	AD	0.001
Monochromats (achromats)		
Typical (rod monochromats)	AR	0.0001
Atypical (cone monochromats)	XR	Unknown
Acquired		
Tritan (blue-yellow)		
Protan-deutan (red-green)		

XR = X-linked recessive; AR = autosomal recessive; AD = autosomal dominant

during meiosis can give rise to a variable number of green-pigment genes, yet still produce a pigment that provides normal color vision. The congenital disorders of color vision can result either from a complete loss of red- and/or green-pigment genes or from a hybrid red-green-pigment gene whose spectral characteristics are anomalous (Fig 8-1).

Achromatopsia

An absence of color discrimination, or *achromatopsia,* means that any spectral color can be matched with any other solely by intensity adjustments. It is classified in 2 forms: blue-cone monochromatism and rod monochromatism. Both disorders present typically with congenital nystagmus, poor visual acuity, and photoaversion. The diagnosis may be missed or misjudged as congenital nystagmus unless an ERG is performed. Characteristically, the ERG shows an absence of conventional cone responses, whereas the rod ERG is relatively normal (see Fig 3-2). Dark adaptometry shows no cone plateau, and no cone–rod break occurs in the dark-adaptation curve.

Rod monochromatism, true color blindness, is inherited as an autosomal recessive trait. Fully affected individuals have no cone function at all and see the world in shades of gray. Patients may have full to partial expression of the disorder, with visual acuity ranging from 20/60 to 20/200. Nystagmus is often present in childhood, and it usually improves with age. The range of severity could imply that allelic or multiple forms of this entity exist. Because these patients may have lightly pigmented fundi and minimal granularity of the macula, they may be misdiagnosed as having ocular albinism; an ERG will quickly distinguish between the 2 diagnoses because the cone responses are normal in albinism.

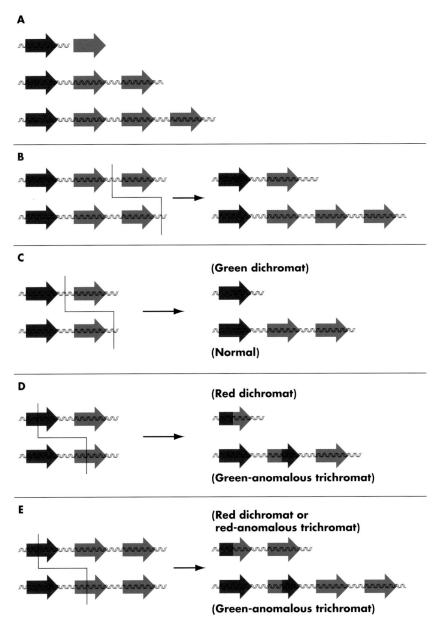

Figure 8-1 Chromosomal variations in normal and color-deficient humans. **A,** X chromosomes derived from normal individuals have 1 red-pigment gene and 1, 2, or 3 green-pigment genes. **B,** Normal variation can arise when a chromosome with 1 red-pigment and 2 green-pigment genes loses one of the green-pigment genes to its mate. **C,** Dichromacy and anomalous trichromacy arise from genetic exchanges that result in the loss of a pigment gene or **(D, E)** the creation of a hybrid gene derived from parts of pigment genes. The severity of the color deficiency in the latter case depends on the crossover point within the hybrid gene and the resultant sensitivity of the hybrid pigment. *(Reprinted with permission from Nathans J. The genes for color vision. Sci Am. 1989;260:42–49.)*

Blue-cone monochromatism is an X-linked recessive congenital cone dysfunction disorder that can be clinically indistinguishable from rod monochromatism in the absence of a family history or of specialized color or ERG testing. These patients have only the blue-sensitive cones, which are so few in number (and normally absent in the central fovea) that visual function mimics rod monochromatism. X-linked recessive inheritance in a male patient with a congenital lack of cone function is the most reliable indicator of this disease. The condition is caused by a loss of function of both red- and green-cone-pigment genes on the X chromosome.

Carr RE. Cone dystrophies. In: Guyer DR, Yannuzzi LA, Chung S, et al. *Retina–Vitreous–Macula*. Philadelphia: Saunders; 1999:942–948.

Nathans J, Piantanida TP, Eddy RL, et al. Molecular genetics of inherited variation in human color vision. *Science*. 1986;232:203–210.

Nathans J, Thomas D, Hogness DS. Molecular genetics of human color vision: the genes encoding blue, green, and red pigments. *Science*. 1986;232:193–202.

Reichel E. Hereditary cone dysfunction syndromes. In: Albert DM, Jakobiec FA, eds. *Principles and Practice of Ophthalmology*. 2nd ed. Philadelphia: Saunders; 2000:2290–2301.

Night Vision (Rod System) Abnormalities

Congenital Night-Blinding Disorders With Normal Fundi

Congenital stationary night blindness (CSNB) is characterized by a lifelong stable abnormality of scotopic vision. Three genetic subtypes of CSNB have been described:

- X-linked, the most common
- Autosomal dominant, typified by the large French Nougaret pedigree
- Autosomal recessive

X-linked CSNB has been mapped to the locus Xp11, and mutations in the rhodopsin gene have been documented in some families with autosomal dominant CSNB.

Snellen visual acuities of CSNB patients range from normal to occasionally as poor as 20/200, but most of the cases of decreased vision are associated with significant myopia. With the exception of myopic changes, the fundus appearance of CSNB patients is usually normal. Children may present with signs of nystagmus, decreased vision, or myopia. Although dark-adaptometry curves are typically 2–3 log units above normal, some CSNB patients never complain of nyctalopia, perhaps being accustomed to it as a way of life (Fig 8-2A).

Electroretinography is important in the diagnosis of CSNB, and there are several classifications of patients based on the test results. The most common ERG pattern is the *negative* ERG (from the Schubert-Bornschein form of CSNB), in which the maximal dark-adapted response has a large a-wave but an absent or much reduced b-wave (Fig 8-3). The photopic (cone) ERG also shows some abnormalities in this disease. A much rarer type of CSNB shows a reduction of both scotopic a- and scotopic b-waves.

Patients with the more prevalent negative ERG pattern have had their conditions further divided into *complete* and *incomplete* types. Patients with the complete type of CSNB have very poor rod function and psychophysical thresholds that are mediated by

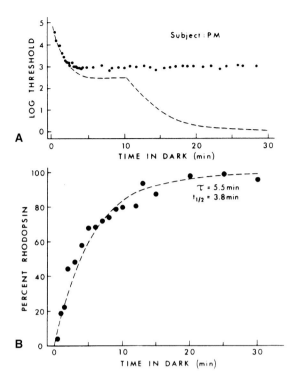

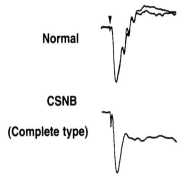

Figure 8-2 Dark adaptation in congenital stationary night blindness. **A,** Dark adaptometry shows no rod adaptation. **B,** Fundus reflectometry shows a normal rate of rhodopsin regeneration. *(Reprinted with permission from Ripps H. Night blindness revisited: from man to molecules. Invest Ophthalmol Vis Sci. 1982;23:588–609.)*

Figure 8-3 Negative-type ERG pattern typical of congenital stationary night blindness (CSNB). The a-wave is of normal amplitude, whereas the b-wave is absent. *(Reprinted with permission from Miyake Y, Yagasaki K, Horiguchi M, et al. On- and off-responses in photopic electroretinogram in complete and incomplete types of congenital stationary night blindness. Jpn J Ophthalmol. 1987;31:81–87.)*

cones. Patients with the incomplete type of CSNB still have some rod function but an elevated dark adaptation threshold.

In spite of poor rod vision in CSNB, both the amount and rate of rhodopsin regeneration following a bright light bleach are normal (Fig 8-2B). Thus, in contrast to retinitis pigmentosa, which involves a loss of photoreceptor cells, the defect in most cases of CSNB appears to be a failure of communication between the proximal end of the photoreceptor and the bipolar cell.

ERG studies have provided insight into the mechanism of CSNB (Fig 8-4). The abnormal cone and rod b-waves in cases with a negative ERG were found to result from a loss of retinal "on-responses." Normally, cones produce a b-wave to both the onset and offset of light, mediated by different neuronal pathways through the retina; and the

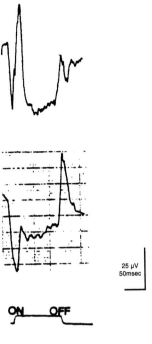

Figure 8-4 On- and off-responses from the human retina. The stimulus here is a long flash of light (about 0.1 second) so that the ERG responses to onset and offset can be seen independently. The normal subject shows an a- and b-wave at the onset of light and a smaller response at the offset. Patients with CSNB have no b-wave at the onset but a large off-response. *(Reprinted with permission from Miyake Y, Yagasaki K, Horiguchi M, et al. On- and off-responses in photopic electroretinogram in complete and incomplete types of congenital stationary night blindness. Jpn J Ophthalmol. 1987;31:81–87.)*

clinical b-wave to a very brief flash of light is a summation of the two responses. Rods, however, stimulate only on-responses. CSNB patients with a selective loss of retinal on-response pathways have no rod vision, therefore, but still have reasonable cone vision by means of the off-responses. A similar negative ERG has been found in some patients with Duchenne muscular dystrophy and systemic malignant melanoma (see Chapter 10).

Congenital Night-Blinding Disorders With Prominent Fundus Abnormality

Fundus albipunctatus is a disorder of the visual pigment regeneration process in which the recovery of normal rhodopsin levels after intense light exposure may take several hours. Affected individuals are symptomatically night blind (and their rod ERG is minimal) until they have spent several hours in a dark environment, but given enough time they adapt to normal sensitivity and the ERG becomes normal. Visual acuity and color vision are typically very good, though often not entirely normal. The fundus shows a striking array of yellow-whitish dots in the posterior pole (except the fovea) that radiate out toward the periphery (Fig 8-5).

Fundus albipunctatus must be distinguished from *retinitis punctata albescens*, which is a variant of retinitis pigmentosa in which the fundus shows yellow-white dots but has narrowed vessels and a severely depressed ERG that does not recover with dark adaptation. Larger, patchlike flecks and less severe impairment of night vision characterize the *fleck retina of Kandori*, a rare disorder.

Patients who have *Oguchi disease* also adapt very slowly to the dark, but their rhodopsin regeneration is normal. The physiologic defect appears to be in the retinal circuitry rather than the visual pigments. Once these patients are dark adapted, just a brief flash of light (too short to bleach the visual pigments) can destroy their dark sensitivity. The fundus in Oguchi disease shows a peculiar yellowish iridescent sheen after light exposure that disappears after dark adaptation (Mizuo-Nakamura phenomenon, Fig 8-6).

The *enhanced S-cone syndrome* (S-cone stands for short-wavelength, or blue-catching, cone) is a rare recessive form of congenital night blindness in which the photopic ERG responses resemble the scotopic ones. These patients lack rod function and have only very weak red- and green-cone function; their ERG behaves like a greatly magnified blue-cone signal. A ring of RPE degeneration is often seen in the region of the vascular arcades, and cystic macular edema may develop (Fig 8-7). Some debate persists as to whether the condition overlaps with the Goldmann-Favre syndrome (see Chapter 9).

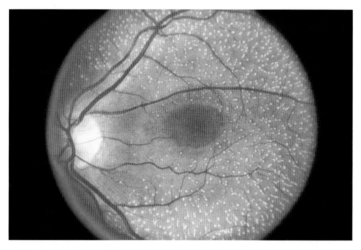

Figure 8-5 Fundus photograph of a patient with fundus albipunctatus, showing multiple spots of unknown material scattered primarily throughout the deep retina. *(Reprinted with permission from Fishman GA, Birch DG, Holder GE, et al. Electrophysiologic Testing in Disorders of the Retina, Optic Nerve, and Visual Pathway. Ophthalmology Monograph 2. 2nd ed. San Francisco: American Academy of Ophthalmology; 2001:51.)*

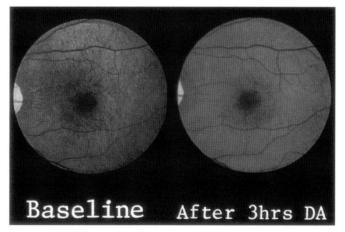

Figure 8-6 The Mizuo-Nakamura phenomenon. The fundus of this patient (with X-linked cone dystrophy) is unremarkable in the dark-adapted state *(right)*, but in the light *(left)*, it has a yellow iridescent sheen.

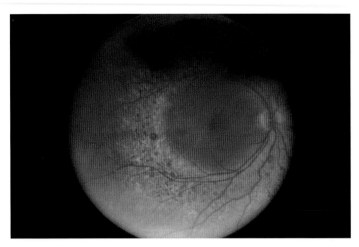

Figure 8-7 Characteristic fundus changes in the enhanced S-cone syndrome. *(Photograph courtesy of Michael F. Marmor, MD.)*

Carr RE. The generalized heredoretinal disorders. In: Regillo CD, Brown GC, Flynn HW Jr, eds. *Vitreoretinal Disease: The Essentials.* New York: Thieme; 1999:307–332.

Dryja TP. Molecular genetics of Oguchi disease, fundus albipunctatus, and other forms of stationary night blindness. LVII Edward Jackson Memorial Lecture. *Am J Ophthalmol.* 2000:547–563.

Marmor MF, Jacobson SG, Foerster MH, et al. Diagnostic clinical findings of a new syndrome with night blindness, maculopathy, and enhanced S cone sensitivity. *Am J Ophthalmol.* 1990;110:124–134.

Noble KG. Congenital stationary night blindness. In: Guyer DR, Yannuzzi LA, Chung S, et al, eds. *Retina–Vitreous–Macula.* Philadelphia: Saunders; 1999:934–941.

CHAPTER 9

Hereditary Retinal and Choroidal Dystrophies

The hereditary dystrophies of the posterior segment constitute a large and potentially confusing group of disorders. Organizing the rapidly expanding genetic information on these disorders into manageable resources is an increasing challenge. Over 500 diseases associated with significant retinal and choroidal disease are listed in *Online Mendelian Inheritance of Man (OMIM)*. Another excellent online resource, *RetNet*, lists over 150 different retinal degenerations in which the chromosomal site and often the specific gene defect have been identified. As the field evolves into molecular diagnosis and a better understanding of disease pathogenesis, ophthalmologists will be less dependent on the clinical phenotype for classification. Clinical characterization is currently helpful in choosing candidate genes for mutational testing and will continue to be necessary in order to counsel patients, assess their level of functioning, and discuss prognosis.

Different levels of organization are useful in approaching these diseases. Traditionally, anatomic classifications have divided the disorders by apparent layer of involvement, such as retina, macula, retinal pigment epithelium, choroid, and vitreous-retina. This approach is not sufficient, however, because many dystrophies overlap and may have multiple layers of involvement. A second level of organization comes from taking a family history to establish the inheritance pattern of the disease. Approximately 60% of thorough pedigrees give useful information. A third approach in diagnostic evaluation is to establish the disease phenotype by clinical examination and electrophysiologic and psychophysical testing. Careful analysis of the information gathered by these 3 approaches allows most patients to be assigned to a disease group, and many can be given a specific clinical diagnosis that can be confirmed by molecular testing.

Hereditary diseases of the eye, with rare exceptions, have bilateral symmetrical involvement. When unilateral ocular involvement is seen, other causes, such as birth defect, intrauterine or antenatal infection, and inflammatory disease, should be considered before a hereditary dystrophy is diagnosed. Occasionally, a patient is seen with clinically uniocular disease, which becomes bilateral after several years. In such cases, the apparently uninvolved eye was presumably in a subclinical state on the initial examination.

Obtaining an accurate family history is essential to determining the inheritance pattern, which in turn is helpful in selecting candidate genes on which to perform mutational testing. The Mendelian patterns of inheritance are well known—namely, autosomal dominant, autosomal recessive, and X-linked recessive. In addition, mitochondrial and X-linked dominant retinal disorders have been described (see RetNet). Approximately 40% of patients have a negative family history on the initial examination.

The search for the gene defects and pathophysiologic mechanisms underlying retinal dystrophies continues at a rapid pace, and some valuable lessons have already been learned. Perhaps the most important insight is that *depending on where a mutation lies in a gene, there may be varying expression or even different phenotypes.* This phenomenon has been seen in a number of different autosomal dominant genes, including *RDS-peripherin*, where cone–rod dystrophy, retinitis pigmentosa, and pattern dystrophy phenotypes have been reported; *rhodopsin*, where stationary night blindness and varying severities of retinitis pigmentosa have been found; and *CRX (cone–rod homeobox-containing gene)*, where Leber congenital amaurosis and cone–rod dystrophy have been observed arising from different mutations. Autosomal recessive genes also have demonstrated varying phenotypes depending on the location and type of mutation within the gene. For example, mutations in the Stargardt gene result in juvenile or adult macular dystrophy, severe progressive cone–rod dystrophy, retinitis pigmentosa (RP), and mild cone–rod dystrophy, depending on the location of the mutation. Another example is the Usher gene, *USH2A*, where 5% of patients have RP without the hearing loss characteristic of Usher syndrome. In some instances, it appears that interaction with secondary expression genes may influence the phenotype.

Until the mechanisms and implications of these genetic variations are understood, it remains important to categorize diseases in a way that helps the clinician recognize patterns of fundus damage and assess prognosis relative to other dystrophy patients. The classification used in this book represents a compromise between several possible approaches. To aid in clinical identification and management, dystrophies with primary diffuse photoreceptor involvement are classed separately from those with predominantly macular involvement, for which the symptoms and prognosis are generally different. Further distinction is made within the diffuse photoreceptor dystrophy category by separating rod-dominant and cone-dominant syndromes. The choroidal and vitreoretinal dystrophies are separated for ease in clinical description.

Heckenlively JR, Daiger SP. Hereditary retinal and choroidal degenerations. In: Rimoin DL, Connor JM, Pyeritz RE, et al, eds. *Emery and Rimoin's Principles and Practice of Medical Genetics.* 3 vols. 4th ed. New York: Churchill Livingstone; 2002:ch 137.

Online Mendelian Inheritance in Man: www.ncbi.nlm.nih.gov/omim

RetNet: http://www.sph.uth.tmc.edu/Retnet/

Sieving PA. Retinitis pigmentosa and related disorders. In: Yanoff M, Duker JS, eds. *Ophthalmology.* 2nd ed. London: Mosby; 2003:813–823.

Webster AR, Brown J, Sheffield VC, et al. Molecular genetics of retinal disease. In: Ryan SJ, ed. *Retina.* 3rd ed. St. Louis: Mosby; 2001:340–361.

Weleber RG, Gregory-Evans K. Retinitis pigmentosa and allied disorders. In: Ryan SJ, ed. *Retina.* 3rd ed. St. Louis: Mosby; 2001:362–460.

Diagnostic and Prognostic Testing

Although a number of tests are helpful in classifying the hereditary retinal and choroidal degenerations, the electroretinogram (ERG) and kinetic visual field examinations have proven to be the most useful. The ERG is an evoked response test in which a signal generated by the retina in response to a flash of light is recorded by a contact lens or foil electrode on the surface of the eye (see Chapter 3). Careful standardization of test conditions is essential in order to obtain interpretable results, and international standards have been published by the International Society for Clinical Electrophysiology of Vision (ISCEV). A kinetic (Goldmann) visual field is needed to correctly interpret the results of the ERG testing, particularly in patients with a cone-predominant (cone–rod) loss, which can be seen in RP, cone–rod dystrophy, Stargardt disease, and even postinflammatory states.

When the ERG is performed in the light-adapted state, the test is called a *photopic ERG* and measures the cone system. The rods in the light-adapted state are bleached out and do not respond to the light stimulus. Cone function can also be measured with a 30-Hz flickering stimulus because rods do not respond over 20 cycles per second. After the patient is dark-adapted for at least 30 minutes, the test is repeated with a dim flash of light below cone threshold. This stimulus evokes a rod-isolated response. A bright flash stimulus in the dark-adapted state tests both photoreceptor systems, giving a mixed cone and rod response. The ERG records the mass response of the photoreceptors and does not correlate with visual acuity, which is a function of macular health. The macula contributes only 10%–15% of the total photopic response. As a general principle, it is important to test the cone and rod systems separately in a standardized fashion, because comparison of the relative changes is used to support or make clinical diagnoses.

The first electroretinographic response to appear following the light stimulus is a negative, or downgoing, waveform called the "a-wave," which represents the response of the photoreceptor layer. The second waveform to appear is a positive, or upgoing, waveform called the or "b-wave," which is derived from bipolar and Müller cells in the middle retinal layers. Certain components of the ERG are lost or altered depending on the disease and severity of involvement. By comparing the cone-isolated, rod-isolated, and mixed cone and rod responses, diagnostic patterns are commonly seen in hereditary retinal disease states and are presented in Table 9-1.

ISCEV ERG Standards: http://www.iscev.org/standards/

Diffuse Photoreceptor Dystrophies

Panretinal degeneration is seen in a large number of different hereditary retinal conditions, most of which are forms of RP. On the electroretinogram, the pattern of loss can be rod predominant (rod–cone) or cone-predominant (cone–rod) or, in more advanced cases, an extinguished ERG.

As noted earlier, *kinetic visual field testing* is needed to further characterize the patient's diagnosis and to assess his or her level of function. Rod–cone RP degenerations show contracted fields, with smaller isopters demonstrating higher thresholds of sensitivity and leaving large spaces between smaller and larger isopters. Partial- to full-ring scotomata are common in midequatorial regions but eventually melt into peripheral isopters, in many cases leaving only a small central island of visual field (Fig 9-1). In cone–rod RP degenerations, contraction of isopters over time occurs, but the isopters

Table 9-1 Basic Guide to Interpreting the Standardized Electroretinogram

ERG change	Disease (or condition)
Nonrecordable ERG	Leber congenital amaurosis
	Retinal aplasia
	Retinitis pigmentosa (RP)
	Total retinal detachment
Abnormal or nonrecordable photopic ERG	
Often mild rod ERG abnormalities	Cone degenerations
	Achromatopsia
	X-linked blue-cone monochromatism
	X-linked cone dystrophy with tapetal-like sheen
Nonrecordable rod ERG	
Abnormal dark-adapted bright-flash ERG	
Normal to near-normal photopic ERG	Congenital stationary night blindness
	Early RP (rare), which is progressive
Barely or nonrecordable scotopic ERG	
Abnormal photopic b-wave ERG	Rod–cone degenerations (RP)
	Leber congenital amaurosis
	Choroideremia
	Chorioretinitis (variable)
	Secondary RP, including some storage diseases
	Progressive retinitis punctata albescens
Abnormal cone and rod b-wave amplitudes	
Cones relatively more affected than the rods	Cone–rod degenerations/dystrophies
	Autosomal dominant
	Autosomal recessive
	X-linked recessive
	Postinflammatory degenerations
Negative waveforms: In the dark-adapted bright-flash ERG, the a-wave is normal to attenuated, but the b-wave does not return to the isoelectric point.	X-linked retinoschisis
	Congenital stationary night blindness
	Enhanced S-cone syndrome (Goldmann-Favre syndrome)
	Some autoimmune retinopathies
Nonspecific abnormalities	Metallic foreign bodies
	Chorioretinitis (acute or old)
	Early panretinal degeneration
	Partial retinal vascular occlusion
	Low serum taurine
	Vasculitis/diabetic retinopathy

(Based on a table in: Rimoin DG, Connor JM, Pyeritz RE, et al, eds. *Emery and Rimoin's Principles and Practice of Medical Genetics*. 3 vols. 4th ed. New York: Churchill Livingstone; 2002:ch 124. Copyright © 2001, with permission from Elsevier.)

tend to be close to each other (like onion rings), and ring scotomata are closer to fixation. In contrast, patients with primary cone degenerations and (non-RP) cone–rod dystrophies maintain full isopters although central scotomata are common. In early cone–rod cases, it may be necessary to do repeated kinetic fields over time to determine if the field is stable or contracting.

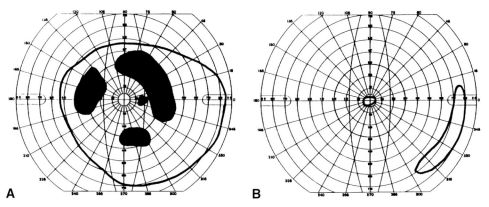

Figure 9-1 Examples of visual fields in retinitis pigmentosa, using a III-4 test object. **A,** Early disease: midperipheral scotomata. **B,** Late disease: severe loss, sparing only a central tunnel and far-peripheral island, which may eventually disappear. *(Illustrations courtesy of Michael F. Marmor, MD.)*

Retinitis Pigmentosa

The term *pigmentary retinopathy* is a generalized reference to a panretinal disturbance of the retinal pigment epithelium and retina. Because of the heterogeneity of the pigmentary retinopathies, an overall definition was established by a working conference of RP specialists in 1984. *Retinitis pigmentosa* was defined as a group of hereditary disorders that diffusely involve photoreceptor and pigment epithelial function characterized by progressive visual field loss and abnormal ERGs. The pigmentary retinopathies can be divided into two large groups: (1) *primary RP*, in which the disease process is confined to the eyes, with no other systemic manifestations, and (2) *secondary pigmentary retinopathy,* in which the retinal degeneration is associated with single or multiple organ system disease. Secondary forms of pigmentary retinopathy are reviewed in Chapter 10.

Clinical features and diagnosis

Typical fundus findings in RP include arteriolar narrowing, variable waxy pallor of the disc, and variable amounts of bone spicule–like pigment changes (Fig 9-2). The peripheral retina and RPE appear atrophic even if spicules are absent *(RP sine pigmento),* and the macula typically shows a loss of the foveal reflex and irregularity of the vitreoretinal interface. Cystoid macular edema is occasionally seen. Vitreous cells and posterior subcapsular cataracts are also commonly observed, although in most patients the cataracts are small and not the main cause of visual loss.

A number of the RP types have distinctive phenotypes, such as the deep retinal white dots or flecks seen in *retinitis punctata albescens* (Fig 9-3), choriocapillaris atrophy in choroideremia, macular RPE atrophy in *RDS-peripherin* mutations, or the preserved para-arteriolar RPE seen in *RP12*. Distinctive phenotypes are the exception, however, and most RP cases have diffuse pigmentary deposits that are secondary effects of the diffuse photoreceptor dysfunction.

In patients newly suspected of having RP, the ERG, in combination with kinetic visual field testing, provides critical diagnostic and prognostic information, as previously noted. The ERG in RP typically shows a loss or marked reduction of both rod and cone

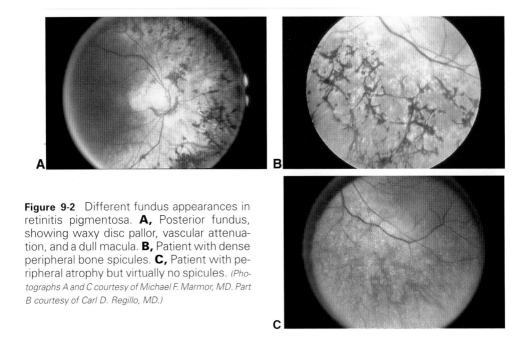

Figure 9-2 Different fundus appearances in retinitis pigmentosa. **A,** Posterior fundus, showing waxy disc pallor, vascular attenuation, and a dull macula. **B,** Patient with dense peripheral bone spicules. **C,** Patient with peripheral atrophy but virtually no spicules. *(Photographs A and C courtesy of Michael F. Marmor, MD. Part B courtesy of Carl D. Regillo, MD.)*

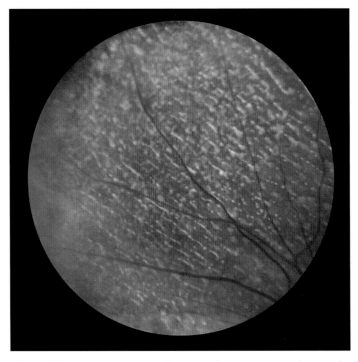

Figure 9-3 Patient with retinitis punctata albescens has numerous deep retinal white dots. *(Photograph courtesy of John R. Heckenlively, MD).*

signals, although rod loss usually predominates. Both a- and b-waves are reduced because the photoreceptors are primarily involved. The b-waves are characteristically prolonged in time as well as diminished in amplitude. The carrier state of X-linked recessive RP often shows a mild reduction or delay in the b-wave responses.

Late in the course of many types of RP, the ERG becomes undetectable with conventional testing. A very small signal can still be recognized in most of these cases by summating a large number of responses, but this is not done routinely in most clinics. An undetectable ERG is not diagnostic of RP but simply documents severe retinal degeneration.

When evaluating suspected RP in a patient with a negative family history (simplex RP), it is important for the clinician to consider acquired causes of retinal degeneration that can mimic RP, including previous ophthalmic artery occlusion, diffuse uveitis, infections such as syphilis, paraneoplastic syndromes, and retinal drug toxicity. Secondary forms of pigmentary retinopathy associated with metabolic or other organ system disease must also be considered (see Chapter 10). The differential diagnosis of RP is important because the prognostic implications of the disease are serious, and an error in diagnosis can be devastating in terms of psychological impact or failure to recognize a treatable entity. The clinician should take a careful history from any new patient and consider evaluating for other conditions by tests or nonocular examination.

Heckenlively JR, Yoser SL, Friedman LF, et al. Clinical findings and common symptoms in retinitis pigmentosa. *Am J Ophthalmol.* 1988;105:504–511.

Sieving PA. Retinitis pigmentosa and related disorders. In: Yanoff M, Duker JS, eds. *Ophthalmology.* 2nd ed. London: Mosby; 2003:813–823.

Weleber RG, Gregory-Evans K. Retinitis pigmentosa and allied disorders. In: Ryan SJ, ed. *Retina.* 3rd ed. St. Louis: Mosby; 2001:362–460.

Regional Variants of RP

Several variants of RP present with unusual or regional distribution of the retinal degeneration. Many of these cases show an unusually sharp demarcation between affected and unaffected areas of the retina, in contrast to the diffuse damage of more typical RP (Fig 9-4). The importance of recognizing these forms is that some are either nonprogressive or very slowly progressive.

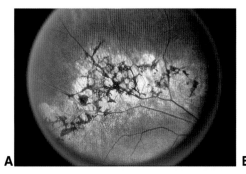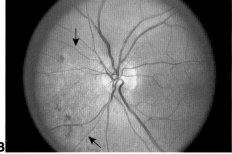

Figure 9-4 Delimited forms of RP. Note the sharp demarcation between the areas of degeneration and other regions of the fundus that appear quite healthy. **A,** Patient with degenerative changes near the arcades. **B,** Patient with sectorial RP *(between arrows),* showing vascular narrowing and spicules only in the inferonasal quadrant. *(Photographs courtesy of Michael F. Marmor, MD.)*

Sectorial RP is the term for disease involving only 1 or 2 sectors of the fundus (Fig 9-4B). The condition is generally symmetric in the 2 eyes, which helps rule out acquired damage (eg, from trauma, vascular insult, or inflammation). Sectorial disease probably comprises a variety of genetic entities, which may account for confusion in the literature about whether sectorial RP is stationary or slowly progressive. Unquestionably, some cases do progress slowly, and all patients should therefore be followed at intervals of 1– 2 years. Carriers of X-linked RP can have fundus findings that appear as a sectorial pigmentary retinopathy. Because there is evidence that the sectorial loss in many cases is related to light toxicity in patients with rhodopsin mutations, UV-light protection and antioxidant vitamins are reasonable recommendations for regional disease.

Some patients with RP-like disease present with macular involvement or markedly reduced acuity very early in the course of disease, which is unusual for RP. Field loss may progress outward from the center rather than inward *(central RP)*. Other patients show a tight ring scotoma within the central 20° or 30° *(pericentral RP)*. This group of regional variants is probably heterogeneous, because most of the cases appear sporadic and few have been well characterized clinically or genetically.

Unilateral RP is a rare disorder that is usually sporadic. In authentic cases, the clinical presentation and findings in the involved eye are similar to those of typical RP. However, the vast majority of unilateral pigmentary retinal degenerations are likely to have an acquired origin such as a previous vascular occlusion, prior retinal detachment, trauma, uveitis, infection (such as diffuse unilateral subacute neuroretinitis), or retained metallic intraocular foreign body. To make a diagnosis of true unilateral RP, the clinician must rule out such secondary causes, document a normal electroretinogram in the unaffected eye, and follow the patient for at least 5 years to rule out bilateral but highly asymmetric disease.

Weleber RG, Gregory-Evans K. Retinitis pigmentosa and allied disorders. In: Ryan SJ, ed. Retina. 3rd ed. St Louis: Mosby; 2001:362–460.

Genetic considerations

Currently, more than 84 different genetic types of RP (or similar degenerations) have been identified. Of these, the gene has been cloned in approximately half. All inheritance patterns are represented. There are currently at least 12 forms of *autosomal dominant RP (ADRP)*, of which 11 have been cloned. ADRP accounts for 10%–20% of RP cases, depending on the country surveyed. Mutations in the rhodopsin gene were the first discovered to cause RP. Rhodopsin is the visual pigment in rods that mediates night vision. The severity of disease resulting from rhodopsin mutations varies considerably. For example, mild disease (a form of stationary night blindness) is associated with codon 90 mutations, whereas severe forms are associated with mutations that interfere with the attachment of vitamin A to the rhodopsin protein. *RDS-peripherin* mutations have wide disease expression, ranging from RP to pattern macular dystrophies (eg, adult vitelliform dystrophy, butterfly dystrophy). Peripherin is a protein present in the peripheral aspect of the rod and cone photoreceptor discs, and the human peripherin gene has sequence homology with a gene in mice that causes a hereditary retinal degeneration. A full listing of dominant forms of RP can be found on RetNet.

Autosomal recessive RP (ARRP) represents about 20% of RP cases, although the number increases if one includes families in which there are several affected siblings (multiplex RP) or consanguinity of parents. At least 15 genetic types of ARRP have been identified, of which over 10 have been cloned. *X-linked RP (XLRP)* accounts for about 10% of RP in the United States and up to 25% in England. Five different forms of XLRP have been identified, of which 2 have been cloned. This number excludes choroideremia, an X-linked childhood onset rod–cone dystrophy, which has visual field loss like that of typical RP.

Up to 40% of cases presenting in the United States have no family history. It is generally assumed that most of these cases represent ARRP, although undoubtedly a few are autosomal dominant with reduced penetrance or X-linked recessive, in which the last affected male was several generations past. Rare cases of mitochondrial and X-linked dominant inheritance have been reported in RP (RetNet).

Bird AC. Retinal photoreceptor dystrophies. LI Edward Jackson Memorial Lecture. *Am J Ophthalmol.* 1995;119:543–562.

RetNet: http://www.sph.uth.tmc.edu/Retnet/

Shastry BS. Retinitis pigmentosa and related disorders: phenotypes of rhodopsin and peripherin/*RDS* mutations. *Am J Med Genet.* 1994;52:467–474.

van Soest S, Westerveld A, de Jong PT, et al. Retinitis pigmentosa: defined from a molecular point of view. *Surv Ophthalmol.* 1999;43:321–334.

Leber congenital amaurosis

The infantile to early childhood forms of RP have been termed *Leber congenital amaurosis (LCA)*, of which there are 7 known causative genes. In many of these forms, mild mutations lead to a later-onset cone–rod dystrophy, and severe mutations result in LCA. Many of the involved genes code for critical proteins in the visual transduction cycles, and most cases have an autosomal recessive inheritance pattern. LCA is typically characterized by severely reduced vision from birth associated with wandering nystagmus and undetectable or severely impaired ERG responses from both cones and rods. In early stages, there are seldom obvious fundus changes. Later, round subretinal black pigment clumps develop in many patients, although some cases will show bone spicule–like pigment changes. Visual function can range from 20/200 vision in some cases to no light perception in others. Some patients with LCA have been observed to rub or poke their eyes (the *oculodigital reflex*), as do other infants with poor vision. Cataracts and keratoconus may be seen in older children.

Most children with LCA have normal intelligence, and some of the psychomotor retardation that has been described may be secondary to sensory deprivation. The systemic disorders that mimic LCA include, among others, the various neuronal ceroid lipofuscinoses and peroxisome disorders (see Chapter 10). The clinician must also rule out other causes of infantile nystagmus such as albinism, achromatopsia, and congenital stationary night blindness (CSNB).

Electrophysiologic testing is essential to establishing the proper diagnosis. The ERG response is typically minimal or undetectable, differentiating LCA from dystrophic diseases in which the ERG response diminishes with age and from syndromes with similar clinical presentation. One caveat is that because the normal ERG response can be small in the first few months of life, infants with apparently abnormal findings in that period should have the ERG repeated at a later time for confirmation.

Dharmaraj SR, Silva ER, Pina AL, et al. Mutational analysis and clinical correlation in Leber congenital amaurosis. *Ophthalmic Genet.* 2000;21:135–150.

Management and therapy

Because of the rarity of these disorders, most ophthalmologists have limited experience working with retinal dystrophy patients. Patients newly diagnosed with RP are inevitably anxious about the possibility of blindness. For most patients, it is reassuring to undergo a complete evaluation by a specialist familiar with hereditary retinal degenerations. Once all the clinical, electrophysiologic, and psychophysical information is assembled, the correct diagnosis should be related to the patient, along with detailed information about the significance of the findings, inheritance pattern, prognosis, and possible treatments.

Popular misconceptions about RP should be dispelled by the ophthalmologist. The most pervasive fear is that of going blind quickly. It is not unusual for RP patients to be told that they will be blind within 1 year, when in fact the disease is a chronic degenerative problem, and the majority of patients do very well for decades. Total blindness is an infrequent endpoint, and estimates of prognosis must be individualized for each patient on the basis of clinical findings. Some RP patients are told not to have children, when in fact careful scrutiny of most pedigrees show that offspring are not at immediate risk unless the patient has autosomal dominant disease. Unless an ophthalmologist is very familiar with inheritance patterns, a genetic counselor should be asked to assist in genetic counseling of patients. Patients need to be reassured that they do not have one of the rare treatable conditions that mimic RP. The risk of deafness may be a concern to some patients, but most of the deafness in Usher syndrome is congenital; RP patients who are not born deaf will not ordinarily develop hearing loss later.

Management of RP includes regular ophthalmologic evaluation at intervals of 1–2 years. Although the death of photoreceptor cells in RP cannot at present be arrested or reversed, ongoing contact allows the clinician to monitor progression with visual field and ERG evaluation; it provides an opportunity to inform patients about new research developments; and it ensures timely recognition of refractive errors or vision-threatening but treatable complications. For example, cataracts can be extracted if they reduce vision, and RP patients do well with intraocular lenses, which give them the broadest possible visual field. Cystoid macular edema is present in a small percentage of RP patients, but when significant, it may respond to oral carbonic anhydrase inhibitors such as acetazolamide (Fig 9-5). Regular follow-up is also important from a research point of view and may help to identify the inheritance type in cases where there is inadequate family history.

Many RP patients benefit from counseling to deal with narrowed visual fields and reduced night vision. Low vision aids frequently help patients with subnormal visual acuity. Advanced cases may need vocational rehabilitation and mobility training. Although many patients maintain reasonable central vision for years, some are legally blind (visual field <20°) and are entitled to more favorable tax treatment and governmental benefits due to this disability.

Various nutritional supplements have been investigated as therapy for RP, and one or more of these may eventually prove to have merit. However, given the diverse biochemical bases of this disease, it seems unlikely that any one nutritional factor will prove

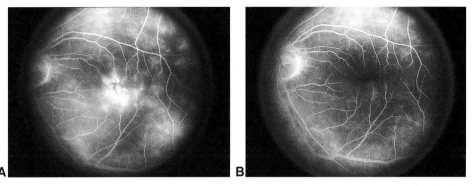

Figure 9-5 Cystoid macular edema in RP. **A,** Dye leakage on fluorescein angiography. **B,** Same patient after 2 weeks of oral acetazolamide. *(Photographs courtesy of Michael F. Marmor, MD.)*

highly beneficial to all RP patients. One large study concluded that high daily doses of vitamin A palmitate (15,000 IU/day) can slow the progression of RP by about 20% per year. However, the use of this treatment must be weighed against the unknown risk of long-term side effects, especially liver toxicity; a safety paper has been reported (Sibulesky et al, 1999). Because of the teratogenicity of vitamin A, high doses should not be used by women who might become pregnant. There is increasing evidence that an antioxidant mix might be helpful in RP patients; at the present time, however, no conclusive epidemiologic or clinical trial data prove that antioxidant supplements are effective against RP.

Light is considered by some to be a source of stress and age-related damage to the retina, as well as a possible accelerator of dystrophic injury. No direct evidence demonstrates that light modifies RP, however, and a study in which one eye was covered with an opaque contact lens failed to show any change in disease progression compared to the fellow eye. Protection from high levels of light exposure, as may occur on the beach or snow, is probably prudent for dystrophy patients, and this is easily achieved with ultraviolet-absorbing sunglasses in combination with a brimmed hat.

Molecular genetics may, in the future, provide a means for modifying the course of RP. As the affected genes for each type of RP are identified and their functions elucidated, it may become possible in some cases to replace or regulate the disease genes or to use the genetic information to employ conventional therapy more effectively. Progress is also being made toward transplantation of retinal cells and the use of humoral factors to slow secondary degenerative changes.

Berson EL, Rosner B, Sandberg MA, et al. A randomized trial of vitamin A and vitamin E supplementation for retinitis pigmentosa. *Arch Ophthalmol.* 1993;111:761–772. Letters by Norton EW, Marmor MF, Clowes DD, Gamel JW, Fielder AR. *Arch Ophthalmol.* 1993;111:1460–1463. Responses by Berson et al. 1993;111:1463–1465.

Fishman GA, Gilbert LD, Fiscella RG, et al. Acetazolamide for treatment of chronic macular edema in retinitis pigmentosa. *Arch Ophthalmol.* 1989;107:1445–1452.

Cone Dystrophies

The cone dystrophies should not be confused with congenital color blindness, in which there are color deficits for specific colors but no associated retinal degeneration. Patients with congenital color blindness (protanopia, deuteranopia, and tritanopia) have normal visual acuity and do not show signs of progressive disease. Congenital color deficiency and other congenital stationary cone dysfunction disorders, including rod monochromatism and blue-cone monochromatism, are discussed in Chapter 8. The progressive cone dystrophies represent a heterogeneous group of diseases with onset in teenage years or later adult life. These disorders are diagnosed by an abnormal or nonrecordable photopic ERG and a normal or near-normal rod-isolated ERG, while peripheral visual fields remain normal. A subset of patients has been described in whom the full-field ERG appears normal, and involvement of only the foveal or central cones has been documented. All 3 Mendelian inheritance patterns have been found in the cone degenerations. Kinetic visual field testing will help separate cone dystrophy patients from patients with RP cone–rod patterns or cone–rod dystrophy, although in early cases perimetry may have to be repeated over several years to ensure that the peripheral fields are stable.

The diagnosis of cone dystrophy is suggested by progressive loss of visual acuity and color discrimination, often accompanied by hemeralopia (day blindness) and photoaversion (light intolerance). Ophthalmoscopy may show a symmetric bull's-eye pattern of macular atrophy (Fig 9-6) or more severe atrophy such as demarcated circular macular lesions. Mild to severe temporal optic atrophy and tapetal reflexes may also be seen.

Dominant cone dystrophy linked to 6p21.1 was found to be due to mutations in guanylatecyclase activator 1A (GUCA1A), a calcium-binding protein that is expressed in photoreceptor outer segments. Mutations of GUCY2D at 17p13.1 were found in another family with autosomal dominant progressive cone degeneration. This same gene with different mutations on both alleles gives autosomal recessive LCA (RetNet). These patients develop foveal atrophy that may be misdiagnosed as Stargardt disease, but the ERG shows severely abnormal photopic responses, whereas the scotopic response is maintained. The Goldmann visual field is full. An adult-onset X-linked recessive cone dystrophy with a tapetal-like sheen (beaten metal appearance) and Mizuo-Nakamura phenomenon (the fundus appearance changes with dark adaptation) has been reported in several pedigrees, but the gene has not yet been determined.

Carr RE. Cone dystrophies. In: Guyer DR, Yanuzzi LA, Chang S, et al. *Retina–Vitreous–Macula*. Philadelphia: Saunders; 1999:942–948.

Nathans J. The evolution and physiology of human color vision: insights from molecular genetic studies of visual pigments. *Neuron*. 1999;24:299–312.

Simunovic MP, Moore AT. The cone dystrophies. *Eye*. 1998;12(pt 3b):553–565.

Cone–Rod Dystrophies

The term *cone–rod* comes from electroretinographic testing, in which the cone-isolated ERG waveform is proportionately worse than the rod-isolated signal, and both are abnormal. A large number of entities can result in this ERG pattern, from old inflammatory damage to well-established genetic diseases such as Stargardt disease. Molecular genetics will help to separate out the specific causes for this group. In the last few years, it has become apparent that a number of the genes in which severe mutations give Leber congenital amaurosis will result in a cone–rod dystrophy if the mutation is less severe or if there is a dominant mutation in one allele. A list of the known genetic causes of cone–

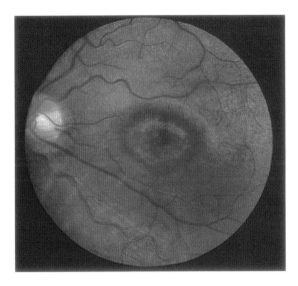

Figure 9-6 Cone dystrophy, showing bull's-eye pattern of central atrophy.

rod dystrophy can be found in RetNet. The more important known genes associated with cone–rod degenerations are the genes for Stargardt disease (*ABCA4*), Alström disease (*ALMS1*), and dominant spinocerebellar ataxia (*SCA7*). Dominant cone–rod dystrophy may result from mutations in *GUCY2D*, whereas recessive mutations cause LCA. Similarly, the *CRX* gene can cause RP, LCA, and cone–rod dystrophy, depending on the type of mutation.

Patients with progressive cone–rod dystrophy demonstrate expanding central scotomata over time and may develop severe visual disability to the point where mobility training may become necessary. Ophthalmoscopy at later stages may show bone spicule–like hyperpigmentation and atrophy in the fundus periphery, and patients may complain of night blindness in addition to poor central acuity and dyschromatopsia. There is a wide variety of expression in this group of disorders, and patients must be followed over time to determine their natural course.

Szlyk JP, Fishman GA, Alexander KR, et al. Clinical subtypes of cone–rod dystrophy. *Arch Ophthalmol.* 1993;111:781–788.

Macular Dystrophies

The macular dystrophies can be difficult to manage for a variety of reasons. The differential diagnosis is sometimes challenging, and several of the conditions cause legal blindness at a relatively young age. The pathophysiologic processes that result in visual loss in these diseases cannot at present be arrested or reversed; yet patients can be reassured that the disease progresses slowly and that they will always retain some useful vision. Patients also need proper refraction and education in the use of an Amsler grid to detect symptoms of a complicating choroidal neovascular membrane. In addition, patients may benefit from referral to a low vision specialist. Children with 20/100 or 20/200 vision usually do very well in regular schools, especially if the ophthalmologist takes the time to communicate with the teacher about the child's visual abilities and limitations.

Stargardt Disease (Fundus Flavimaculatus)

Stargardt disease, or fundus flavimaculatus, is the most common juvenile macular dystrophy and a common cause of central vision loss in adults under the age of 50. The vast majority of cases are autosomal recessive, but some dominant pedigrees have been reported. The gene responsible for most cases of Stargardt disease is the *ABCA4* gene, which encodes an ATP-binding cassette (ABC) transporter protein that is expressed by rod outer segments. Other, less frequent causes of the phenotype include the dominant genes *STGD4* and *ELOVL4* (a photoreceptor-specific component of the fatty acid elongation system), and mutations in the *RDS-peripherin* gene.

The classic Stargardt phenotype is characterized by a juvenile-onset foveal atrophy surrounded by discrete yellowish round or pisciform flecks at the level of the RPE (Fig 9-7). If the flecks are widely scattered throughout the fundus, the condition is commonly referred to as *fundus flavimaculatus*. A clinical diagnosis of Stargardt disease is confirmed by the finding of a "dark choroid" on fluorescein angiography. This phenomenon, in which the retinal circulation is highlighted against a hypofluorescent choroid, is present in at least 80% of patients with the disorder (Fig 9-8). Although the absence of this sign does not rule out Stargardt disease, its presence is quite specific for the disease. The dark choroid sign is believed to represent masking of choroidal fluorescence by an accumulation of lipofuscinlike pigment throughout the RPE (Fig 9-9). The numerous hyperfluorescent lesions seen angiographically in patients with flecks appear to represent transmission defects around the flecks.

The age of onset and presenting clinical features in Stargardt disease are quite variable, sometimes even among individuals within the same family. A patient may present with vision loss and any combination of the clinical triad of macular atrophy, flecks, and

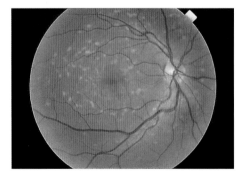

Figure 9-7 Stargardt disease, showing paramacular flecks and central macular atrophy. *(Reproduced with permission from Song M-K, Small KW. Macular dystrophies. In: Regillo CD, Brown GC, Flynn HW Jr, eds. Vitreoretinal Disease: The Essentials. New York: Thieme; 1999:293.)*

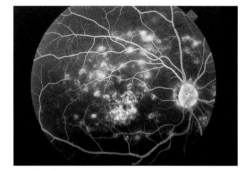

Figure 9-8 Fluorescein angiogram of the eye from Figure 9-7, showing a dark choroid, hyperfluorescent flecks, and early macular RPE atrophy. *(Reproduced with permission from Song M-K, Small KW. Macular dystrophies. In: Regillo CD, Brown GC, Flynn HW Jr, eds. Vitreoretinal Disease: The Essentials. New York: Thieme; 1999:293.)*

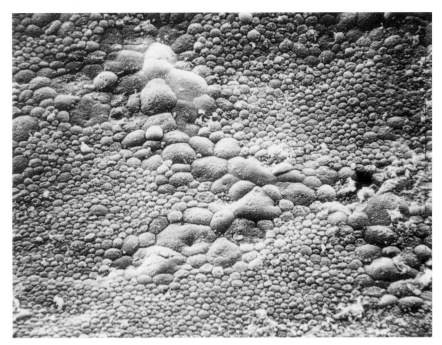

Figure 9-9 Scanning electron micrograph of the RPE in Stargardt disease. The flecks represent regions of RPE cells engorged with abnormal lipofuscinlike material. *(Reproduced with permission from Eagle RC, Lucier AC, Bernardino VB, et al. Retinal pigment abnormalities in fundus flavimaculatus: a light and electron microscopic study. Ophthalmology. 1980;87:1195.)*

a dark choroid. Signs not present on initial presentation may develop later in the course of the disorder. Although in most patients the condition is slowly progressive, the expressivity can range from mild to a progressive cone–rod dystrophy in which there is an expanding central scotoma over time. Peripheral degenerative changes are severe in occasional cases and associated with progressive visual field and ERG loss. The differential diagnosis of Stargardt disease includes those conditions that may cause a bull's-eye atrophic maculopathy (Table 9-2). Although confirmatory molecular testing may become more available in the future, the gene is very large (52 exons) and sequencing techniques currently are not practical for mass screening.

The visual acuity in Stargardt disease typically ranges between 20/50 and 20/200. Most patients retain fair acuity (eg, 20/70–20/100) in at least one eye. Although no

---

Table 9-2 **Differential Diagnosis of Bull's-Eye Maculopathy**

Stargardt disease
Cone and cone–rod dystrophies
Chloroquine retinal toxicity
Age-related macular degeneration
Chronic macular hole
Central aveolar choroidal dystrophy
Olivopontocerebellar atrophy
Ceroid lipofusciniosis

medical treatment is available for this condition, low vision referral is usually quite helpful for these patients.

Armstrong JD, Meyer D, Xu S, et al. Long-term follow-up of Stargardt's disease and fundus flavimaculatus. *Ophthalmology*. 1998;105:448–458.

Fishman GA, Farber M, Patel BS, et al. Visual acuity loss in patients with Stargardt's macular dystrophy. *Ophthalmology*. 1987;94:809–814.

Fishman GA, Stone EM, Grover S, et al. Variation of clinical expression in patients with Stargardt dystrophy and sequence variations in the *ABCR* gene. *Arch Ophthalmol*. 1999; 117:504–510.

Lois N, Holder GE, Bunce C, et al. Phenotypic subtypes of Stargardt macular dystrophy– fundus flavimaculatus. *Arch Ophthalmol*. 2001;119:359–369.

Vitelliform Degenerations

Best disease, or Best vitelliform dystrophy

Best disease is an autosomal dominant maculopathy due to mutations in the *VMD2* gene, located on the long arm of chromosome 11, which encodes the protein *bestrophin*. This protein localizes to the basolateral plasma membrane of the RPE and functions as a novel, transmembrane chloride channel (RetNet). The resulting lipofuscin accumulation may be secondary to abnormal ion flux.

Affected individuals frequently show a yellow yolklike (vitelliform) macular lesion in childhood, which eventually breaks down, leaving a mottled geographic atrophic appearance (Fig 9-10). Late in the disease, the geographic atrophy may be difficult to distinguish from other types of macular degeneration or dystrophy. Some patients—up to 30% in some series—have ectopic vitelliform lesions elsewhere in the posterior fundus. However, the macular appearance in all stages is deceptive, as most patients maintain relatively good vision throughout the course of the disease. Even patients with the "scrambled egg" stage of the maculopathy typically have 20/30 acuity. Approximately 20% of patients will develop a choroidal neovascular membrane in one eye during the course of the disease; although self-limited in most patients, it frequently leaves the patient with

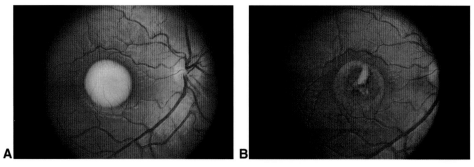

Figure 9-10 Best vitelliform dystrophy. **A,** Characteristic yolk stage, during which acuity is typically good. **B,** Atrophy and scarring after the yolk breaks down. *(Photographs courtesy of Mark W. Johnson, MD.)*

20/200 vision. The visual prognosis generally is good in this group of patients, and guarded but optimistic prognoses can be given to parents.

On electrophysiologic testing, the ERG is characteristically normal and the electrooculogram (EOG) is always abnormal, showing a severe loss of the light response. The Arden ratio (light–dark ratio) is typically less than 1.5 and often near 1.1 (see Chapter 3). The EOG abnormality is always present in Best disease and serves as a marker for the disease, even in individuals who are asymptomatic with normal fundi. Because of its specificity for Best disease, the EOG may be useful in evaluating poorly defined central macular lesions.

Fishman GA, Baca W, Alexander KR et al. Visual acuity in patients with Best vitelliform macular dystrophy. *Ophthalmology.* 1993;100:1665–1670.

Gass JD. *Stereoscopic Atlas of Macular Disease: Diagnosis and Treatment.* 4th ed. St Louis: Mosby; 1997:304–313.

Petrukhin K, Koisti MJ, Bakall B, et al. Identification of the gene responsible for Best macular dystrophy. *Nat Genet.* 1998;19:241–247.

Adult-onset vitelliform lesions

Several types of symmetric yellow deposits that occasionally resemble Best disease may develop in the macula of older adults. The most common disorder, *adult-onset foveomacular vitelliform dystrophy*, belongs to a group called *pattern dystrophies* (discussed later in this chapter), which are usually caused by mutations in the *RDS-peripherin* gene. Adult vitelliform pattern dystrophy is characterized by bilateral, round or oval, yellow subfoveal lesions, typically ⅓ disc diameter in size, and often with a central pigmented spot (Fig 9-11). Occasionally, the lesions may be larger and misdiagnosed as Best disease. This dystrophy generally appears in the fourth to sixth decade in patients who are either visually asymptomatic or have mild blurring and metamorphopsia. Eventually, the lesions may fade, leaving an area of RPE atrophy, but most patients retain reading vision in at

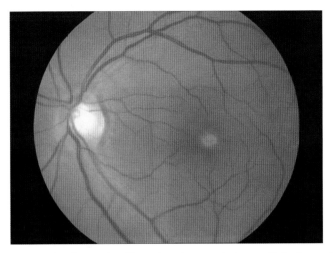

Figure 9-11 Foveomacular dystrophy. Note the characteristic small depigmented lesion with a hyperpigmented core. *(Reproduced with permission from Song M-K, Small KW. Macular dystrophies. In: Regillo CD, Brown GC, Flynn HW Jr, eds.* Vitreoretinal Disease: The Essentials. *New York: Thieme; 1999:296.)*

least one eye throughout their lives. The EOG is these individuals tends to be normal or only mildly subnormal. Autosomal dominant inheritance has been recognized in some families.

Patients with numerous basal laminar (cuticular) drusen may develop an unusual *vitelliform exudative macular detachment* (Fig 9-12). The yellowish subretinal fluid blocks background fluorescence early, often stains late in the angiogram, and may be mistaken for choroidal neovascularization. Patients with yellowish macular detachments often maintain good visual acuity for many months but may eventually lose central vision due to geographic atrophy or choroidal neovascularization and disciform scarring.

Finally, in some patients with large, soft drusen, there is a large central coalescence of drusen, or *drusenoid RPE detachment*, that may occasionally mimic a macular vitelliform lesion (Fig 9-13). Such lesions often have pigment mottling on their surface and are surrounded by numerous other individual or confluent soft drusen. They may remain stable with good vision for many years, but eventually they tend to flatten and evolve into geographic atrophy.

Gass JD, Jallow S, Davis B. Adult vitelliform macular detachment occurring in patients with basal laminar drusen. *Am J Ophthalmol.* 1985;99:445–495.

Lim JI, Enger C, Fine SL. Foveomacular dystrophy. *Am J Ophthalmol.* 1994;117:1–6.

Familial (Dominant) Drusen

Familial drusen typically manifest at younger ages than those seen in typical cases of age-related macular degeneration; it is not uncommon, for example, for affected patients to develop drusen in their 20s. In young patients, drusen are usually numerous and of varying size, typically extending beyond the vascular arcades and nasal to the optic disc (Fig 9-14). Although presumed to be genetically determined, the inheritance pattern in the vast majority of young patients with drusen is never established. In well-described pedigrees, the inheritance pattern has been autosomal dominant. The clinical entities that are well documented in the literature are *Doyne honeycombed dystrophy* and *Malattia Leventinese*. Both forms are caused by mutations in the *EFEMP1* gene on chromosome 2. This gene codes for an epidermal growth factor (EGF)-containing fibrillin-like, extra-

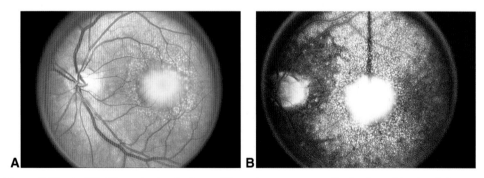

Figure 9-12 **A,** Vitelliform lesion in the setting of numerous cuticular (basal laminar) drusen. **B,** Corresponding late-phase fluorescein angiogram shows staining of drusen and vitelliform lesion. *(Photographs courtesy of Michael F. Marmor, MD.)*

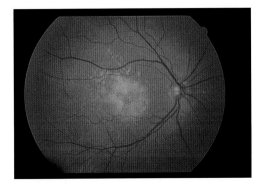

Figure 9-13 Central coalescence of large drusen simulates macular vitelliform lesion. *(Photograph courtesy of Mark W. Johnson, MD).*

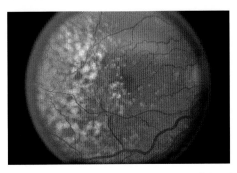 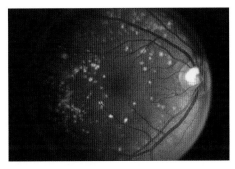

Figure 9-14 Different manifestations of dominant drusen. Variable size and distribution of the drusen are evident. *(Photographs courtesy of Michael F. Marmor, MD.)*

cellular matrix protein. The phenotype is distinctive because the drusen develop in a radiating pattern from the fovea. The many phenotypic variations of drusen suggest that several genetic defects are probably capable of causing them. It may be relevant that drusenlike deposits can be seen in some hereditary renal disorders that involve basement membrane abnormalities, such as Alport syndrome and membranoproliferative glomerulonephritis type II.

The clinical appearance of familial drusen is variable, ranging from a few large, coarse lesions to numerous tiny dots sometimes called *basal laminar* or *cuticular drusen.* Fluorescein angiography will often show more extensive drusen and RPE changes than are evident on ophthalmoscopy. The ERG and EOG are typically normal. Central vision is good as long as the drusen are discrete and extrafoveal. However, these patients may be at a greater than normal risk for macular degeneration as they age.

Kim DD, Mieler WF, Wolf MD. Posterior segment changes in membranoproliferative glomerulonephritis. *Am J Ophthalmol.* 1992;114:593–599.

Marmor MF. Dominant drusen. In: Heckenlively JR, Arden GB, eds. *Principles and Practice of Clinical Electrophysiology of Vision.* St Louis: Mosby; 1991:664–668.

Stone EM, Lotery AJ, Munier FL, et al. A single EFEMP1 mutation associated with both Malattia Leventinese and Doyne honeycomb retinal dystrophy. *Nat Genet.* 1999;22: 199–202.

Pattern Dystrophies

The *pattern dystrophies* are a group of disorders characterized by the development, typically in midlife, of a variety of patterns of yellow, orange, or gray pigment deposition at the level of the RPE in the macular area. They are typically inherited in autosomal dominant fashion. Based on the distribution of pigment deposits, these dystrophies may be subdivided into at least 4 major patterns: *adult-onset foveomacular vitelliform dystrophy* (discussed earlier in this chaper), *butterfly dystrophy* (Fig 9-15), *reticular dystrophy* (Fig 9-16), and *fundus pulverulentus* (coarse pigment mottling). The clinical pattern can vary among affected family members or even between the 2 eyes of one patient, and can evolve from one pattern to another over time. The overlapping ophthalmoscopic features of these patterns and their similar clinical implications suggest that they are either closely related or variable expressions of the same genetic defect. Most forms of autosomal dominant pattern dystrophy have been associated with mutations in the *RDS-peripherin* gene.

The most common presenting symptom of the pattern dystrophies is a slightly diminished visual acuity or mild metamorphopsia. However, patients are often asymptomatic and come to attention with the discovery of unusual macular lesions during routine

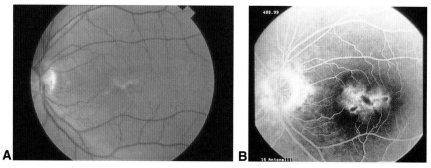

Figure 9-15 Butterfly-type pattern dystrophy. **A,** A 56-year-old female with a typical yellow macular pigment pattern. **B,** Fluorescein angiography shows blocked fluorescence of the pigment lesion itself and a rim of hyperfluorescence from surrounding retinal pigment epithelial atrophy. *(Reproduced with permission from Song M-K, Small KW. Macular dystrophies. In: Regillo CD, Brown GC, Flynn HW Jr, eds.* Vitreoretinal Disease: The Essentials. *New York: Thieme; 1999:297.)*

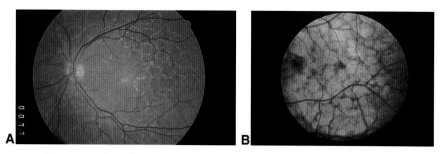

Figure 9-16 Two examples of reticular-type pattern dystrophy, characterized by a fish-net pattern of yellow-orange **(A)** or brown **(B)** pigment deposition in the posterior fundus. *(Photographs courtesy of Mark W. Johnson, MD.)*

ophthalmoscopy. Functional and electrophysiologic testing is generally normal except for a borderline or mildly reduced EOG consistent with a diffuse RPE disorder. These patients have a small risk of developing choroidal neovascularization later in life. Patients over 60 may develop geographic macular atrophy that can eventually compromise central vision. Most patients retain reading vision in at least 1 eye through late adulthood.

Gass JD. *Stereoscopic Atlas of Macular Disease: Diagnosis and Treatment.* 4th ed. St Louis: Mosby; 1997:314–325.

Marmor MF. The pattern dystrophies. In: Heckenlively JR, Arden GB, eds. *Principles and Practice of Clinical Electrophysiology of Vision.* St Louis: Mosby; 1991:700–704.

Nichols BE, Sheffield VC, Vandenburgh K, et al. Butterfly-shaped pigment dystrophy of the fovea caused by a point mutation in codon 167 of the RDS gene. *Nat Genet.* 1993;3: 202–207.

Wells J, Wroblewski J, Keen J, et al. Mutations in the human retinal degeneration slow (RDS) gene can cause either retinitis pigmentosa or macular dystrophy. *Nat Genet.* 1993;3: 213–218.

Sorsby Macular Dystrophy

The characteristic feature of Sorsby macular dystrophy, a dominantly inherited disease, is the development at the age of about 40 years of bilateral subfoveal choroidal neovascular lesions (Fig 9-17). As the macular lesions evolve, they take on the appearance of geographic atrophy, with pronounced clumps of black pigmentation around the central atrophic zone ("pseudo-inflammatory" appearance). An early sign of the disease is the presence of numerous fine drusenlike deposits or a confluent plaque of faintly yellow material beneath the RPE of the posterior pole. Histopathology shows a lipid-containing deposit between the basement membrane of the RPE and the inner collagenous layers of Bruch's membrane that may impede transport and contribute to the pathogenesis. The gene for Sorsby dystrophy, *TIMP3* (chromosome 22), codes for a tissue inhibitor of metalloproteinase, which is involved in extracellular matrix remodeling.

Capon MR, Marshall J, Krafft JI, et al. Sorsby's fundus dystrophy: a light and electron microscopic study. *Ophthalmology.* 1989;96:1769–1777.

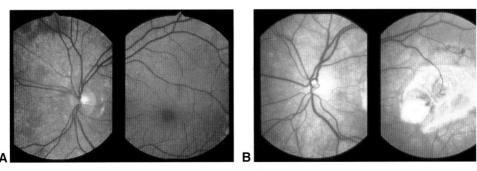

Figure 9-17 Sorsby macular dystrophy. **A,** Characteristic pale drusen. **B,** Late disciform scarring after the development of choroidal neovascularization. *(Photographs courtesy of Alan Bird, MD.)*

Hamilton WK, Ewing CC, Ives EJ, et al. Sorsby's fundus dystrophy. *Ophthalmology.* 1989;96:1755–1762.

Weber BH, Vogt G, Pruett RC, et al. Mutations in the tissue inhibitor of metalloproteinases-3 (TIMP3) in patients with Sorsby's fundus dystrophy. *Nat Genet.* 1994;8:352–356.

Choroidal Dystrophies

There are a number of conditions in which a primary retinal or RPE disease results in atrophy of the choriocapillaris. Historically, these conditions were named based on the clinically obvious choroidal involvement, but these names do not reflect current molecular knowledge.

Diffuse Degenerations

Choroideremia

Choroideremia, a hereditary chorioretinal dystrophy, was first identified as a separate entity from "typical" retinitis pigmentosa by Mauthner in 1871, who reported 2 male patients with pigmentary changes in the fundus, night blindness, and constricted visual fields. The features distinct from typical RP include marked atrophy of the choroid and RPE, normal retinal vessels, and absence of optic atrophy. Choroideremia is an X-linked recessive rod–cone dystrophy that otherwise meets the definition of RP: patients have night blindness and show progressive visual field loss typical of RP over 3 to 5 decades.

The disease is due to mutations in the *CHM* gene at Xq21.2. *CHM* encodes geranylgeranyl transferase Rab escort protein, which attaches isoprenoids to Rab 27. For many years it was assumed that the basic abnormality in choroideremia was a vasculopathy causing primary choriocapillaris atrophy. However, histopathologic studies of choroideremia and studies of the localization of the *CHM* protein place the basic defect in the RPE.

Choroideremia is characterized by diffuse and progressive degeneration of the RPE and choriocapillaris (Fig 9-18). In affected males, the degeneration first manifests as mottled areas of pigmentation in the anterior equatorial region and macula. The anterior areas gradually degenerate to confluent scalloped areas of RPE and choriocapillaris loss, with preservation of larger choroidal vessels. The fluorescein angiographic changes are even more pronounced, with the scalloped areas of missing choriocapillaris appearing hypofluorescent next to brightly hyperfluorescent areas of patent choriocapillaris. The ERG is abnormal early in the course of the disease and is generally extinguished by midlife.

Carriers of X-linked choroideremia often show patches of subretinal black mottled pigment, and, on occasion, older female carriers can show lobular patches of choriocapillaris and RPE loss. Carriers of choroideremia are usually asymptomatic and electrophysiologically normal.

Although choroideremia has a childhood onset, most patients show a slow degenerative course, and good visual acuity is maintained in the majority of patients for 4 or 5 decades. Night blindness usually develops in the first or second decade of life, and the visual field progressively contracts and develops ring scotomata similar to other forms

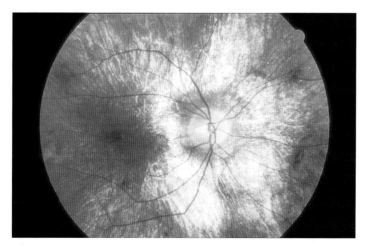

Figure 9-18 Choroideremia. *(Reproduced with permission from Fishman GA, Birch DG, Holder GE, et al.* Electro-physiologic Testing in Disorders of the Retina, Optic Nerve, and Visual Pathways. *2nd ed. Ophthalmology Monograph 2. San Francisco: American Academy of Ophthalmology; 2001:67.*

of RP. The differential diagnosis of choroideremia includes gyrate atrophy (see the following section), thioridazine hydrochloride (Mellaril) retinal toxicity, and Bietti crystalline dystrophy.

Roberts MF, Fishman GA, Roberts DK, et al. Retrospective, longitudinal and cross sectional study of visual acuity impairment in choroideraemia. *Br J Ophthalmol.* 2002;86:658–662.

Seabra MC, Brown MS, Goldstein JL. Retinal degeneration in choroideremia: deficiency of Rab geranylgeranyl transferase. *Science.* 1993;259:377–381.

Gyrate atrophy

Gyrate atrophy is an autosomal recessive dystrophy caused by mutations in the gene for ornithine aminotransferase (*OAT*), located on chromosome 10. Originally thought to be a subtype of choroideremia, the disorder is the result of tenfold elevations of plasma ornithine, which is toxic to the RPE and choroid. Patients with gyrate atrophy have hyperpigmented fundi, with lobular loss of the RPE and choroid. The finding of generalized hyperpigmentation of the remaining RPE helps to clinically distinguish gyrate atrophy from choroideremia. In the early stages, patients have large, geographic peripheral paving stone–like areas of atrophy of the RPE and choriocapillaris, which gradually coalesce to form a characteristic scalloped border at the junction of normal and abnormal RPE (Fig 9-19). Affected patients usually develop night blindness during the first decade of life and experience progressive loss of visual field and visual acuity later in the disease course. The clinical diagnosis can be confirmed by checking plasma ornithine levels; molecular confirmation can be obtained by mutational analysis of the *OAT* gene.

Although dietary restriction of arginine has been used to treat some gyrate atrophy patients, the diet is very difficult to maintain and must be monitored by pediatricians with experience in metabolic disease. Vitamin B_6 treatment lowers the plasma ornithine levels in a small percentage of gyrate atrophy patients. Whether such a reduction improves

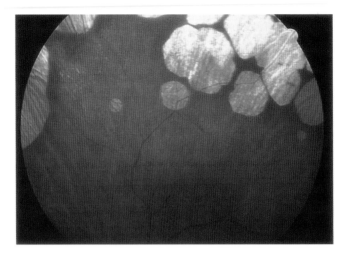

Figure 9-19 Gyrate atrophy.

the long-term visual outcome is unknown, but, unlike arginine restriction, vitamin supplementation is relatively easy to administer. Long-term vitamin therapy should be considered only for patients whose ornithine levels can be shown to drop in response to treatment.

Kaiser-Kupfer MI, Caruso RC, Valle D. Gyrate atrophy of the choroid and retina: long-term reduction of ornithine slows retinal degeneration. *Arch Ophthalmol.* 1991;109:1539–1548.

Ramesh V, McClatchey AI, Ramesh N, et al. Molecular basis of ornithine aminotransferase deficiency in B-6-responsive and -nonresponsive forms of gyrate atrophy. *Proc Natl Acad Sci USA.* 1988;85:3777–3780.

Regional and Central Choroidal Dystrophies

A number of dystrophies have been described that show macular or regional choroidal degeneration. Most distinctive are the central atrophies, including the autosomal dominant disorders central areolar choroidal dystrophy and North Carolina macular dystrophy. It is likely that several genetic types of central choroidal dystrophy exist, with overlapping clinical features. They are all characterized by demarcated atrophy of the RPE and choriocapillaris in the macula and normal full-field electrophysiologic responses; however, there may be differences in onset and progression. The central atrophic lesions must be distinguished from acquired disease such as toxoplasmosis and, in older patients, from age-related macular degeneration or late stages of other macular dystrophies that may cause a central round or bull's-eye pattern of RPE atrophy (see Table 9-2).

Central areolar choroidal dystrophy has been described as showing nonspecific mottled depigmentation within the macula in younger individuals that develops over time into a round or oval area of sharply demarcated geographic atrophy (Fig 9-20). Visual acuity typically stabilizes at approximately 20/200. Associated choroidal neovascularization rarely develops. A gene causing this disorder has been mapped to the short arm of chromosome 17. *North Carolina macular dystrophy* begins in infancy with a cluster of peculiar yellowish white lesions at the level of the RPE in the macular area. These lesions tend to increase in number and confluence, in some patients progressing to a severely atrophic macular lesion that can appear excavated or staphylomatous (Fig 9-21). The process appears to stabilize in most patients by the early teenage years, and visual acuity is usually better than anticipated from the ophthalmoscopic appearance, typically ranging from 20/20 to 20/200. The gene responsible for this disease has been mapped to the long arm of chromosome 6.

Hughes AE, Lotery AJ, Silvestri G. Fine localisation of the gene for central areolar choroidal dystrophy on chromosome 17p. *J Med Genet.* 1998;35:770–772.

Small KW, Hermsen V, Gurney N, et al. North Carolina macular dystrophy and central areolar pigment epithelial dystrophy: one family, one disease. *Arch Ophthalmol.* 1992;110:515–518.

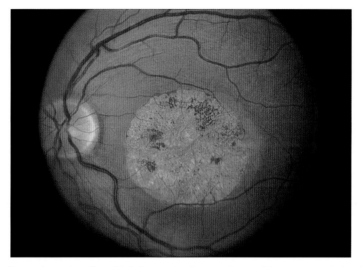

Figure 9-20 Central areolar choroidal dystrophy in a patient with autosomal dominant inheritance. *(Photograph courtesy of Mark W. Johnson, MD.)*

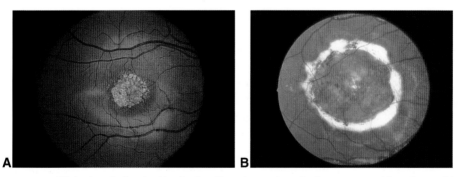

Figure 9-21 Clinical variation in North Carolina dystrophy. **A,** Seven-year-old patient with a cluster of peculiar yellow-white atrophic lesions in the macula. **B,** Patient with a severe, almost colobomatous, macular defect. *(Photograph A courtesy of Mark W. Johnson, MD; photograph B courtesy of Kent Small, MD.)*

Inner Retinal and Vitreoretinal Dystrophies

X-Linked Retinoschisis

The term *retinoschisis* refers to a splitting of the neurosensory retina, which at times may mimic a retinal detachment ophthalmoscopically. There are 3 forms of retinoschisis:

- degenerative peripheral retinoschisis with no known inheritance pattern
- congenital X-linked recessive retinoschisis
- secondary forms associated with vitreoretinal traction, myopic degeneration with staphyloma, or, occasionally, retinal venous occlusion

The phenotype of *congenital X-linked retinoschisis (XLRS)* is somewhat variable, even within families. A constant diagnostic feature, easily seen in pediatric patients, is foveal schisis, which appears as small, cystoid spaces and fine radial striae in the central macula (Fig 9-22). Angiography shows no leakage of fluorescein associated with foveal schisis. The central vision may initially be quite good, but, with time, degeneration occurs and the acuity typically drops to 20/200. Peripheral retinoschisis is not a constant feature but occurs in 50% or more of affected male patients. Histopathologically, the splitting in peripheral XLRS occurs in the nerve fiber layer, whereas in degenerative retinoschisis the level of splitting is variable and usually deeper within the retina. Pigmentary deposits may develop in peripheral areas destroyed by the disease process, so that advanced cases of XLRS can be mistaken for retinitis pigmentosa. The clinical diagnosis may have to be confirmed by evaluating younger affected male family members. Male children with XLRS frequently present with vitreous hemorrhages from broken retinal vessels in areas of retinoschisis. These and other tractional complications such as retinal detachment sometimes require vitreoretinal surgery.

The panretinal involvement and inner retinal location of the disease is reflected in the ERG, where the a-wave is normal or near normal, and the b-wave is attenuated,

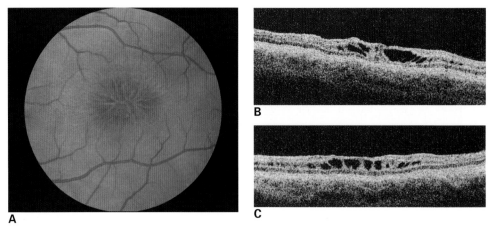

A

B

C

Figure 9-22 Juvenile retinoschisis. **A,** This characteristic pattern of macular schisis is a more constant finding than peripheral changes. Vertical **(B)** and horizontal **(C)** optical coherence tomographic scans show schisis spaces in the middle layers of the macula. *(Photographs courtesy of Mark W Johnson, MD.)*

typically giving a "negative waveform" (see Fig 3-2). Negative waveforms of the dark-adapted, bright-flash ERG occur in diseases in which the middle retina is affected and the photoreceptors are generally unaffected, yielding an a-wave with no effective b-wave (see Table 9-1). The ERG may become extinguished in cases in which there is extensive retinal damage.

The gene for XLRS, *retinoschisin*, was initially found to be localized to the rod photoreceptor; subsequent studies have shown that the protein is transported to Müller cells. Presumably, *retinoschisin* is essential for Müller cell health because mutations in its coding result in degeneration of the Müller cells. Müller cells span the layers of the retina, with their endplates forming the inner limiting membrane and the distal ends forming the outer limiting membrane at the inner segments. Loss of this bridging cellular matrix protein appears to be a key to the pathologic changes seen in congenital retinoschisis.

Molday LL, Hicks D, Sauer CG, et al. Expression of X-linked retinoschisis protein RS1 in photoreceptor and bipolar cells. *Invest Ophthalmol Vis Sci.* 2001;42:816–825.

Regillo CD, Tasman WS, Brown GC. Surgical management of complications associated with X-linked retinoschisis. *Arch Ophthalmol.* 1993;111:1080–1086.

Sieving PA, Yashar BM, Ayyagari R. Juvenile retinoschisis: a model for molecular diagnostic testing of X-linked ophthalmic disease. *Trans Am Ophthalmol Soc.* 1999;97:451–469.

Goldmann-Favre Syndrome

Goldmann-Favre syndrome, also known as the *enhanced S-cone* (or *blue cone*) *syndrome (ESCS)* ["S" for short wavelength] was initially described as a vitreoretinal dystrophy. Its most prominent features include night blindness, increased sensitivity to blue light, pigmentary retinal degeneration, an empty vitreous, unusual ERG abnormalities, and varying degrees of peripheral to midperipheral visual field loss. The posterior pole frequently shows yellow sheenlike round lesions along the arcades, with areas of diffuse degeneration. Macular (and sometimes peripheral) schisis is present, which does not leak on fluorescein angiography. The dark-adapted ERG shows no response to low-intensity stimuli that normally activate the rods, but there are large, slow responses to high-intensity stimuli. These large, slow waveforms persist without change under light adaptation, and there is greater sensitivity to blue light stimuli.

This autosomal recessive disorder results from mutations in the gene *NR2E3*, which codes for a ligand-dependent transcription factor. There is evidence that the disorder is the result of abnormal cell fate determination, leading to excess S cones at the expense of other photoreceptor subtypes. Histopathologic study of the retina from an ESCS patient found that no rods were identified, but cones were increased approximately twofold, and 92% were S cones. Only 15% of the cones expressed L/M-cone opsin ["L/M" for long/medium wavelength], and some of these coexpressed S-cone opsin.

Marmor MF, Jacobson SG, Foerster MH, et al. Diagnostic clinical findings of a new syndrome with night blindness, maculopathy, and enhanced S cone sensitivity. *Am J Ophthalmol.* 1990;110:124–134.

Milam AH, Rose L, Cideciyan AV, et al. The nuclear receptor *NR2E3* plays a role in human retinal photoreceptor differentiation and degeneration. *Proc Natl Acad Sci USA.* 2002;99:473–478.

The authors would like to thank John R. Heckenlively, MD, for his significant contributions to this chapter.

CHAPTER 10

Retinal Degenerations Associated With Systemic Disease

The retina is made up of over 200 highly differentiated cell types, which have an interdependent and cooperative relationship. The metabolic and oxidative requirements of the retina are high, and although the retina and retinal pigment epithelium (RPE) have some protection from systemic toxic elements due to the blood–retinal barrier and the relative isolation inside the scleral shell, the retina remains subject to drug toxicities, infections, trauma, and genetic events that can lead to a secondary retinal degeneration.

The important diagnostic and prognostic questions that arise in evaluating a patient presenting with a retinal degeneration are whether

- it is primary or secondary
- the condition is stable or progressive
- a precise diagnosis can be made

An appropriate treatment plan, whether intervention for the systemic disease or counseling for the condition, is based on the most accurate diagnosis and evidence regarding the speed of progression. The term *pigmentary retinopathy* is a generalized reference to a panretinal disturbance of the retina and RPE, and whereas pigment deposits are common to most pigmentary retinopathies, some diseases have a generalized depigmentation with atrophy and little or no pigment deposition.

Most of the severe secondary pigmentary retinopathies are genetic and many have childhood onsets. The number of pigmentary retinopathies reported in association with systemic genetic or acquired disorders is extensive, and reviews of the hereditary disorders can be found listed as references. Brief summaries of many of these disorders can be found in Table 10-1. Excellent on-line resources include *Online Mendelian Inheritance of Man (OMIM)*, which allows a search based on physical findings to access appropriate syndromes, and *RetNet*, which lists monogenic hereditary disorders.

Drack AV, Traboulsi EI. Systemic associations of pigmentary retinopathy. *Int Ophthalmol Clin.* 1991;31:35–59.

Heckenlively JR, Daiger SP. Hereditary retinal and choroidal degenerations. In: Rimoin DL, Connor JM, Pyeritz RE, et al, eds. *Emery and Rimoin's Principles and Practice of Medical Genetics.* 3 vols. 4th ed. New York: Churchill Livingstone; 2002:ch 137.

Kolb H, Fernandez E, Nelson R. WEBVISION: The organization of the retina and visual system. http://webvision.med.utah.edu/

Table 10-1 Systemic Diseases With Pigmentary Retinopathies (Partial List)

Autosomal dominant disorders

Arteriohepatic dysplasia (Alagille syndrome)

 Intrahepatic cholestatic syndrome, posterior embryotoxon, Axenfeld anomaly, congenital heart disease, flattened facies and bridge of nose, bony abnormalities, myopia, pigmentary retinopathy

Charcot-Marie-Tooth

 Pigmentary retinopathy, degeneration lateral horn spinal cord, optic atrophy

Myotonic dystrophy (Steinert disease)

 Muscle wasting, "Christmas tree" cataract, retinal degeneration, pattern dystrophy; ERG subnormal to abnormal

Oculodentodigital dysplasia syndrome

 Thin nose with hypoplastic alae, narrow nostrils, abnormality of fourth and fifth fingers, hypoplastic dental enamel, congenital cataract, colobomas

Olivopontocerebellar atrophy

 Retinal degeneration (peripheral and/or macular), cerebellar ataxia, possible external ophthalmoplegia

Stickler syndrome (arthroophthalmopathy)

 Progressive myopia with myopic retinal degeneration, joint hypermobility, arthritis; retinal detachment common; ERG subnormal to abnormal

Wagner's hereditary vitreoretinal degeneration

 Narrowed and sheathed retinal vessels, pigmented spots in the retinal periphery and along retinal vessels, choroidal atrophy and optic atrophy, extensive liquefaction and membranous condensation of vitreous body; retinal detachment common; subnormal ERG; overlapping features with Stickler syndrome

Waardenburg syndrome

 Hypertelorism, wide bridge of nose, cochlear deafness, white forelock, heterchromia iridis, poliosis, pigment disturbance of RPE, normal to subnormal ERG

Autosomal recessive disorders

Bardet-Biedl syndrome

 Pigmentary retinopathy, mild mental retardation, polydactyly, obesity, hypogenitalism; barely to nonrecordable ERG, progressive visual field loss

Bietti crystalline retinopathy

 Yellow-white crystals limited to posterior pole, round subretinal pigment deposits, confluent loss of choriocapillaris on fluorescein angiogram; possible crystals in limbal cornea

Friedreich's ataxia

 Spinocerebellar degeneration, limb incoordination, nerve deafness, retinal degeneration, optic atrophy

Homocystinuria

 Fine pigmentary or cystic degeneration of retina, marfanoid appearance, myopia, subluxation or dislocated lenses, cardiovascular abnormalities (thromboses), glaucoma, mental retardation

Mannosidosis

 Resembling Hurler syndrome; macroglossia, flat nose, large head and ears, skeletal abnormalities, possible hepatosplenomegaly, storage material in retina

Mucopolysaccharidosis IH (Hurler syndrome)

 Early corneal clouding, gargoyle facies, deafness, mental retardation, dwarfism, skeletal abnormalities, hepatosplenomegaly, optic atrophy; subnormal ERG

Mucopolysaccharidosis IS (Scheie syndrome)

 Coarse facies, aortic regurgitation, stiff joints, early clouding of the cornea, normal life span, normal intellect, pigmentary retinopathy

Mucopolysaccharidosis III (Sanfilippo syndrome)

 Milder somatic stigmata than Hurler, but severe pigmentary retinopathy

(Continued)

Table 10-1 Systemic Diseases With Pigmentary Retinopathies (Partial List) (Continued)

Neonatal adrenoleukodystrophy
  Pigmentary retinopathy, extinguished ERG, optic atrophy, seizures, hypotonia, adrenal cortical atrophy, psychomotor retardation
  Neuronal ceroid lipofuscinosis (Batten disease)
    Haltia-Santavuori, occurring in infancy with rapid deterioration, fine granular inclusions
    Jansky-Bielschowsky, onset 2–4 years, rapid CNS deterioration, curvilinear body inclusions
    Lake-Cavanagh, onset 4–6 years, ataxia, dementia, curvilinear and fingerprint inclusions
    Spielmeyer-Vogt, onset 6–8 years, slowly progressive, fingerprint inclusions
Refsum disease
  Elevations of phytanic acid, pigmentary retinopathy, optic atrophy, partial deafness, cerebellar ataxia, ichthyosis
Usher syndrome
  Congenital deafness (profound or partial), pigmentary retinopathy
Zellweger (cerebrohepatorenal) syndrome
  Muscular hypotonia, high forehead and hypertelorism, hepatomegaly, deficient cerebral myelination, nystagmus, cataract, microphthalmia, retinal degeneration; nonrecordable ERG

X-linked recessive pigmentary retinopathies
Incontinentia pigmenti (Bloch-Sulzberger syndrome)
  Skin pigmentation in lines and whorls, alopecia, dental anomalies, optic atrophy, falciform folds, cataract, nystagmus, strabismus, patchy mottling of fundi, conjunctival pigmentation
Mucopolysaccharidosis II (Hunter syndrome)
  Little corneal clouding, mild clinical course, mental retardation, some retinal arteriolar narrowing, subnormal ERG
Pelizaeus-Merzbacher disease
  Infantile progressive leukodystrophy, cerebellar ataxia, limb spasticity, mental retardation, possible pigmentary retinopathy with absent foveal reflex

Mitochondrial disorders
Progressive external ophthalmoplegia, ptosis, pigmentary retinopathy, heart block (Kearn-Sayre syndrome); ERG normal to abnormal

---

(From: Rimoin DL, Connor JM, Pyeritz RE, et al, eds. *Emery and Rimoin's Principles and Practice of Medical Genetics*. 3 vols. 4th ed. New York: Churchill Livingston; 2002:ch 124. Copyright © 2001, with permission from Elsevier.)

Online Mendelian Inheritance of Man. http://www.ncbi.nlm.nih.gov/omim
RetNet. http://www.sph.uth.tmc.edu/Retnet/

Disorders Involving Other Organ Systems

Infantile-Onset to Early Childhood–Onset Syndromes

Any infant with retinal dysfunction and a low ERG should be carefully screened for congenital syndromes and metabolic disorders that affect the retina before being diagnosed with Leber congenital amaurosis (LCA). Although there are currently 7 known monogenic or primary forms of LCA, *complicated LCA* is a term used to refer to systemic diseases that result in severe infantile-onset retinal degeneration. Because the site of mutation in a gene may give variance in severity of symptoms and onset, the same disease may have infantile onset with a severe mutation, and a childhood onset with a milder mutation in the same gene. The systemic disorders that mimic LCA include, among others, the various *neuronal ceroid lipofuscinoses (Batten disease)* and peroxisome disorders such as *Refsum disease, Zellweger (cerebrohepatorenal) syndrome,* and *neonatal adrenoleukodystrophy.* Important diagnostic clues that differentiate these LCA-like disorders from primary LCA are seizures and a clear deterioration of neurologic and mental status, usually with an obvious decline in school performance. Frequently, before the storage disease is found, poor eyesight is blamed for declining cognitive and neuromuscular skills, and parents may compensate for their children's reduced cognitive abilities by answering all questions directed by the physician.

Birch DG. Retinal degeneration in retinitis pigmentosa and neuronal ceroid lipofuscinosis: An overview. *Mol Genet Metab.* 1999;66:356–66.

Dharmaraj SR, Silva ER, Pina AL, et al. Mutational analysis and clinical correlation in Leber congenital amaurosis. *Ophthalmic Genet.* 2000;21:135–150.

Bardet-Biedl Complex of Diseases

The *Bardet-Biedl syndrome* comprises a number of different diseases with a similar constellation of findings, including pigmentary retinopathy (with or without pigment deposits), obesity, polydactyly, hypogonadism, and mental retardation. These disorders have previously been classified as autosomal recessive, but recent molecular studies strongly suggest that many are multigenic, with 2 or even 3 different mutations contributing to the phenotype. Macular pigment mottling and peripheral retinal atrophy are present, usually without bone spicule pigment clumping (Fig 10-1). Affected patients are most easily recognized by obesity and the history or presence of polydactyly. It may be necessary to inspect feet or hands for signs of scar tissue from infantile excision of the extra digits. The hands often appear puffy with indistinct knuckles. Because these patients tend to have more a severe retinopathy and learning disabilities, extra attention should be given to supporting the parents in their efforts to obtain special educational support.

Sheffield VC, Nishimura D, Stone EM. The molecular genetics of Bardet-Biedl syndrome. *Curr Opin Genet Dev.* 2001;11:317–321.

Katsanis N, Lupski JR, Beales PL. Exploring the molecular basis of Bardet-Biedl syndrome. *Hum Mol Genet.* 2001;10:2293–2299.

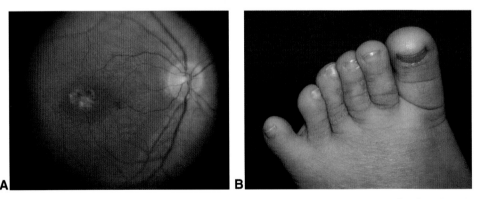

Figure 10-1 Bardet-Biedl syndrome. **A,** Macular pigmentary alterations. **B,** Polydactyly. *(Photographs courtesy of John R. Heckenlively, MD.)*

Hearing Loss and Pigmentary Retinopathy

Usher syndrome

Usher syndrome is the name most commonly given to the association of retinitis pigmentosa (RP) and *congenital* sensorineural hearing loss, whether partial or profound. The disease was first described by Charles Usher, a British ophthalmologist, in 1906. Some RP patients have acquired deafness in later adult years, and this is not usually classified as Usher syndrome. Both the profound (type I) and partial (type II) forms are inherited in an autosomal recessive manner and tend to be stable through adult life. The ophthalmologist should be attuned to patients with RP who present with a nasal intonation to their speech or wear hearing aids, characteristic of Usher type II patients. Recently, a slowly progressive deafness has been identified in one subgroup of Usher patients (gene *USH3A*) due to mutations in clarin-1, a transmembrane protein with a possible role in hair cell and photoreceptor synapses. However, the hearing level of most Usher patients is typically stable over time.

Currently there are 11 types of Usher syndrome in which the chromosomal location is known; of these, 7 have cloned genes (see RetNet for details and references). For example, Usher type 2A is caused by mutations in *usherin* (at chromosome 1q41), which encodes a basement membrane protein found in many tissues, including structural basement membranes in the retina and inner ear. Usher type 1B is caused by a defective myosin, a common component of cilia and microvilli. This finding is intriguing because photoreceptors are modified ciliated cells and cilia are also end organs for otologic function. Usher type 1C is caused by the *harmonin* gene, which encodes a protein expressed in inner ear sensory hair cells.

The exact incidence of Usher syndrome has been difficult to determine, but surveys of RP patients suggest that about 10% are profoundly deaf, and ophthalmologic examinations of children in deaf schools reveal that approximately 6% have RP. The prevalence of Usher syndrome is thought to be 3 cases per 100,000.

In addition to Usher syndrome, a number of other genetic conditions and environmental insults may lead to pigmentary retinopathy and hearing loss, including Alport syndrome, Alström and Cockayne syndromes, dysplasia spondyloepiphysaria congenita, Hurler syndrome, and Refsum disease. By careful study of individual patients and families, the diagnosis of Usher syndrome may be made with relative certainty. Molecular testing for specific forms of Usher syndrome will confirm the diagnosis.

Weil D, Blanchard S, Kaplan J, et al. Defective myosin VIIA gene responsible for Usher syndrome type 1B. *Nature*. 1995;374:60–61.

Kimberling WJ, Weston M, Moller C. Clinical and genetic heterogeneity of Usher syndrome. In: Wright AF, Jay B, eds. *Molecular Genetics of Inherited Eye Disorders*. Chur, Switzerland: Harwood Academic; 1994:359–382.

Neuromuscular Disorders

Pigmentary retinopathy in association with complex neuromuscular pathology is seen in a variety of disorders, including *spinocerebellar degenerations* such as Friedreich's ataxia, some of the *olivopontocerebellar atrophies, Charcot-Marie-Tooth disease, myotonic dystrophy, neuronal ceroid lipofuscinosis (Batten disease), progressive external ophthalmoplegia syndromes,* and *peroxisome disorders* (Zellweger syndrome, Refsum disease, neonatal adrenoleukodystrophy) (see Table 10-1). Mitochondrial, autosomal dominant, and autosomal recessive inheritance patterns can all be found in this group of disorders. These neurologic conditions vary widely in age of onset and retinal findings. The diagnosis is normally made in collaboration with a neurologist or medical geneticist. The role of the ophthalmologist is to confirm the pigmentary retinopathy and to assist in visual rehabilitation of the patient. The ERG abnormalities found in these neurologic disorders only confirm the presence of retinopathy but are not specifically diagnostic for any one disorder.

Duchenne muscular dystrophy has not traditionally been thought of as a disease involving the retina, and patients do not ordinarily have any visual symptoms. However, recent studies have found a striking ERG abnormality in Duchenne patients that may be useful in diagnosis and relevant to understanding retinal function. The ERG shows a negative waveform similar to that in congenital stationary night blindness (CSNB) patients who have a normal a-wave but reduced b-wave (see Chapter 8). This ERG is suggestive of a defective "on-response" pathway, but these Duchenne patients do not have night blindness. It is interesting that Duchenne muscular dystrophy is caused by mutations in the gene for dystrophin, a protein abundant in muscle but also found in neural synaptic regions and in the retina.

Folz SJ, Trobe JD. The peroxisome and the eye. *Surv Ophthalmol.* 1991;35:353–368.

Sigesmund DA, Weleber RG, Pillers DA, et al. Characterization of the ocular phenotype of Duchenne and Becker muscular dystrophy. *Ophthalmology.* 1994;101:856–865.

Other Organ System Disorders

Most retinopathies in association with other organ systems are rare and genetic, and the Online Mendelian Inheritance in Man website (OMIM) can be used to help identify candidate diseases. Collaboration with pediatric and medical geneticists is particularly helpful with these rare diseases.

Renal disease

Several forms of congenital renal disease may be associated with retinal degeneration. *Familial juvenile nephronophthisis* is part of a family of renal-retinal dysplasias, most of which are inherited in the autosomal recessive manner. Juvenile-onset renal failure is accompanied by pigmentary retinal degeneration that may be sectorial. Some of these patients have abnormalities of their bony growth plates, leading to shortness of stature. Patients with the Bardet-Biedl complex disorders commonly have urethral reflux with pyelonephritis and kidney damage. Renal disease is also a component of Alström disease and Alport disease. Type II membranoproliferative glomerulonephritis is associated with a myriad of drusenlike deposits throughout the fundus.

Gastrointestinal disease

Familial adenomatous polyposis (Gardner syndrome) is associated with pigmented lesions similar to congenital hypertrophy of the RPE. The lesions in Gardner syndrome, however, are smaller, ovoid, more variegated, and typically multiple and bilateral (Fig 10-2). This oncogene is inherited in autosomal dominant fashion with incomplete expression. The pigmented retinal lesions constitute an important marker for identifying family members at risk for developing colonic polyps, which have a high malignant potential.

Dermatologic diseases

Ichthyosis is abnormal scaling, dryness, and tightness of the skin that may be found in conjunction with the pigmentary retinopathy of Refsum disease and in Sjögren-Larsson syndrome. *Incontinentia pigmenti (Bloch-Sulzberger syndrome)* is a rare X-linked disorder that causes death in male fetuses and is characterized in females by a peculiar triphasic dermopathy and variable involvement of the eyes, teeth, and central nervous system. Ocular involvement occurs in approximately one third of affected females and includes pigmentary abnormalities as well as peripheral retinal avascularity that may lead to cicatricial retinal detachment (see also BCSC Section 6, *Pediatric Ophthalmology and Strabismus*). Pseudoxanthoma elasticum is associated with angioid streaks and a peau d'orange fundus appearance (see Chapter 4).

Goldberg MF, Custis PH. Retinal and other manifestations of incontinentia pigmenti (Bloch-Sulzberger syndrome). *Ophthalmology.* 1993;100:1645–1654.

Romania A, Zakov ZN, Church JM, et al. Retinal pigment epithelium lesions as a biomarker of disease in patients with familial adenomatous polyposis: a follow-up report. *Ophthalmology.* 1992;99:911–913.

Paraneoplastic Retinopathy (CAR and MAR Syndromes)

Retinal degeneration may occasionally be a complication of cancer through a paraneoplastic immunologic mechanism. BCSC Section 9, *Intraocular Inflammation and Uveitis*, explains the role of the immune system in this process.

The two main paraneoplastic retinopathy syndromes are *cancer-associated retinopathy (CAR)* and *melanoma-associated retinopathy (MAR)*. It is hypothesized that a small

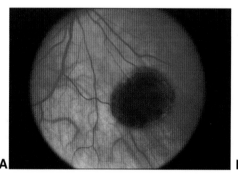 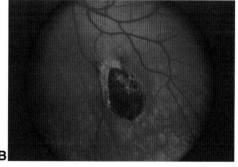

Figure 10-2 Hyperpigmented RPE lesions. **A,** Congenital hypertrophy of the RPE. These isolated lesions typically are rounded, with very dense pigmentation (except for occasional lacunae) and a thin depigmented halo. **B,** Pigmented fundus lesions in Gardner syndrome (familial adenomatous polyposis). These lesions are smaller, more ovoid, more variegated in color, and usually multiple and bilateral. The surrounding RPE may be abnormal. *(Photograph A courtesy of Michael F. Marmor, MD; photograph B courtesy of Elias Traboulsi, MD.)*

number of carcinoma and melanoma tumors express protein antigens that are the same as or cross react with retinal proteins. The body is stimulated to produce antibodies that react to retina causing progressive degeneration. Patients with CAR may complain of rapidly progressive loss of peripheral and even central vision, often accompanied by photopsias and a ring scotoma. Fundus examination shows arterial narrowing but may demonstrate no pigmentary alterations early in the disease course (Fig 10-3). Goldmann visual field examinations document dramatic field loss over a few months, in contrast to RP, which typically shows a chronic, slow loss. The ERG is severely reduced (both a- and b-waves), with both rods and cones affected, but it may have negative waveforms if the middle retina is affected to a greater extent. On occasion, the loss of retinal function may precede the clinical recognition of the cancer. Therefore, any late-onset, rapidly progressive retinal dysfunction should raise suspicion of an underlying malignancy or at least the possibility of autoimmune retinopathy.

Patients with CAR typically have multiple antiretinal antibodies on Western blot studies, but only antirecoverin (23 kD) antibodies have so far been clearly shown to be pathologic to the retina. Immunosuppressive therapy, given in close cooperation with the patient's oncologist, will halt and sometimes reverse the vision loss in patients with CAR. If the patient is too ill for systemic immunosuppression, multiple periocular corticosteroid injections may be effective.

Recently, it was demonstrated that there is a high association between cystoid macular edema and circulating antiretinal antibodies in patients with RP. Overall, it is estimated that 1%–2% of RP patients have antirecoverin antibodies, which may be exacerbating their disease.

Patients with melanoma-associated retinopathy develop visual loss and night blindness and show a negative ERG waveform similar to that seen in CSNB. Their antibodies

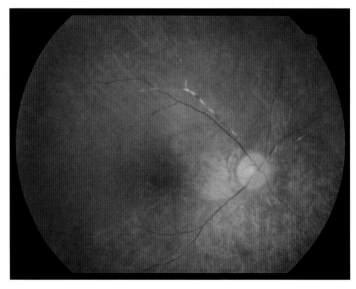

Figure 10-3 Cancer-associated retinopathy in patient with ovarian carcinoma. Note severe vascular attenuation without obvious pigmentary alterations. *(Photograph courtesy of John R. Heckenlively, MD.)*

are directed toward retinal bipolar cells. Confirmation of the diagnosis is by histopathologic staining.

Alexander KR, Barnes CS, Fishman GA, et al. Nature of the cone ON-pathway dysfunction in melanoma-associated retinopathy. *Invest Ophthalmol Vis Sci.* 2002;43:1189–1197.

Heckenlively JR, Jordan BL, Aptsiauri N. Association of antiretinal antibodies and cystoid macular edema in patients with retinitis pigmentosa. *Am J Ophthalmol.* 1999;127:565–573.

Keltner JL, Thirkill CE, Tyler NK, et al. Management and monitoring of cancer-associated retinopathy. *Arch Ophthalmol.* 1992;110:48–53.

Keltner JL, Thirkill CE, Yip PT. Clinical and immunologic characteristics of melanoma-associated retinopathy syndrome: eleven new cases and a review of 51 previously published cases. *J Neuroophthalmol.* 2001;21:173–187.

Metabolic Diseases

It is important to consider metabolic diseases in evaluating patients with retinal degeneration, although a detailed description of the many metabolic disorders that have retinal manifestations is beyond the scope of this book. Some disorders, such as albinism and the central nervous system abnormalities, are covered more fully in BCSC Section 6, *Pediatric Ophthalmology and Strabismus.* Some of these disorders, such as abetalipoproteinemia and Refsum disease, are among the differential diagnostic concerns for RP, although their retinopathy may be granular and atypical.

Albinism

Albinism refers to a group of different genetic abnormalities in which the synthesis of melanin is reduced or absent. The reduction in melanin biosynthesis can effect the eyes, skin, and hair follicles, resulting in *oculocutaneous albinism.* If the skin and hair appear normally pigmented and only the ocular pigmentation is clinically affected, the condition is called *ocular albinism.* This terminology may not be accurate histopathologically, because biopsy of some patients with ocular albinism has shown cutaneous pigmentary dilution as well as giant melanosomes in both the skin and the eye. All forms of albinism have been shown on VEP studies to have abnormal retinogeniculostriate projections, in which the temporal nerve fibers decussate rather than project to the ipsilateral lateral geniculate body. The functional significance of this finding has yet to be elucidated.

Regardless of the type of albinism, the ocular involvement generally conforms to 1 of 2 clinical patterns: (1) congenitally subnormal visual acuity (typically 20/100 to 20/400) and nystagmus, and (2) normal or minimally reduced visual acuity without nystagmus. The first pattern is true albinism; the second has been termed *albinoidism* because of its milder visual consequences. Both patterns share common clinical features of photophobia, iris transillumination, and hypopigmented fundi. They differ by whether the fovea develops: in true albinism, the fovea is hypoplastic, with no foveal pit or reflex and no evident luteal pigment in the fovea (Fig 10-4).

Mutations in at least 7 separate genes can cause a reduction in melanin pigment biosynthesis, producing the various clinical features associated with ocular and oculocutaneous albinism. *Ocular albinism* is usually transmitted as an X-linked recessive

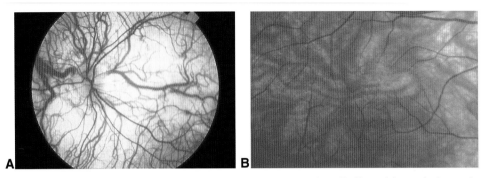

Figure 10-4 Albinism. **A,** Generalized fundus hypopigmentation. **B,** Foveal hypoplasia: no foveal reflex or luteal pigment evident. *(Photographs courtesy of Carl D. Regillo, MD.)*

disorder. Female carriers of X-linked ocular albinism may show partial iris transillumination and fundus pigment mosaicism. There are many types of autosomal recessive *oculocutaneous albinism*, including one tyrosinase-negative and several tyrosinase-positive forms (which have been shown to be nonallelic). In childhood, all patients with oculocutaneous albinism appear similarly hypopigmented. However, with age, patients with tyrosinase-positive forms gradually accumulate more pigment, with some darkening of the skin, hair, and irides over many years. In general, the more pigmentation the patient demonstrates, such as around hair follicles and in the RPE in the posterior pole, the better is the visual prognosis. Many patients demonstrate improvement in their nystagmus and visual acuity as pigmentation increases with age. Genetic counseling depends on carefully establishing the inheritance pattern and may involve molecular testing.

It is important for the clinician to be aware of 2 forms of potentially lethal oculocutaneous albinism. In *Chédiak-Higashi syndrome*, albinism is combined with extreme susceptibility to infections and other complications that often lead to death in childhood or youth. *Hermansky-Pudlak syndrome* is characterized by a platelet defect that causes easy bruising and bleeding. Most Hermansky-Pudlak patients in the United States have been of Puerto Rican origin. If either of these 2 types of albinism is suspected, hematologic consultation is imperative.

International Albinism Center Albinism Database web site: http://www.cbc.umn.edu/tad

King RA, Jackson IJ, Oetting WS. Human albinism and mouse models. In: Wright AF, Jay B, eds. *Molecular Genetics of Inherited Eye Disorders.* Chur, Switzerland: Harwood Academic; 1994:89–122.

Oetting WS, King RA. Molecular basis of albinism: mutations and polymorphisms of pigmentation genes associated with albinism. *Hum Mutat.* 1999;13:99–115.

Central Nervous System Metabolic Abnormalities

A wide range of fundus changes, from pigmentary retinopathy to a cherry-red spot, may be associated with inherited metabolic diseases known to affect the CNS and retina. Although a comprehensive description of them is beyond the scope of this book, the following discussion includes some of the most significant conditions (see Table 10-1).

See also Table 29-1 in BCSC Section 6, *Pediatric Ophthalmology and Strabismus*, for the ocular findings in inborn errors of metabolism.

Neuronal ceroid lipofuscinosis (Batten disease)

The neuronal ceroid lipofuscinoses (NCL) are a group of autosomal recessive diseases caused by the accumulation of waxy lipopigments within the lysosomes of neurons and other cells. The accumulation of lipopigments such as ceroid and lipofuscin activates cellular dysfunction and death, possibly by apoptosis. The disorders are characterized by progressive dementia, seizures, and visual loss with pigmentary retinopathy in early-onset cases. The diagnosis is made on clinical grounds and by demonstrating characteristic curvilinear, fingerprint, or granular inclusions on electron microscopy of a peripheral blood smear or conjunctival or other biopsy tissue.

Several types of NCL have been described, based in part on the age of symptom onset. Gene defects have been proposed for 3 forms of the disorder, but the specific enzyme deficiency is not known for any of the forms. The infantile and juvenile types are associated with pigmentary retinopathies:

- infantile (Haltia-Santavuori) with onset between 8 and 18 months of age
- late infantile (Jansky-Bielschowsky) between 2 and 4 years of age
- early juvenile (Lake-Cavanagh) between 4 and 6 years
- juvenile (Spielmeyer-Vogt-Batten) between 6 and 8 years

Ocular findings in infantile NCL include optic atrophy, macular pigmentary changes with mottling of the fundus periphery, and low or absent ERG. Retinal changes in the infantile forms can lead to confusion with Leber congenital amaurosis. The late infantile and juvenile cases may show macular granularity or a bull's-eye maculopathy, with variable degrees of peripheral RPE change, optic atrophy, and attenuation of the retinal blood vessels (Fig 10-5). The 2 adult forms of NCL do not have ocular manifestations.

Abetalipoproteinemia and vitamin A deficiency

Abetalipoproteinemia is an autosomal recessive disorder in which the apolipoprotein B is not synthesized, leading to fat malabsorption, fat-soluble vitamin deficiencies, and retinal and spinocerebellar degeneration. Red blood cells show acanthocytosis. Therapy with vitamins A and E is needed to prevent or ameliorate the retinal degeneration. Testing for vitamin A levels is useful diagnostically in these and other retinopathies associated with vitamin A deficiency states.

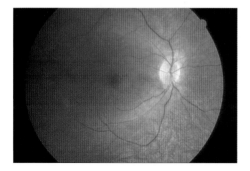

Figure 10-5 Optic atrophy, retinal vascular attenuation, and peripheral pigmentary loss in Batten disease (juvenile neuronal ceroid lipofuscinosis). *(Photograph courtesy of Elias Traboulsi, MD.)*

The most common form of vitamin A deficiency retinopathy occurs in patients who have undergone gastric bypass surgery for Crohn disease or obesity. These patients have malabsorption problems and may develop a blind loop syndrome, where an overgrowth of bacteria consumes vitamin A. The patient notes night blindness and, if untreated, will eventually demonstrate loss of foveal function and diffuse drusenlike spots similar to those in retinitis punctata albescens. Prior to the development of retinal degeneration, the condition is fully reversible by instituting vitamin A therapy.

Peroxisomal disorders and Refsum disease

The peroxisomal disorders are mostly autosomal recessive diseases caused by dysfunction or absence of peroxisomes or peroxisomal enzymes. The biochemical hallmarks are defective oxidation and accumulation of very long chain fatty acids. *Zellweger syndrome* is the prototype of peroxisomal diseases. Severe, infantile-onset retinal degeneration is associated in this disorder with hypotonia, psychomotor retardation, seizures, characteristic facies, renal cysts, and hepatic interstitial fibrosis. Death usually occurs in infancy. Patients with *neonatal adrenoleukodystrophy* (Fig 10-6) also present in infancy but generally survive until 7–10 years of age.

Similar but less severe findings are present in *infantile Refsum disease,* so-called because serum phytanic acid is elevated. Classic *Refsum disease* (phytanic acid storage disease) may not be a peroxisomal disorder. Sometimes not diagnosed until adulthood, it is characterized by pigmentary retinopathy, with reduced ERG, cerebellar ataxia, polyneuropathy, anosmia, hearing loss, and cardiomyopathy (Fig 10-7). Night blindness may be an early symptom. Diagnosis is made by demonstrating elevated plasma levels of phytanic acid or reduced phytanic acid oxidase activity in cultured fibroblasts. Dietary restriction of phytanic acid precursors may slow or stabilize the retinal degeneration.

Mucopolysaccharidoses

The systemic mucopolysaccharidoses (MPSs) are caused by inherited defects in catabolic lysosomal exoenzymes that degrade the glycosaminoglycans dermatan sulfate, keratan

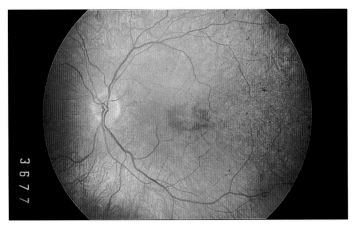

Figure 10-6 Retinal arteriolar attenuation, diffuse pigmentary alterations, and mild optic atrophy in neonatal adrenoleukodystrophy. *(Photograph courtesy of Mark W. Johnson, MD.)*

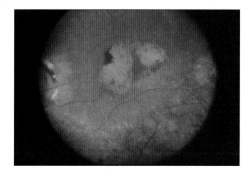

Figure 10-7 Pigmentary retinopathy with macular atrophy in Refsum disease. *(Photograph courtesy of Elias Traboulsi, MD.)*

sulfate, and heparan sulfate. Consequently, excessive quantities of incompletely metabolized acid mucopolysaccharides and/or complex lipids are stored in lysosomes. The MPSs are transmitted as autosomal recessive traits except for type II (Hunter), which is X-linked recessive (see Table 10-1).

Only those MPSs in which heparan sulfate is stored are associated with retinal dystrophy. These include MPS IH *(Hurler syndrome)* and MPS IS *(Scheie syndrome),* the clinical features of which include coarse facies, mental retardation, corneal clouding, and retinal degeneration. The retinal pigmentary changes may be subtle, but an abnormal ERG is recorded. MPS II *(Hunter syndrome)* also features a pigmentary retinopathy but omits corneal clouding; the patients have coarse facies and short stature and may show mental retardation. MPS III *(Sanfilippo syndrome)* shows milder somatic stigmata but severe pigmentary retinopathy.

Other lysosomal metabolism disorders

Tay-Sachs disease (GM$_2$ gangliosidosis type I) is the most common ganglioside storage disease and is caused by deficient subunit A of hexosaminidase A. Glycolipid accumulation in the brain and retina causes mental retardation and blindness, and death generally occurs between the ages of 2 and 5 years. A cherry-red spot is prominent because ganglion cells surrounding the fovea become filled with ganglioside and appear grayish or white (Fig 10-8). The subfoveal RPE and choroidal pigmentation thus contrast to the surrounding white as the cherry-red spot. Sandhoff disease (GM$_2$ gangliosidosis type II) and generalized gangliosidosis (GM$_1$ gangliosidosis type I) can also show cherry red spots.

The chronic nonneuronopathic adult form of *Gaucher disease* does not have cerebral involvement. This disease is characterized by considerable accumulation of glucosylceramide in the liver, spleen, lymph nodes, skin, and bone marrow. Some patients have a cherry-red spot; others show whitish subretinal lesions in the midperiphery of the fundus. The different types of *Niemann-Pick disease* are caused by the absence of different sphingomyelinase isoenzymes. Type B (chronic Niemann-Pick disease, sea-blue histiocyte syndrome) is the mildest, and although there is no functional involvement of the CNS, patients have a macular halo that is considered diagnostic (Fig 10-9). Type A (acute neuronopathic) Niemann-Pick disease shows a cherry-red spot in about 50% of cases.

Cherry-red spots are observed in sialidoses and galactosialidoses. These conditions include mucolipidosis I, the cherry-red spot–myoclonus syndrome, and Goldberg-Cotlier

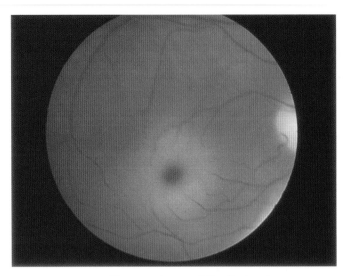

Figure 10-8 Cherry-red spot of Tay-Sachs disease.

syndrome (GM$_1$ gangliosidosis type IV). Mucolipidosis IV causes diffuse retinal degeneration.

Fabry disease (angiokeratoma corporis diffusum) is an X-linked condition caused by mutations in the alpha-galactosidase A gene. Ceramide trihexoside accumulates in the smooth muscle of blood vessels in the kidneys, skin, gastrointestinal tract, CNS, heart, and reticuloendothelial system, leading to various ocular and systemic clinical findings. The first symptom may be burning paresthesias or pain in the extremities in late childhood. Ocular signs include corneal verticillata (whorls), tortuous conjunctiva vessels, tortuous and dilated retinal vessels, and lens changes (Fig 10-10). Vascular tortuosity of conjunctival and retinal vessels is also characteristic of fucosidosis.

Folz SJ, Trobe JD. The peroxisome and the eye. *Surv Ophthalmol.* 1991;35:353–368.

Palmer JD, Mukai S. Metabolic diseases. In: Regillo CD, Brown GC, Flynn HW Jr, eds. *Vitreoretinal Disease: The Essentials.* New York: Thieme; 1999:347–364.

Weleber RG, Gregory-Evans K. Retinitis pigmentosa and allied disorders. In: Ryan SJ, ed. *Retina.* 3rd ed. St. Louis: Mosby; 2001:362–460.

Amino Acid Disorders

In *cystinosis*, intralysosomal cystine accumulates because of a defect in transport out of lysosomes. Three types are recognized, all inherited in autosomal recessive fashion: nephropathic, late-onset (or intermediate), and benign. Cystine crystals accumulate in the cornea and conjunctiva in all 3 types, but only patients with the nephropathic type develop retinopathy. These patients are asymptomatic until 8–15 months of age, when they present with progressive renal failure, growth retardation, renal rickets, and hypothyroidism. The retinopathy is characterized by areas of patchy depigmentation of the RPE alternating with irregularly distributed pigment clumps. Despite the abnormal fundus appearance, no significant visual disturbance occurs. Treatment with cysteamine,

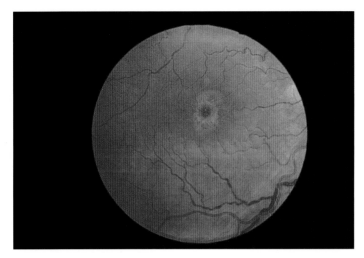

Figure 10-9 Macular halo in chronic Niemann-Pick disease. *(Photograph courtesy of Mark W. Johnson, MD.)*

which reacts with lysosomal cystine to form a mixed disulfide that can leave the lysosome, may be beneficial.

Mitochondrial Disorders

Mutations and deletions in mitochondrial DNA are associated with a number of different retinopathies, many of which are associated with myopathy. *Chronic progressive external ophthalmoplegia* belongs to a group of diseases collectively termed *mitochondrial myopathies,* in which mitochondria are abnormally shaped and increased in number; "ragged-red" fibers may be evident on muscle biopsy. The syndrome is characterized by progressive external ophthalmoplegia, atypical RP, and various systemic abnormalities. When associated with cardiomyopathy, the disorder is known as the *Kearns-Sayre syndrome* (Table 10-2). Onset is usually prior to age 10. The severity of the pigmentary retinopathy is highly variable, often showing mottled macular pigmentary changes early in the course and only rarely involving bone spicule–like changes (Fig 10-11). Many patients retain good visual function and a normal ERG; others, especially those with full-blown Kearns-Sayre syndrome, have severe retinopathy with an extinguished ERG. Other mitochondrial myopathies with pigmentary retinopathy include the *NARP syndrome* (neurogenic muscle weakness, ataxia, and retinitis pigmentosa) and *MELAS* (mitochondrial encephalomyopathy, lactic acidosis, and stroke).

Brown MD, Lott MR, Wallace DC. Mitochondrial DNA mutations and the eye. In: Wright AF, Jay B, eds. *Molecular Genetics of Inherited Eye Disorders.* Chur, Switzerland: Harwood Academic; 1994:469–490.

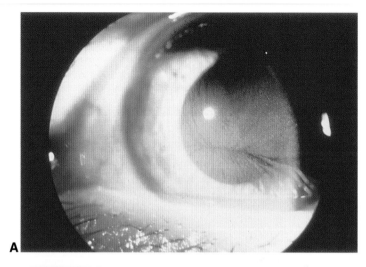

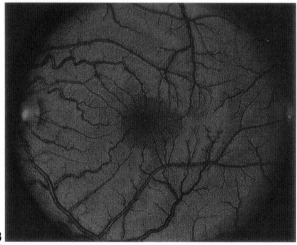

Figure 10-10 Fabry disease. **A,** Corneal whorls (cornea verticillata). **B,** Retinal vascular tortuosity.

Table 10-2 Characteristic Features of Kearns-Sayre Syndrome

Chronic progressive external ophthalmoplegia
Retinal pigmentary degeneration
Heart block

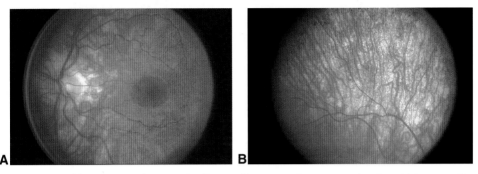

Figure 10-11 Pigmentary changes in Kearns-Sayre syndrome, a mitochondrial myopathy. Retinal function is often quite good. **A,** Macula. **B,** Periphery. *(Photographs courtesy of Michael F. Marmor, MD.)*

Systemic Drug Toxicity

Chloroquine Derivatives

Although retinal toxicity from chloroquine remains a problem in many parts of the world, it is seen infrequently in the United States, where the drug has largely been replaced by hydroxychloroquine for the treatment of rheumatologic and dermatologic conditions. The mechanism of retinal toxicity from these drugs remains unclear. Both agents bind to melanin in the RPE, and this may serve to concentrate the drugs or to prolong their adverse effects. Although the incidence of toxicity is very low, it is of serious concern because associated visual loss rarely recovers and may even progress after the drug is discontinued. Patients and their primary care physicians must be made fully aware of the ophthalmic risks and the need for regular screening examinations to detect retinal toxicity at an early stage (before symptomatic visual loss).

The earliest signs of toxicity include bilateral paracentral visual field changes (best detected with a *red* test object) and a subtle granular depigmentation of the paracentral RPE. With continued drug exposure, there is progressive development of a bilateral atrophic bull's-eye maculopathy (Fig 10-12) and paracentral scotomata, which may in severe cases ultimately spread over the entire fundus, causing widespread retinal atrophy and visual loss. Some patients develop intraepithelial corneal verticillata.

Ophthalmic screening of patients on chloroquine or hydroxychloroquine is aimed primarily at the early detection and minimization of toxicity. As summarized in an Information Statement from the American Academy of Ophthalmology, there appears to be minimal risk of toxicity for individuals using less than 6.5 mg/kg/day of hydroxychloroquine or 3 mg/kg/day of choroquine, particularly in the first 5 years of treatment. In addition to higher daily and cumulative doses, other risk factors for retinal toxicity include obesity ("safe" daily doses are based on lean body weight), kidney or liver disease, older age (ie, over 60 years), and possibly concomitant retinal disease.

Recommendations in screening for chloroquine and hydroxychloroquine retinopathy. Information Statement. San Francisco: American Academy of Ophthalmology; 2002:http://www.aao.org.

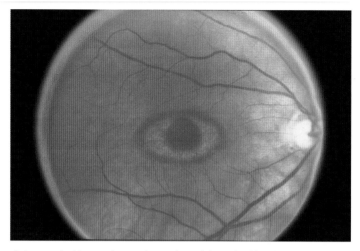

Figure 10-12 Advanced chloroquine retinopathy with typical bull's-eye pattern. *(Photograph courtesy of Michael F. Marmor, MD.)*

Baseline evaluation for patients commencing treatment with a chloroquine derivative should include a complete ophthalmologic examination, with meticulous attention to the macular appearance, test of color vision, examination of the central visual field with Amsler grid and/or static perimetry (eg, Humphrey 10-2 program), and fundus photography for follow-up comparisons. Ideally, central visual field assessments should be performed with a red Amsler grid or a red visual field test object because scotomata detected in this fashion may precede symptomatic visual loss and may even be reversible. Patients should be instructed in the use of the Amsler grid for self-monitoring at home on a regular basis. Annual screening examinations are recommended for everyone in higher-risk categories, including all patients with more than 5 years of usage, and should include a complete ophthalmologic examination and red Amsler grid testing (or Humphrey 10-2 field testing). Cessation of the drug at the first sign of toxicity is recommended.

Phenothiazines

Phenothiazines, including chlorpromazine (Thorazine) and thioridazine (Mellaril), are concentrated in uveal tissue and RPE by binding to melanin granules. High-dose *chlorpromazine* therapy commonly results in abnormal pigmentation of the eyelids, interpalpebral conjunctiva, cornea, and anterior lens capsule; anterior and posterior subcapsular cataracts may develop. However, pigmentary retinopathy from chlorpromazine is rare, if it occurs at all.

In contrast, *thioridazine* causes severe retinopathy that can develop within a few weeks or months of high-dose utilization. Retinopathy is rare at doses of 800 mg/day or less. Initially, patients complain of blurred vision, and the fundus shows coarse retinal pigment stippling in the posterior pole (Fig 10-13A). Over time, the retinopathy evolves to widespread but patchy atrophy of the pigment epithelium and choriocapillaris, with a characteristic nummular pattern of involvement (Fig 10-13B). Fundus changes in the late stages may be confused with choroideremia or Bietti crystalline corneoretinal dystrophy; the symptoms include visual field loss and night blindness.

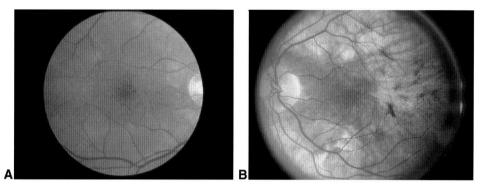

Figure 10-13 Thioridazine toxicity. **A,** The initial change is a coarse, granular maculopathy. **B,** The degeneration evolves into a nummular pattern with patchy areas of hypo- and hyperpigmentation. *(Photographs courtesy of Michael F. Marmor, MD.)*

Visual function may improve after cessation of the drug but will sometimes deteriorate years later if the chorioretinal atrophy progresses slowly. It is not known whether these late atrophic changes after discontinuation of thioridazine or chloroquine represent continued toxicity of the drugs or a decompensation of cells that were injured when the drugs were used initially.

Patients using thioridazine are generally not monitored ophthalmologically because toxicity is rare at standard doses. However, suspected cases or patients who have taken the drug at high doses should have a full evaluation of visual function that includes an ERG and monitoring comparable to that used for the chloroquine derivatives.

Other Agents

Tamoxifen is an antiestrogen drug that has been used for more than 20 years to treat patients with advanced breast cancer. It is also widely used as adjuvant therapy following primary treatment for early-stage breast cancer and continues to be studied for use in preventing breast cancer in women with an increased risk of developing the disease. Retinopathy is rare at the dose levels currently used, but crystalline retinopathy has been reported in patients receiving high-dose therapy (daily doses over 200 mg and over 100 g, cumulatively). The maculopathy is characterized by crystalline deposits and sometimes macular edema (Fig 10-14A). Moderate degrees of both functional loss and anatomic degenerative changes can occur.

A crystalline maculopathy may also be seen after ingestion of high doses of *canthaxanthine*, a carotenoid available in health food stores used to simulate tanning. Canthaxanthine retinopathy is generally asymptomatic, and the deposits resolve when the drug is stopped (Fig 10-14B). Crystalline deposits of oxalate have been seen after the ingestion of *ethylene glycol* and after prolonged *methoxyflurane* anesthesia administered to patients with renal dysfunction (Table 10-3).

Intravenous administration of *desferrioxamine* in doses of 3 to 12 g/24 hours for the treatment of transfusional hemosiderosis can result in rapid bilateral visual loss (usually starting 7 to 10 days after treatment) with nyctalopia, ring scotoma, and reduced ERG responses. The fundi may appear normal initially, with widespread mottled pigmentary changes usually developing within several weeks. Return of visual function occurs over 3 to 4 months, with most patients recovering normal acuity.

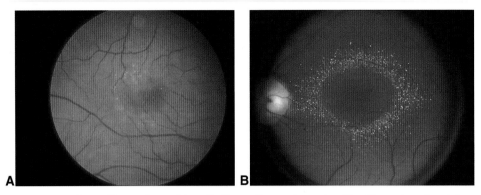

Figure 10-14 Crystalline retinopathies. **A,** Tamoxifen retinopathy. Significant functional damage may be associated with the crystalline changes. **B,** Canthaxanthine retinopathy. Retinal function is usually normal. *(Photograph A courtesy of Michael F. Marmor, MD; photograph B courtesy of William Mieler, MD.)*

Table 10-3 Crystalline Retinopathy

Systemic disease
  Primary hereditary hyperoxaluria
  Cystinosis
  Secondary oxalosis as a result of chronic renal failure and hemodialysis
  Sjögren-Larsson syndrome

Drug induced
  Tamoxifen
  Canthaxanthine
  Talc
  Nitrofurantoin
  Methoxyflurane anesthesia (secondary oxalosis)
  Ethylene glycol ingestion (secondary oxalosis)

Ocular
  Bietti crystalline dystrophy
  Calcific drusen
  Gyrate atrophy
  Retinal telangiectasia

Some patients taking *isotretinoin* (Accutane) for acne have complained of poor night vision and been found to have abnormal dark adaptation curves and ERG responses. Toxicity seems to be infrequent but is more likely in patients undergoing repetitive courses of therapy. The changes are largely reversible.

The use of *rifabutin* in patients with the human immunodeficiency virus (HIV) as prophylaxis against *Mycobacterium avium*–complex infection has been associated with the development of both anterior and posterior uveitis. Hypopyon is sometimes seen. The inflammation is reversible with discontinuation of the medicine.

In rare cases, the cardiac glycosides *(digitalis)* may produce blurred vision, pericentral scotomata, defective color vision, and xanthopsia ("yellow vision"). The drug's ocular effects result from a cone dysfunction syndrome that reverses with cessation of the drug.

Transient blue tinting of vision and temporary abnormal ERG responses have been observed in patients taking high doses of *sildenafil* (Viagra). The visual symptom may occur in up to 50% of patients ingesting more than 100 mg of sildenafil, but no permanent retinal toxic effects have been reported.

Marmor MF. Is thioridazine retinopathy progressive? Relationship of pigmentary changes to visual function. *Br J Ophthalmol.* 1990;74:739–742.

Marmor MF. Sildenafil (Viagra) and ophthalmology [editorial]. *Arch Ophthalmol.* 1999;117:518–519.

Mittra RA, Mieler WF. Drug and light ocular toxicity. In: Regillo CD, Brown GC, Flynn HW Jr, eds. *Vitreoretinal Disease: The Essentials.* New York: Thieme; 1999:545.

Weinberg DV, Jones BE. Retinal toxicity of systemic drugs. In: Albert DM, Jakobiec FA, eds. *Principles and Practice of Ophthalmology.* Philadelphia: Saunders; 2000:2240–2251.

The authors would like to thank John R. Heckenlively, MD, for his significant contributions to this chapter.

CHAPTER 11

Peripheral Retinal Abnormalities

Retinal Breaks

A retinal break is any full-thickness defect in the neurosensory retina. Breaks are clinically significant in that they may provide access for liquefied vitreous to enter the potential space between the sensory retina and the RPE and thus cause a rhegmatogenous retinal detachment. Some breaks are caused by atrophy of inner retinal layers, whereas others result from vitreoretinal traction (tears). Breaks resulting from trauma are discussed separately. Retinal breaks may be classified as

- flap, or horseshoe, tears
- giant retinal tear
- operculated holes
- dialyses
- atrophic retinal holes
- macular holes

A *flap tear* occurs when a strip of retina is pulled anteriorly by vitreoretinal traction, often due to a posterior vitreous detachment or trauma. A tear is considered symptomatic when it is caused by vitreous traction and the patient reports photopsias and/or floaters. A tear that extends 90° or more circumferentially is classified as a *giant retinal tear*. An *operculated hole* occurs when traction is sufficient to tear a piece of retina completely free from the adjacent retinal surface. *Dialyses* are circumferential, linear breaks that occur along the ora serrata, commonly as a consequence of blunt trauma. An *atrophic hole* is generally not associated with vitreoretinal traction and has not been associated with an increased risk of retinal detachment. *Macular hole* is a term that has been used to describe several clinically and histopathologically distinct manifestations varying from minor disturbances in the vitreoretinal interface to full-thickness defects in the neurosensory retina.

Preferred Practice Patterns Committee, Retina Panel. Management of posterior vitreous detachment, retinal breaks, and lattice degeneration. San Francisco: American Academy of Ophthalmology; 1998.

Regillo CD, Benson WE. *Retinal Detachment. Diagnosis and Management.* 3rd ed. Philadelphia: Lippincott-Raven; 1998.

Tiedeman JS. Retinal breaks, holes, and tears. *Focal Points: Clinical Modules for Ophthalmologists.* San Francisco: American Academy of Ophthalmology; 1996, module 3.

Traumatic Breaks

Open or closed eye trauma, including penetrating or perforating injuries, can cause retinal breaks by direct retinal perforation, contusion, or vitreous traction. Fibrocellular proliferation occurring later at the site of an injury may cause vitreoretinal traction and subsequent detachment. See also Chapter 13, Posterior Segment Trauma.

Blunt trauma can cause retinal breaks by direct contusive injury to the globe through 2 mechanisms:

1. Coup: adjacent to the point of trauma
2. Contrecoup: opposite the point of trauma

Blunt trauma compresses the eye along its anterior–posterior diameter and expands it in the equatorial plane. Because the vitreous body is relatively elastic, slow compression of the eye has no deleterious effect on the retina. However, rapid compression of the eye results in severe traction at the vitreous base that may cause retinal breaks.

Contusion injury may cause large, ragged equatorial breaks, dialysis, or a macular hole. Traumatic breaks are often multiple, and they are commonly found in the inferotemporal and superonasal quadrants. The most common injuries are dialyses, which may be as small as 1 ora bay or extend 90° or more. Dialyses are usually located at the posterior border of the vitreous base but can also be found at the anterior border (Fig 11-1, part 1). Avulsion of the vitreous base (anterior vitreous detachment) may be associated with dialysis and is considered pathognomonic of ocular contusion. The vitreous base can be avulsed from the underlying retina and nonpigmented epithelium of the pars plana without tearing either one; generally, however, either or both are also torn in the process.

Less common types of breaks caused by blunt trauma are horseshoe-shaped tears (which may occur at the posterior margin of the vitreous base, at the posterior end of a meridional fold, or at the equator), and operculated holes (Fig 11-1, part 3).

Trauma in young eyes

Although young patients have a higher incidence of eye injury than other age groups, they rarely develop an acute rhegmatogenous retinal detachment following blunt trauma because their vitreous has not yet undergone syneresis, or liquefaction. The vitreous, therefore, provides an internal tamponade to the retina in spite of retinal tears or dialyses. However, with time, the vitreous may liquefy over a tear, allowing fluid to pass through the break to detach the retina. The clinical presentation of the retinal detachment is usually delayed, as follows:

- 12% of detachments are found immediately
- 30% are found within 1 month
- 50% are found within 8 months
- 80% are found within 24 months

Traumatic retinal detachments in young patients may be shallow and often show signs of chronicity, including multiple demarcation lines, subretinal deposits, and intraretinal cysts.

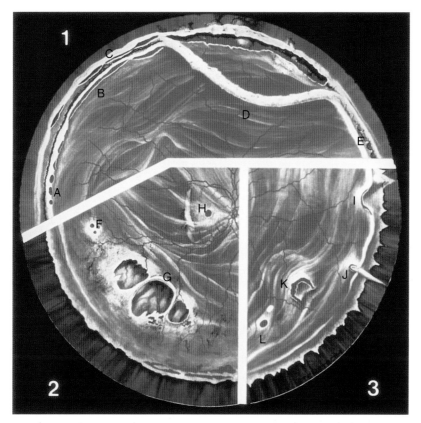

Figure 11-1 *Part 1.* Retinal breaks at borders of vitreous base. *A,* Small breaks at posterior border of vitreous base. *B,* Retinal dialysis at posterior border of vitreous base. *C,* Dialysis at anterior border of vitreous base. *D,* Avulsion of vitreous base that lies free in vitreous cavity. *E,* Tenting-up of retina and epithelium of pars plana ciliaris, forming ridges at posterior and anterior borders of vitreous base.

Part 2. Retinal breaks with no apparent vitreoretinal attachment. *F,* Round holes in atrophic retina. *G,* Irregular retinal hole in equatorial zone, associated with chorioretinal degeneration and vitreous and retinal hemorrhage. *H,* Atrophic macular hole associated with pigmentary changes and a choroidal rupture.

Part 3. Retinal breaks associated with abnormal vitreoretinal attachments. *I,* Horseshoe-shaped tear associated with an anomalous posterior extension of the vitreous base. *J,* Horseshoe-shaped tear at posterior end of meridional fold. *K,* Horseshoe-shaped tear in equatorial zone. *L,* Tear with operculum in overlying vitreous.

(Figure reproduced with permission from Cox MS, Schepens CL, Freeman HM. Retinal detachment due to ocular contusion. Arch Ophthalmol. 1966;76:678–685. Copyright 1966, American Medical Association.)

When posterior vitreous separation is present or occurs later following trauma, retinal breaks are often associated with abnormal vitreoretinal attachments and may resemble nontraumatic breaks. Retinal detachments may occur acutely in these patients.

Balles MW. Traumatic retinopathy. In: Albert DM, Jakobiec FA, eds. *Principles and Practice of Ophthalmology.* Philadelphia: Saunders; 2000:2221–2226.

Cox MS, Schepens CL, Freeman HM. Retinal detachment due to ocular contusion. *Arch Ophthalmol.* 1966;76:678–685.

Dugel PU, Ober RR. Posterior segment manifestations of closed-globe contusion injury. In: Ryan SJ, ed. *Retina.* 3rd ed. St Louis: Mosby; 2001:2386–2399.

Smiddy WE, Green WR. Retinal dialysis: pathology and pathogenesis. *Retina.* 1982;2:94–116.

Posterior Vitreous Detachment

The vitreous gel is attached most firmly at the *vitreous base,* a circumferential zone straddling the ora serrata that extends approximately 2 mm anterior and 4 mm posterior to the ora. Vitreous collagen fibers at this base are so firmly attached to the retina and pars plana epithelium that the vitreous cannot be separated easily without tearing these tissues. The vitreous is also firmly attached at the margin of the optic disc, at the macula, along major vessels, at the margin of lattice degeneration, and at sites of chorioretinal scars.

Most retinal tears result from traction caused by spontaneous or traumatic posterior vitreous detachment (PVD; Fig 11-2). The initial event is syneresis of the central vitreous. There is growing evidence that age-related PVD is insidious and slowly progressive over many years. A PVD typically begins in the perifoveal macula and extends throughout the macular region. The early stages are usually asymptomatic and occult; in most eyes, the evolving PVD remains subclinical for years until separation from the disc occurs (this separation from the disc is often accompanied by symptoms and signs of a Weiss ring). The vitreous gel remains attached at the vitreous base, and the resulting vitreous traction, commonly at the posterior margin of the vitreous base or other zones of firm attachment, can produce a retinal break (Fig 11-3.)

The prevalence of PVD increases with the axial length of the eye and with the patient's age. Other conditions associated with vitreous syneresis and PVD include aphakia, inflammatory disease, trauma, and myopia. It may be clinically difficult to determine whether the vitreous is attached to or separated from the surface of the retina. Clinical studies typically reveal a low incidence of PVD in patients less than 50 years of age. Autopsy studies demonstrate PVD in less than 10% of patients under the age of 50 years but in 63% of those over age 70 years.

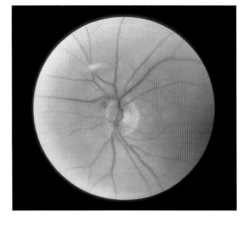

Figure 11-2 Posterior vitreous detachment. This patient has a glial floater (Weiss ring) overlying the optic disc. A peripapillary hemorrhage is visible at the nasal margin of the disc. *(Photograph courtesy of M. Gilbert Grand, MD.)*

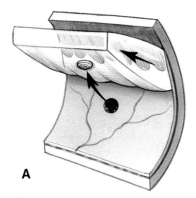

A

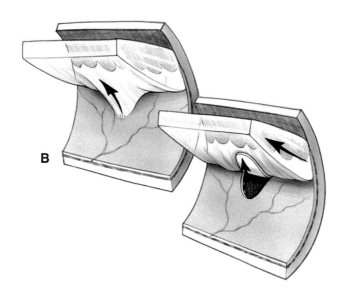

B

Figure 11-3 Mechanism of retinal tear formation associated with posterior vitreous separation. **A,** Round or oval hole. **B,** Flap tear: posterior extension of vitreous base with firm vitreoretinal attachment. *(Illustration by Christine Gralapp after illustrations by Tim Hengst.)*

Aphakia is commonly accompanied by PVD, which occurs in 66%–100% of aphakic eyes. Foos found in an autopsy study (1972) that 93% of surgically aphakic eyes had a PVD. The frequency of PVD was similar in patients undergoing intracapsular cataract extraction (ICCE) (84%) and extracapsular cataract extraction (ECCE) with an open capsule (76%), but it was much lower in eyes undergoing ECCE with an intact posterior capsule (40%).

Many patients do not report acute symptoms when a PVD occurs. Symptoms of PVD include the entoptic phenomena of photopsias (flashing lights) and floaters. Patients with these symptoms should be seen promptly, and office staff should be made aware of the urgency of these symptoms. Flashing lights are caused by the physical stimulus of vitreoretinal traction on the retina. Floaters are caused by vitreous opacities such as blood, glial cells torn from the optic disc, or aggregated collagen fibers, all of which can cast shadows on the retina.

Vitreous hemorrhage may arise from rupture of retinal vessels that cross retinal tears or from avulsion of superficial retinal or prepapillary vessels. Vitreous hemorrhage is an ominous sign. Approximately 15% of all patients with acute symptomatic PVD have a retinal tear. However, 50%–70% of PVD patients who have associated vitreous hemorrhage have retinal tears, whereas only 10%–12% with no vitreous hemorrhage have retinal tears.

Examination and Management of PVD

Indirect ophthalmoscopy with scleral depression and slit-lamp biomicroscopy with a 60- to 90-diopter indirect lens or corneal contact lens are used to make the definitive diagnosis of PVD and to rule out retinal breaks or detachment. The presence of hemorrhage or pigment in the vitreous suggests a possible retinal break and demands a thorough examination. Even in the absence of hemorrhage, pigment, or detectable retinal break, the ophthalmologist may wish to reexamine the patient in 3–4 weeks, depending on clinical circumstances such as aphakia or myopia, because breaks may evolve over time. All patients should be instructed to return to the ophthalmologist immediately if they notice a change in symptoms, such as increasing floaters or the development of visual field loss.

If a large vitreous hemorrhage precludes a complete examination, bilateral ocular patching and bed rest with the patient's head elevated 45° for 1 or 2 days may clear the vitreous sufficiently to allow breaks in a superior location to be found. This approach is especially important for patients at high risk of retinal detachment—for example, those with high myopia, aphakia, detachment in the fellow eye, or a family history of detachment. Echography may be performed to rule out retinal detachment and other fundus lesions. If the cause of the hemorrhage cannot be found, the patient should be reexamined at frequent regular intervals until the cause is identified.

Byer NE. Natural history of posterior vitreous detachment with early management as the premier line of defense against retinal detachment. *Ophthalmology.* 1994:101:1503–1514.

Green WR, Sebag J. Vitreoretinal interface. In: Ryan SJ, ed. *Retina.* 3rd ed. St Louis: Mosby; 2001:1882–1960.

Uchino E, Uemura A, Ohba N. Initial stages of posterior vitreous detachment in healthy eyes of older persons evaluated by optic coherence tomography. *Arch Ophthalmol.* 2001;119:1475–1479.

Lesions Predisposing to Retinal Detachment

Lattice Degeneration

Lattice degeneration, a vitreoretinal abnormality, is found in 6%–10% of the general population and is bilateral in one third to one half of affected patients. It occurs more commonly in—but is not limited to—myopic eyes; a familial predilection is present.

Lattice degeneration may predispose to retinal breaks and detachment. The most important histopathologic features include discontinuity of the internal limiting membrane of the retina, an overlying pocket of liquefied vitreous, condensation and adherence of vitreous at the margin of the lesion, and varying degrees of atrophy of the inner layers of retina (Figs 11-4, 11-5, 11-6).

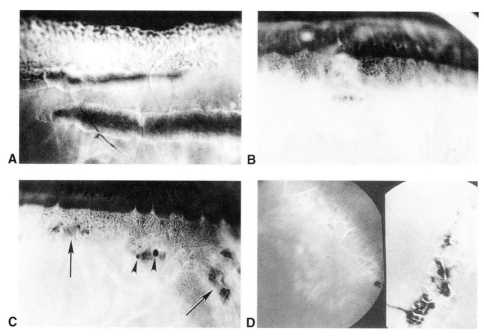

Figure 11-4 Various appearances of lattice degeneration of the retina. **A,** Overlapping linear areas of retinal thinning. Condensed vitreous at margin is apparent. (EP 31974.) **B,** Small area of retinal thinning, with vitreous condensation at margin and pocket of fluid vitreous centrally. (EP 30295). **C,** Several areas of retinal thinning *(arrows).* One area has 2 holes *(arrowheads)* within area of thinning. (EP 30979). **D,** Ophthalmoscopic appearance of lattice degeneration *(left)* with a linear area of lattice "wicker" caused by sclerotic blood vessels. In addition, photograph at right shows secondary RPE hyperplasia with migration into the retina. *(From Green WR. Retina. In: Spencer WH, ed. Ophthalmic Pathology: An Atlas and Textbook. 3rd ed. Philadelphia: Saunders; 1985:866.)*

Although only a small number of patients with lattice degeneration develop a detachment, it is found in 20%–30% of all eyes with rhegmatogenous retinal detachments. Lattice degeneration progresses to retinal detachment either by means of a tractional tear at the lateral or posterior margin of the lattice lesion or, less commonly, by means of an atrophic hole within the zone of lattice itself (Figs 11-7, 11-8).

Byer NE. Lattice degeneration of the retina. *Surv Ophthalmol.* 1979;23:213–248.
Byer NE. Long-term natural history of lattice degeneration of the retina. *Ophthalmology.* 1989;96:1396–1402.

Vitreoretinal Tufts

Peripheral retinal tufts are small, peripheral retinal elevations caused by focal areas of vitreous or zonular traction. Tractional tufts are classified on the basis of anatomic, pathogenetic, and clinical distinctions into the following:

- noncystic retinal tufts (Fig 11-9)
- cystic retinal tufts (Fig 11-10)
- zonular traction retinal tufts (Fig 11-11)

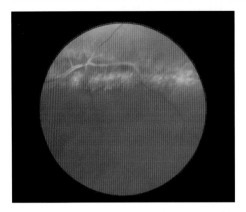

Figure 11-5 Lattice degeneration seen without scleral indentation. Vascular sheathing is visible where the vessel crosses the area of lattice. Characteristic white lattice lines are seen. *(Reproduced with permission from Byer NE. Peripheral Retina in Profile: A Stereoscopic Atlas. Torrance, CA: Criterion Press; 1982.)*

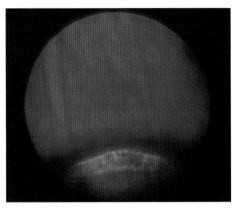

Figure 11-6 Lattice degeneration as viewed with scleral indentation. *(Reproduced with permission from Byer NE. Peripheral Retina in Profile: A Stereoscopic Atlas. Torrance, CA: Criterion Press; 1982.)*

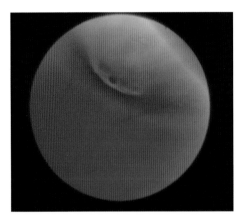

Figure 11-7 Lattice with a small atrophic hole. *(Photograph courtesy of Norman E. Byer, MD.)*

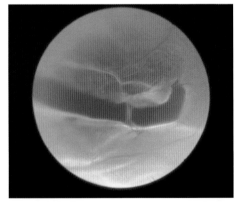

Figure 11-8 Lattice with a large, posteriorly located flap tear and associated detachment. Note vessel bridging the tear. *(Reproduced with permission from Byer NE. Peripheral Retina in Profile: A Stereoscopic Atlas. Torrance, CA: Criterion Press; 1982.)*

Retinal pigment epithelial hyperplasia may surround the tuft. Cystic and zonular traction retinal tufts, both with firm vitreoretinal adhesions, may predispose to retinal detachment. Flap tears and operculated holes may occur as a result of traction associated with PVD.

Byer NE. Cystic retinal tufts and their relationship to retinal detachment. *Arch Ophthalmol.* 1981;99:1788–1790.

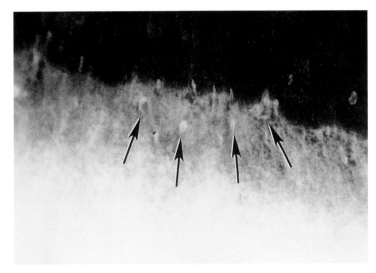

Figure 11-9 Gross appearance of noncystic retinal tufts *(arrows)*. *(From Green WR. Retina. In: Spencer WH, ed. Ophthalmic Pathology: An Atlas and Textbook. 3rd ed. Philadelphia: Saunders; 1985:894.)*

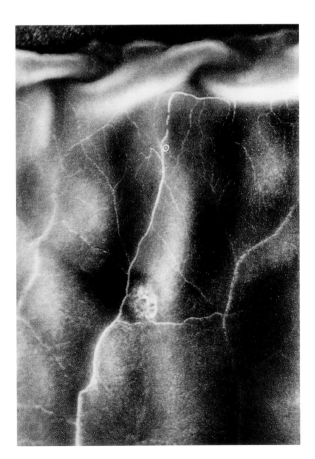

Figure 11-10 Cystic retinal tuft in peripheral retina of 14-year-old boy. Tuft measures 0.47 mm at its circular base, is 3.7 mm from ora serrata, and contains many microcysts with dense walls (75% of ×19). *(From Duane TD Jaeger EA, eds. Clinical Ophthalmology. Philadelphia: Lippincott; 1990, vol 3, ch 26:24. Photograph courtesy of Robert Y. Foos, MD.)*

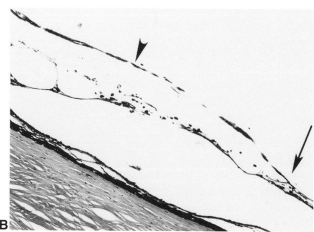

Figure 11-11 A, Zonular traction tuft *(arrow)* extending over pars plana from peripheral retina. **B,** Tuft is attached to peripheral retina *(arrow)* and extends *(arrowhead)* over retina. *(From Green WR. Retina. In: Spencer WH, ed. Ophthalmic Pathology: An Atlas and Textbook. 3rd ed. Philadelphia: Saunders; 1985:897.)*

Meridional Folds, Enclosed Ora Bays, and Peripheral Retinal Excavations

Meridional folds are folds of redundant retina, usually found superonasally. They are most commonly associated with dentate processes but may also extend posteriorly from ora bays. Occasionally, tears associated with PVD occur at the most posterior limit of the folds. Retinal tears can also occur at or near the posterior margins of *enclosed ora bays,* oval islands of pars plana epithelium located immediately posterior to the ora serrata and completely or almost completely circumscribed by peripheral retina (Fig 11-12). Occasionally, tears may occur at the site of *peripheral retinal excavations.* These lesions may represent atypical lattice degeneration. The excavations may have firm vitreoretinal adhesions and are found adjacent to or up to 4 disc diameters posterior to the ora serrata. They are often aligned with meridional folds.

Glasgow BJ, Foos RY, Yoshizumi MO. Degenerative diseases of the peripheral retina. In: Tasman W, Jaeger EA, eds. *Duane's Clinical Ophthalmology.* Philadelphia: Lippincott; 1994; vol 3; chap 26:1–30.

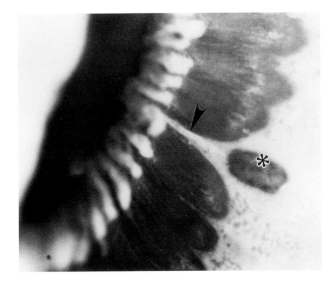

Figure 11-12 Meridional complex, consisting of a dentate process *(arrowhead)* that is continuous with pars plicata and an area of entrapped pars plana *(asterisk)*. *(EP 39305 from Green WR. Pathology of the retina. In: Frayer WC, ed.* Lancaster Course in Ophthalmic Histopathology, *unit 9. Philadelphia: FA Davis; 1981.)*

Lesions Not Predisposing to Retinal Detachment

Paving-stone, or Cobblestone, Degeneration

Paving-stone (cobblestone) degeneration is characterized by peripheral, small, discrete areas of atrophy of the outer retina that appear in 22% of persons over 20 years of age (Fig 11-13). They may occur singly or in groups and sometimes are confluent. Histopathologically, paving stones are characterized by attenuation or absence of the choriocapillaris, loss of the RPE and outer retinal layers, and adhesions between the remaining inner layers and Bruch's membrane. These lesions are most common in the inferior quadrants, anterior to the equator. Ophthalmoscopically, they appear yellowish white and are sometimes surrounded by a rim of hypertrophic RPE. Because the RPE is absent, large choroidal vessels can be seen beneath the lesions.

Paving-stone degeneration is never the site of a primary retinal break, but some observers have reported that a secondary tear may occur if a retinal detachment caused by an unrelated break puts traction on a paving stone. Such breaks appear to be exceedingly rare. In fact, a zone of paving stones usually prevents the spread of a detachment.

> Glasgow BJ, Foos RY, Yoshizumi MO. Degenerative diseases of the peripheral retina. In: Tasman W, Jaeger EA, eds. *Duane's Clinical Ophthalmology.* Philadelphia: Lippincott; 1994; vol 3; chap 26:1–30.

Retinal Pigment Epithelial Hyperplasia

When stimulated by chronic low-grade traction, the RPE cells proliferate abnormally. Diffuse RPE hyperplasia can be seen straddling the ora serrata with dimensions that correspond roughly to the vitreous base or occurring focally on the pars plana and peripheral retina, especially at areas of focal traction such as vitreoretinal tufts and lattice degeneration. Old areas of inflammation and trauma may also be sites of RPE hyperplasia.

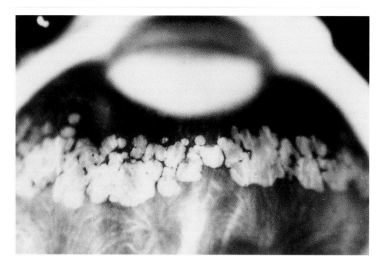

Figure 11-13 Gross appearance of paving-stone degeneration. *(From Green WR. Pathology of the retina. In: Frayer WC, ed. Lancaster Course in Ophthalmic Histopathology, unit 9. Philadelphia: FA Davis; 1981.)*

Retinal Pigment Epithelial Hypertrophy

Acquired RPE hypertrophy is an aging and degenerative change that commonly occurs in the periphery. Histopathologically, it is characterized by large cells and by large, spherical melanin granules. Hypertrophy is usually seen just posterior to the ora serrata. Similar histopathologic features are seen in congenital hypertrophy of the RPE (grouped pigmentation, or "bear tracks").

Peripheral Cystoid Degeneration

Typical peripheral cystoid degeneration, characterized by zones of microcysts in the far peripheral retina, is present in almost all adults after the age of 20 years. Although retinal holes may form in these areas, they rarely lead to a retinal detachment. Reticular peripheral cystoid degeneration is almost always located posterior to typical peripheral cystoid degeneration. It presents with a linear or reticular pattern following the retinal vessels. This form is found in about 20% of adults and may in a few instances develop into reticular degenerative retinoschisis.

Prophylactic Treatment of Retinal Breaks

Any retinal break can cause a retinal detachment by allowing liquid vitreous to separate the sensory retina from the RPE. However, the vast majority of retinal breaks do not cause a detachment. Approximately 6% of all eyes have a break, but only 1 person per 10,000–15,000 a year develops a detachment. Assuming an average life expectancy of 74 years in the United States, it is estimated that 0.07% of the population will develop a retinal detachment over their lifetime.

The ophthalmologist may consider prophylactic treatment of breaks in an attempt to reduce the risk of retinal detachment. The inherent risk of treatment must be weighed against the potential benefit of the procedure. Furthermore, it must be recognized that treatment may not eliminate the risk of new tears or detachment.

The goal of prophylactic treatment of retinal breaks is to create a chorioretinal scar around each break to prevent fluid vitreous from entering the subretinal space. Either cryotherapy or photocoagulation can be used. Operculated or atrophic holes may be surrounded with 2–3 mm of coagulation. However, flap tears require a larger treatment area, extending farther anteriorly (preferably to the ora serrata), because continuing vitreous traction can pull the flap through a cryotherapy or laser scar and cause detachment. If subretinal fluid is present, treatment must extend beyond the fluid to reach attached retina. In treating lattice degeneration, the ophthalmologist should take care to treat the entire lesion, paying particular attention to its posterior margin and lateral extent.

Many clinical series have demonstrated that acute breaks are more dangerous than old breaks. Acute breaks are typically associated with vitreous hemorrhage or punctate hemorrhage at the margin of the tear. Some retinal breaks, such as round atrophic holes, operculated holes, and macular holes, have a minimal risk of progressing to retinal detachment, whereas other breaks, such as acute symptomatic flap tears, may have a substantial risk.

The ophthalmologist must consider multiple factors, including symptoms, residual traction, location of the break, phakic status, refractive error, status of the fellow eye, family history, the presence of subretinal fluid, and the potential for follow-up evaluation. The following discussion serves only as a guideline, because recommendations may vary, depending on multiple clinical factors. (See also the discussion of hereditary hyaloideoretinopathies with optically empty vitreous in Chapter 12.)

Hilton GF, McLean EB, Brinton DA. *Retinal Detachment: Principles and Practice.* 2nd ed. Ophthalmology Monograph 1. San Francisco: American Academy of Ophthalmology; 1995.

Preferred Practice Patterns Committee, Retina Panel. *Management of Posterior Vitreous Detachment, Retinal Breaks, and Lattice Degeneration.* San Francisco: American Academy of Ophthalmology: 1998.

Smiddy WE, Flynn HW Jr, Nicholson DH, et al. Results and complications in treated retinal breaks. *Am J Ophthalmol.* 1991;112:623–631.

Straatsma BR, Foos RH, Feman SS. Degenerative diseases of the peripheral retina. In: Duane TD, ed. *Clinical Ophthalmology.* Philadelphia: Harper & Row; 1983; vol 3; chap 26:1–29.

Symptomatic Retinal Breaks

Approximately 15% of eyes with a symptomatic PVD are found to have one or more breaks, and retinal breaks in symptomatic eyes have a high risk of causing retinal detachment. Therefore, *acute symptomatic flap tears* are commonly treated prophylactically.

Acute operculated holes are less likely to cause detachment because there is no residual traction on the adjacent retina; therefore, such breaks may not require treatment. However, if slit-lamp biomicroscopy reveals persistent vitreous traction at the margin of an operculated hole, that hole is truly comparable to a flap tear, and prophylaxis should be considered. Additional factors that may mitigate toward treatment are large holes, a superior location, and the presence of vitreous hemorrhage.

Atrophic holes are often incidental findings in a patient who presents with an acute PVD. If no associated traction occurs, treatment is generally not required.

Macular holes are believed to be caused by vitreomacular and perifoveal vitreous detachment. Macular holes usually cause visual symptoms but rarely lead to retinal detachment, with the exception of those associated with high myopia or persistent vitreoretinal traction. Treatment of macular holes may be considered in order to improve visual acuity rather than to prevent detachment (Table 11-1).

Asymptomatic Retinal Breaks

Asymptomatic flap tears infrequently cause retinal detachment and generally are not treated in emmetropic, phakic eyes. However, asymptomatic flap tears accompanied by lattice degeneration, myopia, subclinical detachment, or aphakia associated with detachment in the fellow eye may increase a patient's risk of retinal detachment, and, under these circumstances, treatment may be considered. Asymptomatic operculated and atrophic holes rarely cause retinal detachment and are generally not treated (Table 11-2).

> Byer NE. What happens to untreated asymptomatic retinal breaks, and are they affected by posterior vitreous detachment? *Ophthalmology.* 1998;105:1045–1050.

Prophylaxis of Lattice Degeneration

As mentioned earlier in this chapter, lattice degeneration occurs in approximately 6%–10% of eyes but is found in 20%–30% of eyes with a retinal detachment. Limited data are available, but an 11-year follow-up of untreated lattice degeneration patients with no symptomatic tears showed that retinal detachment occurred in approximately 1%. Thus, the presence of lattice, with or without atrophic holes on routine examination, generally does not require prophylaxis in the absence of other risk factors. High myopia, presence of retinal detachment in the fellow eye, presence of flap tears, and aphakia are risk factors that may suggest prophylactic treatment.

Table 11-1 Indications for Treatment of Retinal Tears and Holes in Symptomatic Patients

Type of Lesion	Treatment
Horseshoe tears	Almost always
Dialysis	Almost always
Operculated tear	Sometimes
Atrophic hole	Rarely
Lattice degeneration without horseshoe tears	Rarely

(Modified with permission from Preferred Practice Patterns Committee, Retina Panel. *Management of Posterior Vitreous Detachment, Retinal Breaks, and Lattice Degeneration.* San Francisco: American Academy of Ophthalmology; 1998:13.)

Table 11-2 Indications for Treatment of Retinal Tears and Holes in Asymptomatic Patients

Type of Lesion	Types of Eyes			
	Phakic	Highly Myopic	Fellow Eye*	Aphakic or Pseudophakic
Retinal dialysis	Almost always[†]	Almost always[†]	Almost always[†]	Almost always[†]
Horseshoe tears	Sometimes	Sometimes	Sometimes	Sometimes
Operculated tears	No	Rarely	Rarely	Rarely
Atrophic holes	Rarely	Rarely	Rarely	Rarely
Lattice degeneration with or without holes	No	No	Sometimes	Rarely

* Applies to patients who have had a retinal detachment in the other eye.

[†] Indications for therapy may be modified if subretinal fluid associated with a dialysis is contained by a demarcation line.

(Modified with permission from Preferred Practice Patterns Committee, Retinal Panel. *Management of Posterior Vitreous Detachment, Retinal Breaks, and Lattice Degeneration.* San Francisco: American Academy of Ophthalmology; 1998:14.)

Byer NE. Long-term natural history of lattice degeneration of the retina. *Ophthalmology.* 1989;96:1396–1402.

Wilkinson CP. Evidence-based analysis of prophylactic treatment of asymptomatic retinal breaks and lattice degeneration. *Ophthalmology.* 2000;107:12–18.

Aphakia and Pseudophakia

Because aphakic and pseudophakic patients have a higher risk of retinal detachment (1%–3%) compared to phakic patients, they should be warned of potential symptoms and carefully examined if symptoms occur. The value of prophylactic treatment of asymptomatic breaks is uncertain. Flap tears or eyes with subclinical detachments are sometimes treated in aphakic or pseudophakic patients.

Fellow Eye in Patient With Retinal Detachment

Approximately 10% of phakic patients who have retinal detachment in one eye and 20%–36% of aphakic patients with detachment in one eye will develop detachment in their second eye. Prophylactic treatment of flap tears is often considered, whereas the benefit of treatment of round holes has not been conclusively determined. A retrospective study found that the risk of retinal detachment in the fellow eye of patients with phakic lattice retinal detachments was reduced over 7 years of follow-up from 5.1% in untreated eyes to 1.8% in those with full treatment of their lattice. However, it is noteworthy that the incidence of retinal detachment was low in both groups; therefore, prophylaxis is not universally recommended.

Folk JC, Arrindell EL, Klugman MR. The fellow eye of patients with phakic lattice retinal detachment. *Ophthalmology.* 1989;96:72–79.

Subclinical Retinal Detachment

The definition of a *subclinical retinal detachment* varies. Although the term may refer to an asymptomatic retinal detachment, it more commonly describes a detachment in which subretinal fluid extends more than 1 disc diameter from the break but not more than 2 disc diameters posterior to the equator. Because approximately 30% of such detachments will progress, treatment is often recommended. Treatment is particularly advised for symptomatic patients or those with traction on the break. Patients with demarcation lines may be observed but should not be considered secure, as progression may occur through the demarcation line.

> Brod RD, Flynn HW Jr, Lightman DA. Asymptomatic rhegmatogenous retinal detachments. *Arch Ophthalmol.* 1995;113:1030–1032.

Retinal Detachment

Retinal detachments are classified as

- rhegmatogenous
- tractional
- exudative

The most common type, *rhegmatogenous retinal detachment (RRD)*, is caused by liquefied vitreous passing through a retinal break into the potential space between the sensory retina and the RPE. The term is derived from the Greek *rhegma*, meaning "break." The less common *tractional detachments* are caused by proliferative membranes that contract and elevate the retina. Combinations of tractional and rhegmatogenous causes may lead to a detachment. *Exudative*, or *secondary, detachments* are caused by retinal or choroidal diseases in which leakage of fluid accumulates beneath the sensory retina. Although they commonly occur in limited areas associated with choroidal neovascularization, exudative detachments rarely become extensive, unlike rhegmatogenous or tractional detachments.

The differential diagnosis of retinal detachment includes retinoschisis, choroidal tumors, and retinal elevation secondary to detachment of the choroid. Diagnostic features of the 3 forms of retinal detachment are shown in Table 11-3.

Rhegmatogenous Retinal Detachment

In 90%–97% of RRDs, a definite retinal break can be found (Fig 11-14). In the others, one is presumed to be present. If no break can be found, the ophthalmologist must rule out all other causes of retinal elevation. Fifty percent of patients with RRD have photopsias or floaters. The IOP is usually lower in the affected eye than in the fellow eye but may occasionally be higher. Shafer's sign, descriptively termed "tobacco dust" for small clumps of pigmented cells, is frequently present in the vitreous or anterior segment. The detached retina usually has a corrugated appearance, especially in recent retinal detachments, and undulates with eye movements. In a long-standing RRD, however, the retina may appear smooth and thin. Fixed folds resulting from *proliferative vitreoretinopathy (PVR)* almost always indicate a rhegmatogenous retinal detachment. Shifting fluid may occur but is uncommon.

Table 11-3 Diagnostic Features of the Three Types of Retinal Detachments

	Rhegmatogenous (Primary)	Tractional	Nonrhegmatogenous (Secondary) Exudative
History	Aphakia, myopia, blunt trauma, photopsia, floaters, field defect; generally healthy	Diabetes, prematurity, penetrating trauma, sickle cell disease	Systemic factors such as malignant hypertension, eclampsia, renal failure
Retinal break	Identified in 90%–95% of cases	No primary break; may develop secondary break	No break, or coincidental
Extent of detachment	Extends to ora early	Frequently does not extend to ora	Gravity-dependent; extension to ora is variable
Retinal mobility	Undulating bullae or folds	Taut retina, concave surface, peaks to traction points	Smoothly elevated bullae, usually without folds
Evidence of chronicity	Demarcation lines, intraretinal macrocysts, atrophic retina	Demarcation lines	Usually none
Pigment in vitreous	Present in 70% of cases	Present in trauma cases	Not present
Vitreous changes	Frequently syneretic, posterior vitreous detachment, traction on flap of tear	Vitreoretinal traction	Usually clear, except in uveitis
Subretinal fluid	Clear	Clear, no shift	May be turbid and shift rapidly to dependent location with changes in head position
Choroidal mass	None	None	May be present
Intraocular pressure	Frequently low	Usually normal	Varies
Transillumination	Normal	Normal	Blocked transillumination if pigmented choroidal lesion present
Examples of conditions causing detachment	Retinal break	Proliferative diabetic retinopathy, ROP, toxocariasis, sickle cell retinopathy, posttraumatic vitreous traction	Uveitis, metastatic tumor, malignant melanoma, Coats disease, Eales disease, VKH syndrome, retinoblastoma, choroidal hemangioma, senile exudative maculopathy, optic pit, exudative detachment after cryotherapy or diathermy

(Reproduced with permission from Hilton GF, McLean JB, Brinton DA, eds. *Retinal Detachment: Principles and Practice.* 2nd ed. Ophthalmology Monograph 1. San Francisco: American Academy of Ophthalmology; 1995.)

PVR is the most common cause of failure to repair RRD. In PVR, retinal pigment epithelial, glial, and other cells grow on both the inner and outer retinal surfaces and on the vitreous face, forming membranes. Contraction of these membranes causes fixed retinal folds, equatorial traction, detachment of the nonpigmented epithelium of the pars plana, and generalized retinal shrinkage (Fig 11-15). As a result, the causative retinal breaks may reopen, new breaks may occur, or a tractional detachment may develop.

To better compare research data, a generally accepted classification of PVR was developed and subsequently updated (Tables 11-4, 11-5). The new classification has 3 grades of PVR describing increasing severity of the disease. Posterior and anterior contractions are now classified according to focal, diffuse, subretinal, circumferential, and anterior displacement. The extent of the pathology is described with clock hours.

The classification of retinal detachment with proliferative vitreoretinopathy. Retina Society Terminology Committee. *Ophthalmology.* 1983;90:121–125.

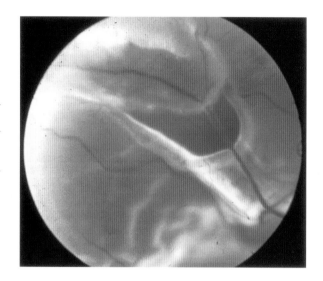

Figure 11-14 Horseshoe retinal tear with associated retinal detachment. Intact retinal vessel bridges tear. Some vessels crossing flap tears rupture, and, along with photopsia, initial symptoms may include black spots from a localized vitreous hemorrhage.

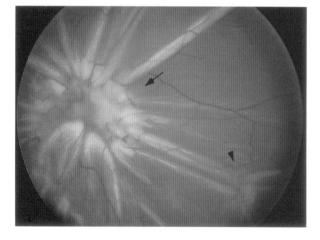

Figure 11-15 Retinal detachment with proliferative vitreoretinopathy. Revised Retina Society classification CP-12 with diffuse retinal contraction in posterior pole *(arrow)* and single midperipheral starfold *(arrowhead)*. See Table 11-5.

Table 11-4 Classification of Retinal Detachment with Vitreoretinopathy, 1983

Grade	Name	Clinical Signs
A	Minimal	Vitreous haze, vitreous pigment clumps
B	Moderate	Wrinkling of inner retinal surface, rolled edge of retinal break, retinal stiffness, vessel tortuosity
C	Marked	Full-thickness fixed retinal folds C-1 One quadrant C-2 Two quadrants C-3 Three quadrants
D	Massive	Fixed retinal folds in four quadrants D-1 Wide funnel shape D-2 Narrow funnel shape* D-3 Closed funnel (optic nerve head not visible)

* Existence of narrow funnel shape is evidenced by indirect ophthalmoscopy when anterior end of funnel can be seen within 45° field of +20 D condensing lens (Nikon or equivalent).

(Retina Society Terminology Committee. The classification of retinal detachment with proliferative vitreoretinopathy. *Ophthalmology.* 1983;90:121–125.)

Table 11-5 Classification of Proliferative Vitreoretinopathy, 1991

Grade	Features
A	Vitreous haze, vitreous pigment clumps, pigment clusters on inferior retina
B	Wrinkling of inner retinal surface, retinal stiffness, vessel tortuosity, rolled and irregular edge of retinal break, decreased mobility of vitreous
CP 1–12	Posterior to equator: focal, diffuse, or circumferential full-thickness folds,* subretinal strands*
CA 1–12	Anterior to equator: focal, diffuse, or circumferential full-thickness folds,* subretinal strands,* anterior displacement,* condensed vitreous with strands

* Expressed in number of clock-hours involved.

(Machemer R, Aaberg TM, Freeman HM, et al. An updated classification of retinal detachment with proliferative vitreoretinopathy. *Am J Ophthalmol.* 1991;112:159–165.)

Lean JS. Proliferative vitreoretinopathy. In: Albert DM, Jakobiec FA, eds. *Principles and Practice of Ophthalmology.* Philadelphia: Saunders; 1994:1110–1121.

Machemer R, Aaberg TM, Freeman HM, et al. An updated classification of retinal detachment with proliferative vitreoretinopathy. *Am J Ophthalmol.* 1991;112:159–165.

Management of rhegmatogenous retinal detachment

The principles of surgery for retinal detachment are the following:

1. Find all breaks.
2. Create a chorioretinal irritation around each break.
3. Bring the retina and choroid into contact for sufficient time to produce a chorioretinal adhesion to permanently close the break.

One of the most important elements in management is a careful retinal examination, first preoperatively and then intraoperatively.

The retinal break can be closed by a number of methods. A scleral buckle, which indents the sclera beneath the retinal break, promotes reapposition of the retina to the RPE by reducing vitreous traction and diminishing the flux of vitreous fluid through the retinal tear (Fig 11-16). With PVR, epiretinal membranes exert traction that tends to pull retinal breaks away from the RPE. The indentation of the scleral buckle may change the vector of tractional forces exerted by epiretinal membranes and thus reduce traction on the breaks.

Whereas most buckling procedures produce a permanent indentation, some breaks, particularly those with minimal or no vitreous traction, can be treated by means of a temporary tamponade. *Pneumatic retinopexy,* used in selected retinal detachments caused by breaks in the superior two thirds of the fundus, is a procedure in which a gas bubble is injected into the vitreous cavity to tamponade the retinal breaks until the retina is reattached. A balloon device can be used to create a temporary scleral buckle to close retinal breaks. All retinal reattachment procedures must produce a firm chorioretinal adhesion by cryotherapy, laser, or diathermy. *Vitrectomy* is useful in selected retinal detachments to internally relieve vitreoretinal traction. See Chapter 16.

Brinton DA, Hilton GF. Pneumatic retinopexy and alternative retinal attachment techniques. In: Ryan SJ, ed. *Retina.* 3rd ed. St Louis: Mosby; 2001:2047–2062.

Haller JA. Retinal detachment. *Focal Points: Clinical Modules for Ophthalmologists.* San Francisco: American Academy of Ophthalmology; 1998, module 5.

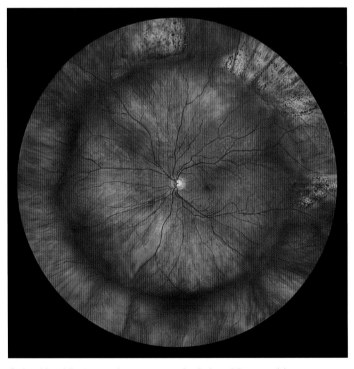

Figure 11-16 Scleral buckle 1 month postoperatively in a 28-year-old woman. *(Photograph courtesy of Mark W. Johnson, MD, and Richard Hackel, CRA.)*

Hilton GF, McLean EB, Brinton DA. *Retinal Detachment: Principles and Practice*. 2nd ed. Ophthalmology Monograph 1. San Francisco: American Academy of Ophthalmology; 1995.

Meredith TA. *Atlas of Retinal and Vitreous Surgery*. St Louis: Mosby; 1999:9–43.

Regillo CD, Benson WE. *Retinal Detachment: Diagnosis and Management*. 3rd ed. Philadelphia: Lippincott-Raven; 1998:100–134.

Williams GA, Aaberg TM Sr. Techniques of scleral buckling. In: Ryan SJ, *Retina*. 3rd ed. St Louis: Mosby; 2001:2010–2046.

Young LHY, D'Amico DJ. Retinal detachment. In: Albert DM, Jakobiec FA, eds. *Principles and Practice of Ophthalmology*. Philadelphia: Saunders; 1994:1084–1092.

Anatomic reattachment

The overall rate of anatomic reattachment with current techniques is 90%. The prognosis is better for reattachment in patients whose detachments are caused by dialyses or small holes or who have detachments associated with demarcation lines. Aphakic and pseudophakic eyes have a slightly less favorable prognosis. Detachments caused by giant tears or associated with PVR, uveitis, choroidal detachments, or posterior breaks secondary to trauma have the worst prognosis for anatomic reattachment.

Regillo CD, Benson WE. *Retinal Detachment: Diagnosis and Management*. 3rd ed. Philadelphia: Lippincott-Raven; 1998:100–134.

Williams GA, Aaberg TM. Techniques of scleral buckling. In: Ryan SJ, *Retina*. 2nd ed. St Louis: Mosby; 1994:1979–2017.

Postoperative visual acuity

The status of the macula—whether it was detached and for how long—is the primary presurgery determinant of postoperative visual acuity. If the macula was detached, degeneration of photoreceptors may prevent good postoperative visual acuity. Although 87% of eyes with retinal detachment sparing the macula recover visual acuity of 20/50 or better, only one third to one half with a detached macula attain that level. Among patients with a macular detachment of less than 1 week's duration, 75% will obtain a final visual acuity of 20/70 or better, as opposed to 50% with a macular detachment of 1–8 weeks' duration.

In 10%–15% of successfully repaired retinal detachments with the macula attached preoperatively, visual acuity does not return to the preoperative level. This loss of acuity occurs secondary to factors such as macular edema or macular pucker. Intraoperative complications and preexisting visual loss as a result of underlying ocular pathology may also limit visual recovery.

Hilton GF, McLean EB, Brinton DA. *Retinal Detachment: Principles and Practice*. 2nd ed. Ophthalmology Monograph 1. San Francisco: American Academy of Ophthalmology; 1995:161–166.

Tractional Retinal Detachment

Vitreous membranes caused by penetrating injuries or by proliferative retinopathies such as diabetic retinopathy can pull the neurosensory retina away from the RPE, causing a tractional retinal detachment. The retina characteristically has a smooth surface and is immobile. The detachment is concave toward the front of the eye and rarely extends to the ora serrata. In most cases, the causative vitreous membrane can be seen biomicroscopically with a 3-mirror contact lens or a 60- to 90-diopter indirect lens.

If the traction can be released by vitrectomy, the detachment may resolve. In some cases, traction may tear the retina and cause a rhegmatogenous retinal detachment that is convex toward the front of the eye. The retina then becomes more mobile and has the irregular folds and corrugations characteristic of a rhegmatogenous detachment. Treatment may require a combination of vitrectomy to release the traction and a scleral buckling procedure to seal the break.

Exudative Retinal Detachment

It is critical to recognize a large exudative retinal detachment because, unlike other types of retinal detachment, its management is usually not surgical. Exudative detachment occurs when either retinal blood vessels or the RPE is damaged, allowing fluid to pass into the subretinal space (Fig 11-17). Neoplasia and inflammatory diseases are the leading causes of large exudative detachments.

The presence of shifting fluid is highly suggestive of a large exudative retinal detachment. Because the subretinal fluid responds to the force of gravity, it detaches the area of the retina in which it accumulates. For example, when the patient is sitting, the inferior retina is detached. However, when the patient becomes supine, the fluid moves posteriorly in a matter of seconds or minutes, detaching the macula. Another characteristic of exudative detachments is the smoothness of the detached retina, in contrast to the corrugated appearance seen in rhegmatogenous retinal detachment. Fixed retinal folds, usually indicative of PVR, are rarely if ever seen in exudative detachments. Occasionally, the retina is sufficiently elevated in exudative detachments to be seen directly behind the lens, a rare occurrence in rhegmatogenous detachments.

Regillo CD, Benson WE. *Retinal Detachment: Diagnosis and Management.* 3rd ed. Philadelphia: Lippincott; 1998:60–66.

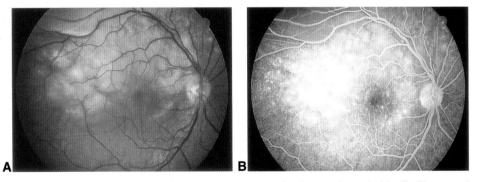

Figure 11-17 A, Exudative retinal detachment as a result of posterior scleritis. **B,** Fluorescein angiogram shows multifocal leakage through RPE into subretinal space. *(Photographs courtesy of William F. Mieler, MD.)*

Differential Diagnosis of Retinal Detachment

Retinoschisis

Typical peripheral cystoid degeneration is seen in virtually all adults. Contiguous with and extending up to 2–3 mm posterior to the ora serrata, the area of degeneration has a bubbly appearance and is best seen with scleral depression (Fig 11-18). The cystoid cavities in the outer plexiform layer contain a hyaluronidase-sensitive mucopolysaccharide. The only known complication of typical cystoid degeneration is coalescence and extension of the cavities and progression to typical degenerative retinoschisis.

Reticular peripheral cystoid degeneration is almost always located posterior to and continuous with typical peripheral cystoid degeneration, but it is considerably less common. It has a linear or reticular pattern that corresponds to the retinal vessels and a finely stippled internal surface. The cystoid spaces are in the nerve fiber layer. This condition may progress to reticular degenerative retinoschisis (bullous retinoschisis).

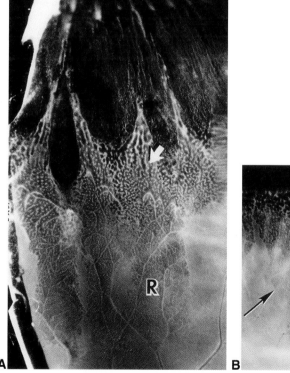
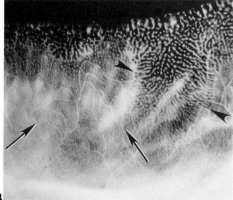

Figure 11-18 A, Typical *(arrow)* and reticular (R) cystoid degeneration of the peripheral retina, posterior to an enclosed ora bay (×12). **B,** Reticular peripheral cystoid degeneration (RPCD) *(between arrows)* and typical peripheral cystoid degeneration *(between arrowheads)*. RPCD has reticular pattern and finely stippled appearance. *(Part A from Duane TD, Jaeger EA, eds.* Clinical Ophthalmology. *Philadelphia: Lippincott; 1990, vol 3, ch 26:13. Photograph courtesy of Robert Y. Foos, MD. Part B from Green WR. Retina. In: Spencer WH, ed.* Ophthalmic Pathology: An Atlas and Textbook. *3rd ed. Philadelphia: Saunders; 1985:817. Photograph courtesy of Robert Y. Foos, MD.)*

Although degenerative retinoschisis is sometimes subdivided into typical and reticular forms, clinical differentiation is difficult. The complications of posterior extension and progression to retinal detachment are associated with the reticular form. Retinoschisis is bilateral in 50%–80% of affected patients, often occurs in the inferotemporal quadrant, and is commonly associated with hyperopia.

In *typical degenerative retinoschisis,* the retina splits in the outer plexiform layer. The outer layer is irregular and appears pockmarked on scleral depression. The inner layer is thin and is seen clinically as a smooth, oval elevation, most commonly found in the inferotemporal quadrant but sometimes located superotemporally (Fig 11-19). Occasionally, small, irregular white dots (snowflakes) can be seen; these are remnants of Müller cells and neurons that bridge or formerly bridged the cavity. The retinal vessels appear sclerotic. In all cases, typical bubbly-appearing peripheral cystoid degeneration can be found anterior to the schisis cavity. The schisis may extend posteriorly to the equator, but complications such as hole formation, retinal detachment, or marked posterior extension are rare. The split in retina almost never extends as far posteriorly as the macula.

In *reticular degenerative retinoschisis,* the splitting occurs in the nerve fiber layer. The very thin inner layer may be markedly elevated. As in typical retinoschisis, the outer layer appears pockmarked and the retinal vessels sclerotic. Posterior extension is more common in reticular than in typical retinoschisis. Approximately 23% of cases have outer wall holes that may be large and have rolled edges.

Differentiation of retinoschisis from RRD

Retinoschisis must be differentiated from rhegmatogenous retinal detachment (Table 11-6). Retinoschisis causes an absolute scotoma, whereas RRD causes a relative scotoma. "Tobacco dust" and/or hemorrhage are rarely found in the vitreous with retinoschisis,

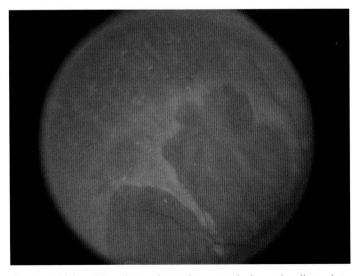

Figure 11-19 Retinoschisis with a large, irregular outer hole and yellow dots on the inner surface. *(From Lee BL, van Heuven WAJ. Peripheral lesions of the fundus.* Focal Points: Clinical Modules for Ophthalmologists. *San Francisco: American Academy of Ophthalmology; 2000, module 8.)*

Table 11-6 Differentiation of Retinal Detachment and Retinoschisis

Clinical Feature	Retinal Detachment	Schisis
Surface	Corrugated	Smooth-domed
Hemorrhage or pigment	Present	Usually absent
Scotoma	Relative	Absolute
Reaction to photocoagulation	Absent	Generally present
Shifting fluid	Variable	Absent

whereas they are commonly seen with RRD. Retinoschisis has a smooth surface and usually appears dome-shaped; in contrast, RRD often has a corrugated, irregular surface. In long-standing RRD, however, the retina also may appear smooth and thin, similar to retinoschisis. Whereas long-standing RRD may also show atrophy of the underlying RPE, demarcation line(s), and macrocysts, in retinoschisis the underlying RPE is normal.

Retinoschisis is associated with about 3% of full-thickness retinal detachments. Two types of schisis-related detachments occur. In the first type, if holes are present in the outer but not in the inner wall of the schisis cavity, the contents of the cavity can migrate through an outer wall hole and slowly detach the retina. Demarcation lines and degeneration of the underlying RPE are common. A demarcation line in an eye with retinoschisis suggests that a full-thickness detachment is or was formerly present and has spontaneously regressed. This type of schisis detachment usually does not progress, or it progresses slowly and seldom requires treatment.

In the second type of schisis detachment, holes are present in both the inner and outer layers. The schisis cavity may collapse, and a progressive RRD may result. Such detachments often progress rapidly and usually require treatment. The causative breaks may be located very posteriorly and thus may be difficult to repair. Vitrectomy techniques may be required.

Byer NE. Long-term natural history study of senile retinoschisis with implications for management. *Ophthalmology.* 1986;93:1127–1137.

Regillo CD, Benson WE. *Retinal Detachment: Diagnosis and Management.* 3rd ed. Philadelphia: Lippincott; 1998:68–70.

Straatsma BR, Foos RH, Feman SS. Degenerative diseases of the peripheral retina. In: Duane TD, ed. *Clinical Ophthalmology.* Philadelphia: Harper & Row; 1983; vol 3; chap 26:1–29.

Tiedeman JS. Retinal breaks, holes, and tears. *Focal Points: Clinical Modules for Ophthalmologists.* San Francisco: American Academy of Ophthalmology; 1996, module 3.

CHAPTER 12

Diseases of the Vitreous

Normal Anatomy

The vitreous is a gel structure that fills the posterior cavity of the globe. Collagen is the major structural protein component of the vitreous; the other major component is hyaluronic acid. The *vitreous base* straddles the ora serrata, extending 1.5–2.0 mm anteriorly and 1.0–3.0 mm posteriorly. It cannot be separated mechanically from the underlying retina. The *vitreous cortex* is the outer lining of the vitreous. Anterior to the vitreous base it is called the anterior vitreous cortex. Posterior to the vitreous base it is called the posterior vitreous cortex and is adherent to the basal lamina of the internal limiting membrane of the retina.

Posterior Vitreous Detachment

With age, the vitreous liquefies in parallel with a loss of hyaluronic acid, a mucopolysaccharide that separates the collagen fibers of the vitreous. The more liquid vitreous accumulates in lacunae within the vitreous; these lacunae are surrounded by displaced collagen fibers. With loss of the gel volume, a contractile force appears to develop. There are several possible reasons for this force to develop, including an age-related loss of hyaluronic acid, electrostatic attraction of adjacent collagen fibers in the absence of hyaluronic acid, and possible cross-linking of collagen fibers. If a defect develops in the posterior vitreous face, the liquid vitreous escapes posteriorly. The anterior collagen fibers are anchored in the vitreous base. With contraction of the vitreous, the posterior section detaches, as the vitreous in the vitreous base cannot. The vitreous detachment occurs at the outer portion of the cortical vitreous, where the collagen fibers course in a direction parallel to the retinal surface. The prevalence increases in patients who have had cataract extractions, particularly if the posterior capsule's integrity has been violated, and in patients with a history of inflammation of the vitreous body.

The imaging of posterior vitreous detachments (PVDs) may be made by a variety of techniques. The easiest way is through biomicroscopic examination with a wide-field lens. The posterior vitreous face may be seen a few millimeters above the retinal surface. A fine ring of tissue, a Weiss ring, frequently is torn loose from the surface of the nerve and serves as a marker for PVD over the nerve. The use of additional modalities has broadened our concepts about the initiation and progression of PVD. The posterior vitreous face may also be seen during contact B-scan ultrasonography as a thin white line bounding the vitreous gel. It is common to see partial detachments of the posterior vitreous face by contact B-scan ultrasonography. Optical coherence tomography (OCT) has shown that PVDs often start as localized detachments of the vitreous over the perifoveal macula, called a *posterior perifoveal vitreous detachment.* This detachment may spread radially to involve larger areas. Persistent traction by the vitreous may induce a number of different pathologic abnormalities in the retina. This sets the stage for the combined effects of static traction from the contracting vitreous as well as dynamic traction from ocular saccades acting through the vitreous to place stress on the affected retina. Focal traction on the peripheral retina may lead to breaks and detachments. Persistent attachment to the macula may lead to tractional distortion and elevation of the macula called *vitreous macular traction syndrome.* Persistent attachment to the central macula can lead to traction on the fovea, causing foveal deformation, including macular holes (Fig 12-1).

Remnants of the vitreous often remain on the inner retina after a posterior vitreous "detachment." These plaques of vitreous can participate in the genesis of tractional retinopathies.

Spaide RF, Wong D, Fisher Y, et al. Correlation of vitreous attachment and foveal deformation in macular hole states. *Am J Ophthalmol.* 2002;133:226–229.

Developmental Abnormalities

Tunica Vasculosa Lentis

Remnants of the tunica vasculosa lentis and hyaloid system are commonly seen, none of them visually significant. *Mittendorf dot,* an anterior remnant, is a small and dense white round dot attached to the lens capsule slightly nasally and inferiorly to the posterior pole of the lens. A posterior remnant known as *Bergmeister's papilla* is a fibroglial tuft of tissue extending into the vitreous for a short distance at the margin of the optic nerve head. The entire hyaloid artery, either patent or occluded, may also persist from disc to lens within Cloquet's canal.

Prepapillary Vascular Loops

Initially thought to be remnants of the hyaloid artery, prepapillary vascular loops are now known to be normal retinal vessels that have grown into Bergmeister's papillae before returning to the disc. The loops are typically less than 5 mm in height. These vessels may supply one or more quadrants of retina. Fluorescein angiography has shown that 95% are arterial and 5% are venous. Complications include branch retinal artery obstruction, amaurosis fugax, and vitreous hemorrhage (Fig 12-2).

Persistent Hyperplastic Primary Vitreous, or Persistent Fetal Vasculature

Persistent hyperplastic primary vitreous (PHPV) was historically thought to result from failure of the primary vitreous to regress. More recently, the term *persistent fetal vasculature (PFV)* has been proposed to provide an integrated interpretation of the signs and

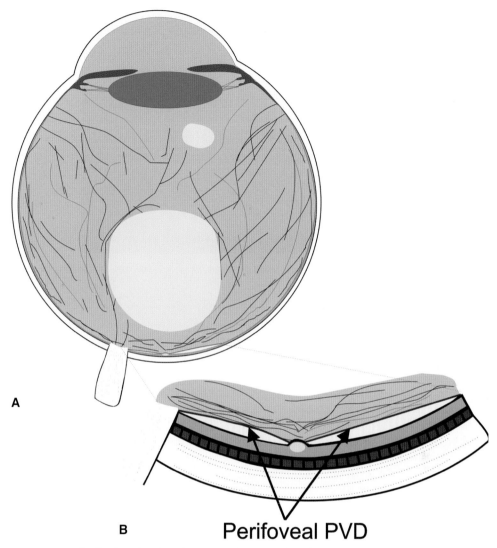

Perifoveal PVD

Figure 12-1   A, During the development of a posterior vitreous detachment, the perifoveal vitreous starts to detach first, producing a perifoveal posterior vitreous detachment. **B,** Persistent attachment of the vitreous to a more localized area in the central macula can lead to deformation and structural failure in the fovea. *(Illustrations by Richard Spaide, MD.)*

symptoms associated with PHPV. This disease, which is unilateral in 90% of cases, may have serious visual consequences. There are usually no associated systemic findings. Anterior, posterior, and combined forms of this developmental abnormality have been described.

Anterior PHPV

In anterior PHPV, the hyaloid artery remains, and a white vascularized fibrous membrane is present behind the lens. Associated findings include microphthalmos, a shallow anterior chamber, and long ciliary processes that are visible around the small lens. Leukocoria

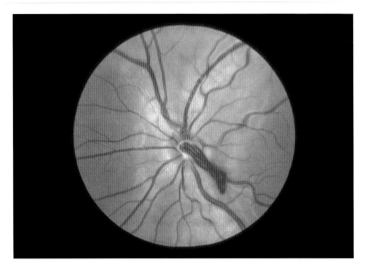

Figure 12-2 Prepapillary vascular loop. *(Photograph courtesy of M. Gilbert Grand, MD.)*

often is noted at birth. A dehiscence of the posterior lens capsule may, in many cases, cause swelling of the lens, cataract, and secondary angle-closure glaucoma. In addition, glaucoma may result from incomplete development of the chamber angle.

The natural course of anterior PHPV may lead to blindness in the most advanced cases. Lensectomy and removal of the fibrovascular retrolental membrane will prevent angle-closure glaucoma; however, growth of a secondary cataract is common. Deprivational and refractive amblyopia is a serious postoperative challenge in these patients (Fig 12-3).

Anterior PHPV should be considered in the differential diagnosis of leukocoria. Differentiating PHPV from retinoblastoma is particularly important. Unlike PHPV, retinoblastoma is usually not obvious at birth, is more often bilateral, and is almost never associated with microphthalmos or cataract. PHPV is anterior in the eye at birth; retinoblastomas do not appear in the anterior fundus until well after birth. Ancillary testing such as diagnostic echography and x-ray techniques to look for calcification within retinoblastoma can be helpful in differentiating the two.

Posterior PHPV

Posterior PHPV may occur in association with anterior PHPV or as an isolated finding. The eye may be microphthalmic, but the anterior chamber is usually normal and the lens typically clear, without a retrolenticular membrane. A stalk of tissue emanates from the optic disc and courses toward the retrolental region, often running along the apex of a retinal fold that may extend anteriorly from the disc, usually in an inferior quadrant. The stalk fans out circumferentially toward the anterior retina. Posterior PHPV should be differentiated from retinopathy of prematurity, ocular toxocariasis, and familial exudative vitreoretinopathy.

Goldberg MF. Persistent fetal vasculature (PFV): an integrated interpretation of signs and symptoms associated with persistent hyperplastic primary vitreous (PHPV). LIV Edward Jackson Memorial Lecture. *Am J Ophthalmol.* 1997;124:587–626.

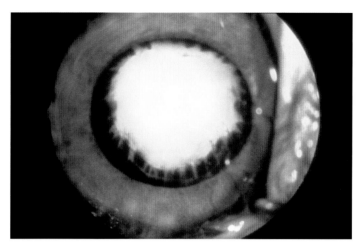

Figure 12-3 PHPV as seen in a 4-month-old male. Note cataract secondary to retrolental mass. Blood vessels on the iris represent persistent vascularized pupillary membranes. *(Photograph courtesy of Jerry A. Shields, MD.)*

Mittra RA, Huynh LT, Ruttum MS, et al. Visual outcomes following lensectomy and vitrectomy for combined anterior and posterior persistent hyperplastic primary vitreous. *Arch Ophthalmol.* 1998;116:1190–1194.

Reese AB. Persistent hyperplastic primary vitreous. *Am J Ophthalmol.* 1955;40:317–331.

Hereditary Hyaloideoretinopathies With Optically Empty Vitreous

The hallmark of this group of conditions, known as hereditary hyaloideoretinopathies, is vitreous liquefaction that results in an optically empty cavity except for a thin layer of cortical vitreous behind the lens and whitish, avascular membranes that adhere to the retina. Fundus abnormalities include equatorial and perivascular (radial) lattice (Fig 12-4). The electroretinogram may be subnormal.

These conditions can be classified into 2 main groups: those with ocular signs and symptoms exclusively, and those with associated systemic findings. The first group includes *Jansen disease,* which has a high incidence of retinal detachment, and *Wagner disease,* which is not associated with retinal detachment. Both diseases are transmitted as autosomal dominant traits. Additional ocular abnormalities include myopia, strabismus, and cataract.

The second group, with associated systemic abnormalities, includes hereditary arthroophthalmopathy (marfanoid variety) of the Stickler syndrome, hereditary arthroophthalmopathy with stiff joints (Weill-Marchesani–like variety), and 4 varieties with frank dwarfism.

Stickler syndrome, the most common variety, is transmitted as an autosomal dominant trait. Most patients with Stickler syndrome have a mutation in the gene encoding type II procollagen. Varying mutations may produce Stickler syndrome phenotypes of differing severity. Additional ocular abnormalities include myopia, open-angle glaucoma,

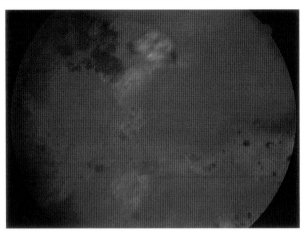

Figure 12-4 Extensive lattice degeneration and pigmentary change in patient with Stickler syndrome. *(Photograph courtesy of William F. Mieler, MD.)*

and cataract. Orofacial findings include midfacial flattening and the Pierre Robin malformation complex of micrognathia, cleft palate (which may be submucosal), and glossoptosis. These skeletal abnormalities may not be that obvious and require a high index of clinical suspicion. Generalized skeletal abnormalities include joint hyperextensibility and enlargement, arthritis, and mild spondyloepiphyseal dysplasia. It is very important to recognize this syndrome because of the high incidence of retinal detachment. The detachments may be difficult to repair because of multiple, posterior, or large breaks and because of a tendency toward proliferative vitreoretinopathy. These patients typically have flattened vitreous condensations adherent to the retina. For this reason, the ophthalmologist should strongly consider prophylactic therapy of retinal breaks. (See Prophylactic Treatment of Retinal Breaks in Chapter 11.)

Blair NP, Albert DM, Liberfarb RM, et al. Hereditary progressive arthro-ophthalmopathy of Stickler. *Am J Ophthalmol*. 1979;88:876–888.

Maumenee IH. Vitreoretinal degeneration as a sign of generalized connective tissue diseases. *Am J Ophthalmol*. 1979;88:432–449.

Familial Exudative Vitreoretinopathy

Familial exudative vitreoretinopathy (FEVR) is characterized by failure of the temporal retina to vascularize and by retinal exudation, tractional detachment, and retinal folds (Fig 12-5). It is usually inherited as an autosomal dominant trait, but X-linked transmission also occurs. Several different gene loci have been associated with the FEVR phenotype. The X-linked variant of FEVR is linked to the Norrie disease gene locus. Peripheral fibrovascular proliferation and tractional retinal detachment are often associated. Tractional retinal detachments with subretinal lipid exudate and exudative detachments may be seen in the neonatal period or in adolescence, and late-onset rhegmatogenous retinal detachments may occur. There is dragging of the macula and vascular

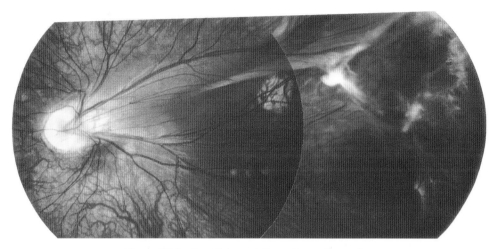

Figure 12-5 Familial exudative vitreoretinopathy.

arcades temporally. The condition is generally bilateral, although the severity of ocular involvement may be asymmetric. Affected individuals with FEVR, unlike those with retinopathy of prematurity (ROP), are full term and have normal respiratory status. There is no peripheral mesenchymal shunt. Differentiation of FEVR from ROP is also aided by family history and careful examination of all family members; the only finding in some family members with FEVR may be straightening of vessels and peripheral nonperfusion. Fluorescein angiography with peripheral sweeps is indispensable in examining family members.

Shubert A, Tasman W. Familial exudative vitreoretinopathy: surgical intervention and visual acuity outcomes. *Graefes Arch Clin Exp Ophthalmol.* 1997;235:490–493.

Tasman W, Augsburger JJ, Shields JA, et al. Familial exudative vitreoretinopathy. *Trans Am Ophthalmol Soc.* 1981;79:211–226.

Asteroid Hyalosis

Minute white opacities composed of calcium-containing phospholipids are found in the otherwise normal vitreous in asteroid hyalosis (Fig 12-6). Clinical studies have confirmed a relationship between asteroid hyalosis and diabetes and hypertension. Asteroid hyalosis has an overall incidence of 1 in 200 persons, most frequently in those over 50 years of age. The condition is unilateral in 75% of cases, and it only rarely causes a significant decrease in visual acuity. When asteroid hyalosis blocks the view of the posterior fundus and retinal pathology is suspected, fluorescein angiography is usually successful in imaging abnormalities. Occasionally, vitrectomy may be necessary to remove visually significant opacities or to facilitate treatment of underlying retinal abnormalities such as proliferative retinopathy or choroidal neovascularization.

Bergren RL, Brown GC, Duker JS. Prevalence and association of asteroid hyalosis with systemic diseases. *Am J Ophthalmol.* 1991;111:289–293.

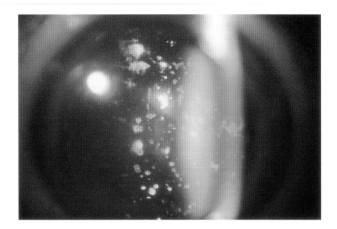

Figure 12-6 Asteroid hyalosis.

Spencer WH, ed. *Ophthalmic Pathology: An Atlas and Textbook.* 4 vols. 4th ed. Philadelphia: Saunders; 1996.

Cholesterolosis (Hemophthalmos, Synchysis Scintillans)

Numerous yellowish white, gold, or multicolored cholesterol crystals are seen in the vitreous and anterior chamber in cholesterolosis. This condition appears almost exclusively in eyes that have undergone repeated or severe accidental or surgical trauma with large intraocular hemorrhages. The descriptive term *synchysis scintillans* refers to the highly refractile appearance of the crystals. In contrast to eyes with asteroid hyalosis, in which the opacities are evenly distributed throughout the vitreous cavity, eyes with cholesterolosis frequently have a PVD, which allows the crystals to settle inferiorly.

Spencer WH, ed. *Ophthalmic Pathology: An Atlas and Textbook.* 4 vols. 4th ed. Philadelphia: Saunders; 1996.

Amyloidosis

Bilateral vitreous opacification can occur as an early manifestation of the dominantly inherited form of familial amyloidosis. Amyloidosis involving the vitreous has rarely been observed in nonfamilial cases. In addition to the clinically apparent vitreous deposition, amyloid can be deposited in the retinal vasculature, the choroid, and the trabecular meshwork.

Reported retinal findings include hemorrhages, exudates, cotton-wool spots, and peripheral retinal neovascularization. In addition, abnormalities of the orbit, extraocular muscles, eyelids, conjunctiva, cornea, and iris may present. Nonocular manifestations of amyloidosis include upper and lower extremity polyneuropathy and CNS abnormalities. Amyloid can be deposited in multiple organs, including the heart and skin, and in the gastrointestinal tract.

The extracellular vitreous opacities initially appear to lie adjacent to retinal vessels posteriorly; they later develop anteriorly. At first, the opacities appear granular with wispy fringes, but as they enlarge and aggregate, the vitreous takes on a "glass wool" appearance. With vitreous liquefaction or PVD, the opacities may be displaced into the visual axis, causing reduced visual acuity and photophobia.

The differential diagnosis includes chronic (dehemoglobinized) vitreous hemorrhage. Vitrectomy may be indicated for vitreous opacities when symptoms warrant intervention, but recurrent opacities may develop in residual vitreous. Histologic examination of removed vitreous has shown material with a fibrillar appearance and staining reaction characteristic of amyloid. Electron microscopic studies are confirmatory. Immunocytochemical studies have shown the major amyloid constituent to be a protein resembling prealbumin.

Bhistikul RB, Mukai S. Vitreous amyloidosis. In: Albert DM, Jakobiec FA, eds. *Principles and Practice of Ophthalmology*. Philadelphia: Saunders; 2000:2530–2539.

Spencer WH, ed. *Ophthalmic Pathology: An Atlas and Textbook*. 3rd ed. Philadelphia: Saunders; 1985:571–572.

Spontaneous Vitreous Hemorrhage

The decreased vision and floaters caused by nontraumatic spontaneous vitreous hemorrhages are common causes of emergency visits to ophthalmologists' offices. The most frequent underlying etiology in adults is diabetic retinopathy (39%–54%). Other major causes include

- retinal break without detachment (12%–17%)
- posterior vitreous detachment (7.5%–12.0%)
- rhegmatogenous retinal detachment (7%–10%)
- retinal neovascularization following branch vein and central vein occlusion (3.5%–10.0%)

Any cause of peripheral neovascularization may cause a vitreous hemorrhage (see Table 5-6). In children, trauma should always be considered in the differential diagnosis of a vitreous hemorrhage (see Chapter 13). Congenital retinoschisis and pars planitis are other causes of vitreous hemorrhage in children as well as in adults.

In most cases of vitreous hemorrhage, the underlying cause can be detected by retinal examination. If the hemorrhage is too dense to permit ophthalmoscopy or biomicroscopy, suggestive clues can be obtained from the history and from examination of the fellow eye. Diagnostic echography should be performed to rule out retinal detachment or tumor. If the cause still cannot be determined, 2 days of bed rest with elevation of the head of the bed and bilateral patches may permit the blood to settle. If the etiology still cannot be established, the ophthalmologist should consider frequent reexamination with repeat echography until the cause is found.

Morse PH, Aminlari A, Scheie HG. Spontaneous vitreous hemorrhage. *Arch Ophthalmol*. 1974;92:297–298.

Winslow RL, Taylor BC. Spontaneous vitreous hemorrhage: etiology and management. *South Med J*. 1980;73:1450–1452.

Pigment Granules

In a patient without uveitis, retinitis pigmentosa, or a history of surgical or accidental eye trauma, the presence of pigmented cells in the anterior vitreous ("tobacco dust"), known as *Shafer's sign,* is highly suggestive of a retinal break (see Chapter 11).

Vitreous Abnormalities Secondary to Cataract Surgery

Incarceration of vitreous in the wound during cataract surgery can lead to many post-operative complications:

- It contributes to faulty wound closure, possibly permitting entry of microorganisms into the eye and subsequent endophthalmitis.
- An insecure wound may allow epithelial or fibrous ingrowth, with the incarcerated vitreous serving as a scaffold for the proliferating cells, especially in the presence of other complicating factors such as inflammation and hemorrhage.
- A wound leak may lead to hypotony, partial or complete collapse of the anterior chamber, peripheral anterior synechiae, and/or secondary glaucoma.

Incarcerated vitreous in the wound and iridovitreal adhesions may cause chronic ocular discomfort with inflammation, cystoid macular edema, and disc edema (Irvine-Gass syndrome). These complications have reportedly been reduced by sectioning discrete anterior vitreous bands with the Nd:YAG laser or by vitrectomy. Retinal detachment is another complication caused by contraction of the incarcerated vitreous. Such detachments may be rhegmatogenous or a combination of tractional and rhegmatogenous types and may require vitrectomy techniques in addition to scleral buckling (see Chapter 16). The risk of complications from vitreous loss can be greatly reduced, first by careful anterior vitrectomy and then by meticulous closure of the wound at the time of cataract surgery.

For further discussion of the complications of cataract surgery see BCSC Section 11, *Lens and Cataract.* For postoperative endophthalmitis see BCSC Section 9, *Intraocular Inflammation and Uveitis.*

Fung WE. Vitrectomy for chronic aphakic cystoid macular edema: results of a national, collaborative, prospective, randomized investigation. *Ophthalmology.* 1985;92:1102–1111.

Harbour JW, Smiddy WE, Rubsamen PE, et al. Pars plana vitrectomy for chronic pseudophakic cystoid macular edema. *Am J Ophthalmol.* 1995;120:302–307.

CHAPTER 13

Posterior Segment Trauma

Ocular trauma is an important cause of visual impairment in the United States. The types of posterior segment injuries can be classified as follows:

- blunt trauma (no break in ocular tissues)
- penetrating trauma (entrance break, no exit break)
- perforating trauma (entrance and exit breaks)
- intraocular foreign bodies

Microsurgical techniques have improved the ability to repair corneal and scleral lacerations, and vitrectomy techniques allow management of severe intraocular injuries (see Chapter 16). Ocular trauma is also discussed in BCSC Section 6, *Pediatric Ophthalmology and Strabismus;* Section 7, *Orbit, Eyelids, and Lacrimal System;* and Section 8, *External Disease and Cornea.*

Evaluation of the Patient Following Ocular Trauma

A complete history is crucial when the patient with ocular trauma is first examined. The following important information should be obtained:

- How and when was the patient injured?
- Was the injury work related?
- What emergency measures were taken (eg, tetanus shot given, antibiotics administered)?
- Are there concomitant systemic injuries?
- When was the patient's last oral intake?
- What was the status of the eye before the injury?
- Is the presence of an intraocular foreign body possible?
- Was the patient hammering metal on metal or working near machinery that could have caused a projectile to enter the eye?
- Was the patient wearing spectacles or was he or she close to shattered glass?
- How forceful was the injury?
- Was the patient wearing eye protection?

Initial caution is required to avoid more damage to the eye. Evaluation should be made to determine if there is a closed-globe or open-globe injury. In an open-globe injury, the eyewall has a full-thickness wound. This eyewall defect may be caused by rupture, which is mechanical failure from hydrostatic overload, or by laceration, which is caused by a sharp object cutting the eyewall.

If an open-globe injury is suspected, the eye should be covered with a shield. The physician should avoid prying open the eye of an uncooperative patient. If severe chemosis or eyelid edema prevents a thorough examination, this is best postponed until the time of surgery. Examination under anesthesia should be considered for children or anyone unable to cooperate.

If the patient is able to cooperate, the examiner should measure visual acuity of both eyes and evaluate the pupil for an afferent pupillary defect. Careful slit-lamp examination can reveal an entrance wound, hyphema, iris damage or incarceration, cataract, or other anterior segment pathology, although a scleral entrance wound is sometimes obscured by hemorrhagic conjunctiva. Intraocular pressure should be checked. Reduced IOP may suggest a posterior scleral rupture; however, normal IOP does not exclude an occult penetration.

It is important to examine the eye with the indirect ophthalmoscope as soon as possible. A posterior penetration or an intraocular foreign body is less difficult to detect if the patient is examined before synechiae, cataract, dispersed vitreous hemorrhage, or infection can develop. If the examiner suspects that the eye may possibly harbor an intraocular foreign body that is not seen on examination, an imaging study should be considered.

Ultrasound examination may be useful in eyes with opaque media following trauma, although it may be necessary to defer ultrasonography until an open wound is closed surgically. To increase the efficacy of the ultrasonographic examination, it is best to assure the patient that the examination is not painful. Sterile gonioscopic gel is used as a coupling agent for the ultrasound. When copious amounts are used, the ultrasonographic examination can be performed with minimal pressure on the closed lid. Intraocular air may cause artifacts that complicate the interpretation of ultrasonography. Computed tomography is very helpful in evaluating patients suspected of having intraocular foreign bodies. Metal foreign bodies may introduce artifacts that make them appear larger than they really are, making exact localization difficult. On occasion, wood and certain types of plastic may be very difficult to detect by computed tomography. These types of foreign bodies may be identified and localized with magnetic resonance imaging (MRI). MRI should be used only after the presence of ferromagnetic foreign bodies has been absolutely ruled out because of the possibility that such foreign bodies may be moved by the magnetic field, causing ocular damage.

Blunt Trauma

The object that causes the injury in a blunt trauma does not penetrate the eye but may cause rupture of the eyewall. Blunt trauma can have a number of serious sequelae:

- angle recession
- hemorrhage into the anterior chamber (hyphema) or vitreous
- retinal tears or detachment
- subluxated or dislocated lens

- commotio retinae
- choroidal rupture
- macular hole
- avulsed optic nerve
- scleral rupture

See Chapter 11 for discussion of traumatic retinal breaks and retinal detachment and BCSC Section 11, *Lens and Cataract*, for discussion of dislocated lenses.

It is essential that a complete ophthalmologic examination be performed following blunt trauma, because an eye with minimal or no anterior damage may have a severe posterior injury. For example, a patient without hyphema or iritis may nonetheless have a large retinal tear, choroidal rupture, or blowout fracture.

Vitreous Hemorrhage

Vitreous hemorrhage can result from damage to blood vessels of the iris, ciliary body, retina, or choroid and can also be caused by retinal tears. The cause of the vitreous hemorrhage should always be sought. Sometimes a hemorrhage that is limited at presentation later becomes diffuse; thus, the eye should be carefully examined with the indirect ophthalmoscope as soon as possible. If the posterior segment cannot be visualized through a vitreous hemorrhage, ultrasound examination is indicated. Retinal or choroidal detachment, most retinal tears, and posterior vitreous detachment can be detected by ultrasound techniques. Echographic signs of an occult scleral rupture include vitreous strands that lead to a posterior or peripheral rupture site.

Sometimes bed rest with elevation of the patient's head causes the hemorrhage to settle sufficiently to allow ophthalmoscopic examination. If the source of the hemorrhage still cannot be determined, frequent follow-up and repeat ultrasound examination should be carried out until the hemorrhage clears. In the absence of complications, a unilateral hemorrhage can be observed until it clears. Macular hole, choroidal rupture in the macula, traumatic maculopathy, retinal detachment, or other traumatic injuries can limit visual recovery.

Commotio Retinae

The term *commotio retinae* describes the damage to the outer retinal layers caused by shock waves that traverse the eye from the site of impact following blunt trauma. Ophthalmoscopically, a sheenlike retinal whitening appears some hours following injury (Fig 13-1). It is most commonly seen in the posterior pole but may occur peripherally as well. Several mechanisms for the retinal opacification have been proposed, including extracellular edema, glial swelling, and photoreceptor outer segment disruption. With foveal involvement, a cherry-red spot may appear, because the cells involved in the whitening are not present in the fovea. Commotio retinae in the posterior pole, also called *Berlin edema*, may decrease visual acuity to as low as 20/200. Fortunately, the prognosis for visual recovery is good, as the condition clears in 3–4 weeks. In some cases, however, visual recovery is limited by associated macular pigment epitheliopathy, choroidal rupture, or macular hole formation. There is no acute treatment.

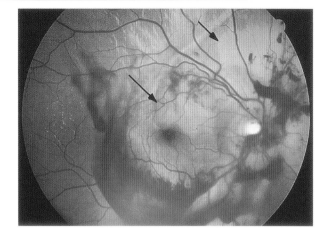

Figure 13-1 Commotio retinae *(arrows)* and vitreous hemorrhage following blunt trauma.

Choroidal Rupture

When the eye is compressed along its anterior-posterior axis, the eyewall becomes stretched in its horizontal axis because of hydraulic displacement of the vitreous. Bruch's membrane, which has little elasticity, may tear, along with the overlying RPE and underlying choriocapillaris. Associated adjacent subretinal hemorrhage is common. Choroidal ruptures may be single or multiple, commonly in the periphery, and may be concentric to the optic disc (Fig 13-2). Ruptures that extend through the central macular area may cause permanent visual loss. There is no immediate treatment.

Occasionally, choroidal neovascularization (CNV) develops as a late complication in response to the damage to Bruch's membrane (Fig 13-3). A patient with choroidal rupture near the macula should be alerted to the risk of CNV and advised to use an Amsler grid for self-testing. Treatment may be indicated if the CNV does not involve the foveal center. Despite treatment, CNV may recur. The natural outcome of CNV in the foveal center associated with a choroidal rupture may not be as poor as in AMD; however, photodynamic therapy may be indicated. Subfoveal surgery may be considered for these cases. See Chapter 4 for guidelines on treatment of CNV.

Posttraumatic Macular Hole

The fovea is extremely thin, and blunt trauma may cause a full-thickness macular hole by either one or a combination of mechanisms, including contusion necrosis and vitreous traction (Fig 13-4). Holes may be noted immediately or soon after blunt trauma that causes severe Berlin edema, after a subretinal hemorrhage caused by a choroidal rupture, following severe cystoid macular edema, or after a whiplash separation of the vitreous from the retina. In addition, central abnormal depressions or macular pits (similar to those found in patients following sun gazing) have been described following blunt trauma to the eye and whiplash injuries. (Lightning and electrical injury can cause macular holes; these patients usually have signs of cataract and can have acute peripapillary retinal whitening.) Posttraumatic macular holes may be successfully closed with vitrectomy and gas injection.

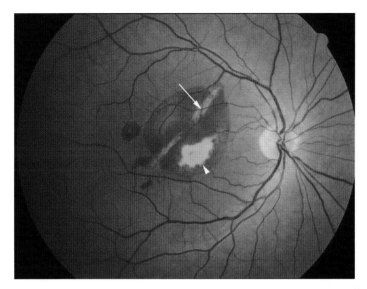

Figure 13-2 Following trauma, this patient had a submacular hemorrhage. The hemorrhage started to clear, revealing a choroidal rupture *(arrow)*. The yellow material located at the infer-onasal portion of the macula *(arrowhead)* is dehemoglobinized blood. *(Photograph courtesy of Mark Johnson, MD.)*

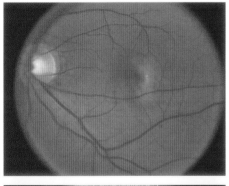

Figure 13-3 A, Choroidal rupture with CNV 10 weeks after blunt trauma. **B,** Fluorescein angiogram demonstrates lacy choroidal neo-vascular membrane bordering foveal avas-cular zone. **C,** Laser scar 6 months after laser surgery; no recurrence; visual acuity is 20/20.

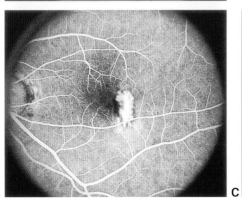

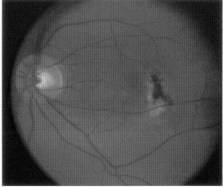

Retinitis Sclopetaria

An unusual retinal picture can be produced by high-speed missile injuries to the orbit. Large areas of choroidal and retinal rupture and necrosis are combined with extensive subretinal and retinal hemorrhage, often involving as much as 2 quadrants of the retina. As the blood resorbs, the injured area is filled in by extensive scar formation and widespread pigmentary alteration. (Fig 13-5) The macula is almost always involved, leading

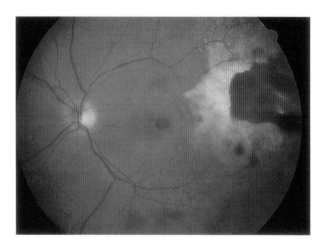

Figure 13-4 Posttraumatic macular hole 15 days after ocular contusion by a BB pellet. Posttraumatic pigment metaplasia and hemorrhage are also present.

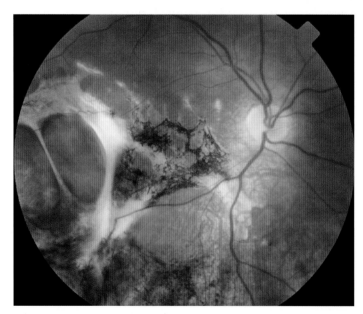

Figure 13-5 This patient was shot in the right inferotemporal orbit with a bullet. The path of the bullet missed the globe by several millimeters. The patient acutely lost visual acuity. This photograph was taken 2 months after her injury and shows large areas of subretinal proliferation and retinal pigment epithelial hyperplasia. Her visual acuity returned to 20/70. *(Photograph courtesy of Richard F. Spaide, MD.)*

to significant visual loss, but secondary retinal detachment rarely develops. The pattern of damage is ascribed to shock waves generated by the object passing close to the sclera, but a similar fundus picture may develop from blunt trauma to the eyelids from paintball injuries.

Scleral Rupture

Severe blunt injuries can rupture the globe. The 2 most common locations for rupture are at the limbus (under intact conjunctiva) or parallel to and under the insertions of the rectus muscles, a region where the sclera is thinnest. Important diagnostic signs of rupture include marked decrease in ocular ductions, a very boggy conjunctival chemosis with hemorrhage, deepened anterior chamber, and severe vitreous hemorrhage. The IOP is usually reduced but may be normal or even elevated. An intraocular foreign body must be ruled out in all cases of ruptured globe. The principles of surgical management of ruptured and lacerated globes are discussed in the following section.

Lacerating and Penetrating Injuries

Lacerating and penetrating injuries result from cutting or tearing of the eyewall by a sharp object. A penetrating injury is caused by a laceration at a single site on the globe. The prognosis is related to the location and extent of the wound, as well as the associated damage and degree of hemorrhage. Any corneal laceration that crosses the limbus must be explored until its posterior extent has been visualized. See also BCSC Section 8, *External Disease and Cornea*. If a posterior rupture is suspected, a 360° peritomy should be carefully performed with cautious exploration under the rectus muscles.

The principles of initial management of a penetrating injury include meticulous microsurgical wound closure in which incarcerated uvea is reposited or excised. Corneal lacerations may be closed with 10-0 nylon interrupted sutures, and scleral wounds may be closed with strong 7-0 or 8-0 nonabsorbable sutures. Vitreous should be excised from the wound and the anterior chamber re-formed. The ophthalmologist should take care not to apply excessive pressure to the eye during wound closure. Small posterior wounds may be allowed to heal without treatment because attempts at wound closure may increase the risk of posterior vitreous extrusion. BCSC Section 4, *Ophthalmic Pathology and Intraocular Tumors,* discusses wound healing in detail in Chapter 2, Wound Repair.

Late complications following a penetrating injury (tractional retinal detachment, cyclitic membrane formation, and phthisis bulbi) result from intraocular cellular proliferation and tractional membrane formation. Removal of the vitreous may reduce the risk of late tractional retinal detachment by eliminating the scaffold on which the membranes grow. The optimal timing of vitrectomy after penetrating injuries is unknown. Some surgeons favor immediate vitrectomy before cellular proliferation can begin; however, most prefer initial primary repair of the wound to decrease the risk of endophthalmitis. Depending on the circumstances, vitrectomy may be postponed for 4–14 days for the following reasons:

- to decrease the risk of intraoperative hemorrhage in acutely inflamed and congested eyes

- to allow the cornea to clear and improve intraoperative visualization
- to permit spontaneous separation of the vitreous from the retina, which may facilitate a more complete vitrectomy

Although there are some theoretical reasons for early vitrectomy, the overruling priority at the time of the acute injury is to close the globe. Primary wound closure should not be delayed by uncertainty of whether or not an early vitrectomy should be performed. Immediate vitrectomy may be necessary in some circumstances—for example, if evidence suggests infectious endophthalmitis or a retained intraocular foreign body at the time of primary repair. See also Chapter 16.

> Mieler WF, Mittra RA. The role and timing of pars plana vitrectomy in penetrating ocular trauma. *Arch Ophthalmol.* 1997;115:1191–1192.

Perforating Injuries

Whereas a penetrating injury has a wound through the eyewall into the globe, a perforating injury has both entrance and exit wounds. Perforating injuries may be caused by sharp objects such as needles or knives or by high-velocity pellets or small fragments of metal. An important iatrogenic cause is needle perforation during retrobulbar anesthesia for cataract surgery. Experimental studies have shown that fibrous proliferation after perforating injuries occurs along the scaffold of damaged vitreous between the entrance and exit wounds. The wounds are closed by fibrosis within 7 days after the injury. Small-gauge injuries with only a small amount of hemorrhage and no significant ancillary damage often heal without serious sequelae. Anterior wounds are usually cleared of externalized vitreous and closed with sutures, but small posterior wounds are best left unrepaired to avoid extruding vitreous through the wound during attempted closure. Vitrectomy may be considered for the following:

- the presence of moderate to severe vitreous hemorrhage
- ancillary damage requiring repair
- signs of developing transvitreal traction

Vitrectomy is usually delayed 7 days to allow the posterior wounds to close by proliferation so that posterior suturing will not be necessary.

It is important to attempt to separate the posterior hyaloid during vitrectomy to prevent later proliferation and contraction that can lead to retinal detachment. Development of a PVD may be difficult, however, in children, young adults, and in eyes with retinal breaks and/or a retinal detachment. Retinal detachment usually may be caused by the primary injury itself or by traction transmitted by vitreous and proliferating cells to other retinal areas.

Intraocular Foreign Bodies

Most cases involving intraocular foreign bodies create a visible entry wound, or the object itself can be seen. Even without such evidence, however, an intraocular foreign body should be suspected and ruled out after any ocular or orbital trauma. A detailed history should be taken. Small, high-velocity pieces of steel, such as might be broken off in hammering steel on steel or thrown by high-speed machinery, are often overlooked, but they can lead to severe visual impairment. If possible, a sample of the suspected foreign body should be examined to see whether it is magnetic and radiopaque.

Frontal and lateral skull x-rays are usually sufficient to determine the presence, although not the precise location, of most radiopaque foreign bodies. In an eye with opaque media, both plain-film x-rays to detect the number and size of foreign bodies and other imaging studies (CT scans without contrast or echography) to locate the foreign bodies are often indicated (Fig 13-6). CT is better than plain-film x-rays at pinpointing the location of radiopaque foreign bodies and at detecting and locating less radiopaque foreign bodies. When very small or less radiopaque foreign bodies are suspected, bone-free

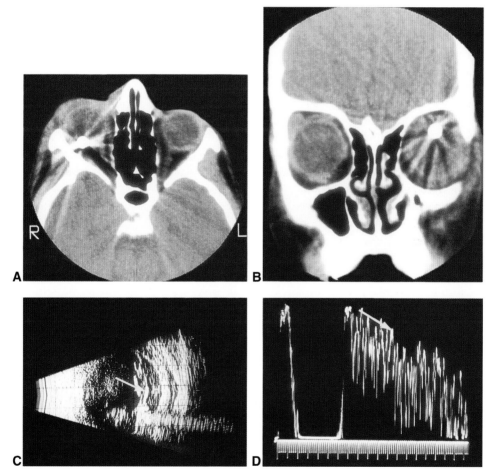

Figure 13-6 Intraocular BB pellet. Axial **(A)** and coronal **(B)** CT views show the BB to be in the superior and posterior globe. B-scan echography **(C)** shows retinal detachment *(arrow)* and subretinal hemorrhage *(H)*. A characteristic reverberation of echoes between the front and back surfaces of the round BB gives a "trail of echoes" artifact that extends posterior to the foreign body on B-scan *(asterisk)*, and on A-scan **(D)** *(arrow)*.

x-ray studies may be helpful. The presence of nonradiopaque foreign bodies and their relationship to intraocular structures may be determined by an experienced ultrasonographer. The possibility of multiple foreign bodies should not be overlooked. MRI is contraindicated if the foreign body is metallic because the magnetic force may move metallic foreign bodies, causing ocular damage.

Surgical Techniques for Removal of Intraocular Foreign Bodies

The surgeon planning removal of a magnetic intraocular foreign body must consider the following:

- location of the foreign body in the eye
- surgeon's ability to visualize the foreign body
- size and shape of the foreign body
- composition of the foreign body
- whether the foreign body is encapsulated

Pars plana vitrectomy allows removal of the vitreous and controlled extraction of the intraocular foreign body.

A pars plana magnet extraction can be considered for small, nonencapsulated ferromagnetic foreign bodies that can be easily seen in the vitreous cavity, are not embedded in or adherent to retina or other structures, and have no associated significant retinal pathology such as a retinal tear. After an incision is made through the pars plana pigmented epithelium, the magnet is aligned with its long axis pointing directly at the foreign body and its short blunt tip against the gaped sclerotomy site. When the magnet is pulsed, the foreign body will be pulled through the pars plana to the magnet.

If the media are opaque because of cataract or hemorrhage, if the foreign body is encapsulated and adherent to vitreous or retina, or if it is large or nonmagnetic, vitrectomy (with lensectomy if necessary) and forceps extraction of the foreign body are indicated. Before forceps extraction is attempted, the foreign body should be freed of all attachments. A small rare earth magnet may be used to engage the foreign body and mobilize it from the retinal surface. Although small foreign bodies can be removed through the pars plana sclerotomy site, some large foreign bodies may be extracted more safely through the corneoscleral limbus or the initial wound to minimize peripheral retinal damage.

Retained Intraocular Foreign Bodies

The reaction of the eye to a retained foreign body varies greatly depending on the foreign body's chemical composition, sterility, and location. Inert, sterile foreign bodies such as stone, sand, glass, porcelain, plastic, and cilia are generally well tolerated. If found several days after the injury, they may be left in place if they are not obstructing vision. Evaluation for retinal toxicity with electroretinography may be helpful in some cases.

Common reactive foreign bodies are zinc, aluminum, copper, and iron. Zinc and aluminum tend to cause minimal inflammation and may become encapsulated. If very large, however, any foreign body may incite inflammation, causing glial and/or fibrovascular proliferation into the vitreous preretinally and along the ciliary processes. Tractional retinal distortion and detachment and phthisis bulbi may result in loss of useful vision. Migration of the foreign body also can occur, especially with copper.

Pure copper (eg, wire, percussion cap) is especially toxic, and prompt removal is required. Pure copper causes acute chalcosis with severe inflammation and may lead to loss of the eye. Late removal may not cure the chalcosis, which has been reported to increase after surgery in some cases because of dissemination of the metal. If copper is alloyed with another metal for a final copper content of less than 85% (brass, bronze), chronic chalcosis may occur. Copper has an affinity for limiting membranes. Typical findings in chalcosis are deposits in Descemet's membrane (similar to the Kayser-Fleischer ring of Wilson disease), greenish aqueous particles, green discoloration of the iris, "sunflower" cataract, brownish red vitreous opacities and strand formation, and metallic flecks on retinal vessels and in the macular region.

Iron from intraocular foreign bodies is mostly deposited in epithelial tissues such as the iris sphincter and dilator muscles, the nonpigmented ciliary epithelium, the lens epithelium, the retina, and the RPE. Oxidation and dissemination of ferric ions through-out the eye promotes the Haber-Weiss reaction, in which transition metal ions catalyze the generation of powerful oxidants such as hydroxyl radicals. These cause lipid peroxidation, sulfhydryl oxidation, and depolymerization, with cell membrane damage and enzyme inactivation. BCSC Section 2, *Fundamentals and Principles of Ophthalmology,* and Section 9, *Intraocular Inflammation and Uveitis,* discuss these reactions in greater detail with illustrations.

Retinal photoreceptors and RPE cells are especially susceptible to siderosis (Table 13-1). Electroretinogram changes in siderosis include an increased a-wave and normal b-wave during the very early phase of toxicity, with a diminishing b-wave amplitude later. Eventually, the ERG may become extinguished. Serial ERGs can be helpful for following eyes with small retained foreign bodies. If the b-wave amplitude decreases, removal of the foreign body generally is recommended.

Table 13-1 Symptoms and Signs of Siderosis

Symptoms
Nyctalopia
Concentrically constricted visual field
Decreased vision

Signs
Rust-colored corneal stromal staining
Iris heterochromia
Pupillary mydriasis and poor reactivity
Brown deposits on the anterior lens
Cataract
Vitreous opacities
Peripheral retinal pigmentation (early)
Diffuse retinal pigmentation (late)
Narrowed retinal vessels
Optic disc discoloration and atrophy
Secondary open-angle glaucoma from iron accumulation in the trabecular meshwork

Posttraumatic Endophthalmitis

Endophthalmitis occurs following 2%–7% of penetrating injuries; the incidence is higher in association with intraocular foreign bodies and higher in rural settings. Posttraumatic endophthalmitis can progress rapidly; its clinical signs include marked inflammation with fibrin, hypopyon, and vitreous infiltration and corneal opacification. The risk of endophthalmitis after penetrating ocular injury may be reduced by prompt wound closure and early removal of intraocular foreign bodies. Prophylactic subconjunctival, intravenous, and sometimes intravitreal antibiotics are often recommended.

Bacillus cereus, which rarely causes endophthalmitis in other settings, accounts for almost 25% of cases of traumatic endophthalmitis. *B cereus* endophthalmitis has a rapid and severe course and, once established, leads to severe visual loss and often loss of the eye. *B cereus* endophthalmitis most commonly occurs following soil-contaminated injuries, especially those involving foreign bodies. Anterior chamber and vitreous cultures should be obtained, and antibiotics should be injected if endophthalmitis is suspected. *B cereus* is sensitive to vancomycin or clindamycin given intravitreally. For gram-negative organisms, a frequent pathogen in posttraumatic endophthalmitis, ceftazidime may be an effective therapy that avoids the toxicities associated with aminoglycosides. Because choices for antibiotic selection may be revised often, ophthalmologists should consult a recent reference for current guidelines.

The role of prophylactic antibiotics in cases without signs of endophthalmitis is controversial. Caution should be exercised in their use because of reports of retinal vascular infarction following intravitreal injection of aminoglycoside antibiotics. Intravitreal antibiotics are generally limited to cases at high risk for infection. See also BCSC Section 9, *Intraocular Inflammation and Uveitis*.

Reynolds DS, Flynn HW Jr. Endophthalmitis after penetrating ocular trauma. *Curr Opin Ophthalmol*. 1997;8:32–38.

Sympathetic Ophthalmia

If no hope of visual recovery in a recently lacerated or ruptured eye remains, enucleation should be considered to reduce the risk of sympathetic ophthalmia. Modern estimates suggest an incidence of 1 in 500 cases of penetrating injury. Because the extent of intraocular damage is often difficult to determine initially, it is usually best to close the wound and retain the eye if at all possible. In general, primary enucleation should be performed only if the globe cannot be repaired. After the primary wound repair, management of a severely injured eye that maintains a visual acuity of light perception may be problematic. The viability of the globe should be assessed within the first 7 to 14 days.

One strategy sometimes used following careful preoperative evaluation is to explore the eye using a vitrectomy approach. If the eye shows potential for anatomic and possibly visual recovery, it is repaired and retained. If the eye has no potential for recovery, it should be enucleated within 2 weeks of the initial injury in order to reduce the risk of sympathetic ophthalmia. The patient and surgeon should decide preoperatively whether enucleation (if necessary) will be performed at the time of exploratory vitrectomy or in a later surgery. See also BCSC Section 9, *Intraocular Inflammation and Uveitis.*

A large proportion of patients with sympathetic ophthalmia present between 3 months and 1 year after trauma, but many show initial signs and symptoms of the disease over a very wide time interval. If the injured eye is still present, it is common for inflammation to flare up in that eye, followed by signs and symptoms of inflammation in the fellow eye. Symptoms can include loss of acuity, loss of accommodation, photophobia, and pain. Signs include panuveitis, multifocal infiltrates at the level of the RPE (Dalen-Fuchs nodules) or choroid, exudative detachment, optic nerve swelling, and thickening of the uveal tract as detected by contact B-scan ultrasonography. Early aggressive treatment is required to save the sympathizing eye, which is often the only functional eye the patient has.

Albert DM, Diaz-Rohena R. A historical review of sympathetic ophthalmia and its epidemiology. *Surv Ophthalmol.* 1989;34:1–14.

Power WJ, Foster CS. Update on sympathetic ophthalmia. *Int Ophthalmol Clin.* 1995;35: 127–137.

Shaken Baby Syndrome/Child Abuse

Severe shaking of infants, a form of child abuse, is the cause of shaken baby syndrome. The typical baby is almost always less than 1 year and frequently less than 6 months of age. Systemic signs and symptoms include

- bradycardia, apnea, and hypothermia
- lethargy, irritability, seizures, hypotonia
- signs of failure to thrive
- full or bulging fontanelles and increased head size
- skin bruises, particularly on the upper arms, chest, or thighs
- spiral fractures of the long bones
- subdural and subarachnoid hemorrhages

Ocular signs include

- retinal hemorrhages and cotton-wool spots (Fig 13-7)
- retinal folds
- hemorrhagic schisis cavities

The retinal hemorrhages in shaken baby syndrome often have a hemispheric contour. They start to resolve with amazing rapidity, so it is important to examine suspected shaken baby syndrome infants on presentation. The retinopathy may resemble that found in Terson syndrome, Purtscher retinopathy, or central retinal vein occlusion. None of these conditions are common in infants. Retinal hemorrhages may be caused by accidental trauma, but they are not seen in typical accidental trauma, such as sustained through falls at home. The physician should report cases of suspected child abuse to the proper governmental child welfare agency for further investigation. See also BCSC Section 6, *Pediatric Ophthalmology and Strabismus.*

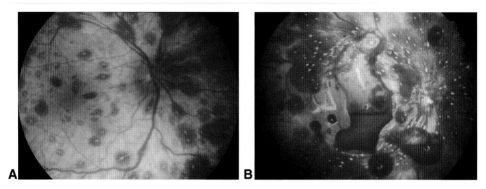

Figure 13-7 Shaken baby syndrome with preretinal and retinal hemorrhages. **A,** This photograph was taken several days after admission, at a time when many of the smaller hemorrhages had started to resorb. **B,** A large number of hemorrhages are located on and within the retina. There are regions of hemorrhagic retinoschisis centrally. Because the baby was upright, the red blood cells sank down into a dependent position within the larger regions of hemorrhagic retinoschisis. Note that some of the hemorrhages were white-centered, whereas others have reflections of the flash from the fundus camera on them. *(Photographs from Spaide RF, Swengel RM, Scharre DW, et al. Shaken baby syndrome.* Am Fam Physician. *1990;41:1145–1152.)*

Matthews GP, Das A. Dense vitreous hemorrhages predict poor visual and neurological prognosis in infants with shaken baby syndrome. *J Pediatr Ophthalmol Strabismus.* 1996;33: 260–265.

Avulsion of the Optic Disc

A forceful backward dislocation of the optic nerve from the scleral canal can occur under several circumstances, including

- extreme rotation and forward displacement of the globe
- penetrating orbital injury, causing a backward pull on the optic nerve
- sudden increase in intraocular pressure, causing rupture of the lamina cribrosa

Total visual loss usually occurs. Findings may vary from a pitlike depression of the optic nerve head to posterior hemorrhage and contusion necrosis (Fig 13-8); however, hemorrhage is usually seen acutely.

Gass JD. *Stereoscopic Atlas of Macular Diseases: Diagnosis and Treatment.* 4th ed. St Louis: Mosby; 1997.

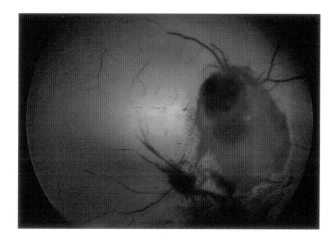

Figure 13-8 Avulsion of the optic nerve. Nerve is obscured by hemorrhage, and a mixed vascular occlusion is present.

CHAPTER 14

Adverse Effects of Electromagnetic Energy on the Retina

Radiation Retinopathy

Exposure to ionizing radiation can damage the retinal vasculature. Radiation retinopathy typically has a delayed onset, is slowly progressive, and clinically causes microangiopathic changes that resemble diabetic retinopathy. Radiation retinopathy can occur following either external beam or local plaque therapy, typically within months to years after radiation treatment. In general, radiation retinopathy is seen around 18 months after treatment with external beam radiation, and a little earlier with brachytherapy. Because radiation retinopathy is very similar to other vascular diseases, eliciting a history of radiation treatment is important to verify the diagnosis. Exposure to doses of 30–35 grays (Gy) or more is usually required; occasionally, however, retinopathy may develop after as little as 15 Gy of external beam radiation. Studies have shown retinal damage in 50% of patients receiving 60 Gy and in 85%–95% of patients receiving 70–80 Gy. The total dose, volume of retina irradiated, and fractionation scheme are important in determining the threshold dose for radiation retinopathy. See BCSC Section 4, *Ophthalmic Pathology and Intraocular Tumors*, for further discussion of these therapies, including sample dosages.

Clinically, affected patients may be asymptomatic or may complain of decreased acuity. Ophthalmologic examination may reveal signs of retinal vascular disease, including cotton-wool spots, retinal hemorrhages, microaneurysms, perivascular sheathing, capillary telangiectasis, macular edema, and disc edema. Capillary nonperfusion documented by fluorescein angiography is commonly present, and extensive retinal ischemia can lead to neovascularization of the retina, iris, and disc (Figs 14-1, 14-2). Other complications may occur, such as optic atrophy, central retinal artery occlusion, central retinal vein occlusion, choroidal neovascularization, vitreous hemorrhage, neovascular glaucoma, and tractional retinal detachment. Visual outcome is primarily related to macular involvement with cystoid macular edema, exudative maculopathy, or capillary nonperfusion. Occasionally, visual loss may be caused by acute optic neuropathy. Although no clinical trials have been performed, management of radiation retinopathy is similar to that for diabetic retinopathy and includes focal laser therapy to reduce macular edema or panretinal photocoagulation to treat zones of ischemia and neovascularization.

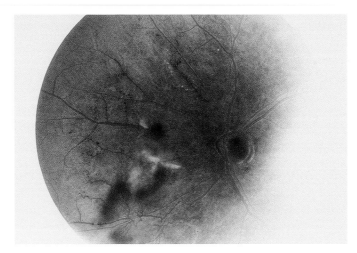

Figure 14-1 Fluorescein angiogram of a patient who has been treated with external-beam radiation to the contralateral eye. The nasal retina in this fellow eye shows microvascular abnormalities, including capillary nonperfusion, microaneurysm formation, neovascularization of the surface of the retina, and neovascularization of the disc. *(Photograph courtesy of M. Gilbert Grand, MD.)*

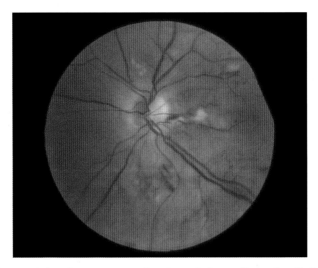

Figure 14-2 Microvascular changes secondary to radiation retinopathy. Patient received external-beam radiation for metastatic intracranial tumors. Note microvascular changes including nerve fiber layer infarctions and intraretinal hemorrhages. *(Photograph courtesy of M. Gilbert Grand, MD.)*

Brown GC, Shields JA, Sanborn G, et al. Radiation retinopathy. *Ophthalmology.* 1982;89: 1494–1501.

Mukai S, Guyer DR, Gragoudas ES. Radiation retinopathy. In: Albert DM, Jakobiec FA, eds. *Principles and Practice of Ophthalmology.* 2nd ed. Philadelphia: Saunders; 2000:2232–2235.

Photic Damage

The eye has several protective mechanisms against light damage, including constriction of the pupils, light absorption by melanin in the RPE, and antioxidants. Light injures the retina by 3 basic mechanisms:

- mechanical
- thermal
- photochemical

Mechanical injury occurs when the power of the absorbed light is intense enough to form gas or water vapor or to produce acoustic shock waves that mechanically disrupt retinal tissue. The absorbed energy may be so great that it strips electrons from molecules in the target tissue, producing a collection of ions and electrons referred to as *plasma*. For example, a Q-switched neodymium:ytrrium-aluminum-garnet (Nd:YAG) laser produces its therapeutic effect through mechanical light damage and uses this effect to disrupt a cloudy posterior capsule behind an intraocular lens.

Thermal injury occurs when excessive light absorption by the RPE and surrounding structures causes local elevation of temperature, leading to inflammation and scarring of the RPE and the surrounding neurosensory retina and choroid. The end result of this temperature elevation is protein denaturation and tissue disruption. A therapeutic application of thermal light injury is the retinal burn caused by laser photocoagulation. See Chapter 15 for discussion of photocoagulation.

Photochemical injury occurs due to biochemical reactions that cause retinal tissue destruction without elevation of temperature. In general, photochemical injury is less severe; it produces acute and chronic degenerative changes through biochemical reactions not yet fully understood but felt to be due to tissue oxidation from free radical formation. Such changes are seen primarily at the level of the outer segments of the photoreceptors, which are more sensitive than the inner segments. Solar retinopathy and photic retinopathy after exposure to operating microscope illumination are examples of photochemical injury.

De La Paz MA, D'Amico DJ. Photic retinopathy. In: Albert DM, Jakobiec FA, eds. *Principles and Practice of Ophthalmology*. 2nd ed. Philadelphia: Saunders; 2000:2226–2231.

Mainster MA, Khan JA. Photic retinal injury. In: Ryan SJ, ed. *Retina*. 3rd ed. St Louis: Mosby; 2001:1797–1809.

Tso MO, Woodford BJ. Effect of photic injury on the retinal tissues. *Ophthalmology* 1983;90:952–963.

Solar Retinopathy

Solar retinopathy, also known as *foveomacular retinitis, eclipse retinopathy,* and *solar retinitis,* is photochemical retinal injury caused by direct or indirect viewing of the sun; it usually occurs after viewing a solar eclipse or gazing directly at the sun. The damage is felt to be secondary to visible blue light and shorter wavelengths of ultraviolet A or near-UV radiation. Younger patients with clearer lenses and patients taking drugs that photosensitize the eye, including tetracycline and psoralens, are at a higher risk of solar retinopathy, and patients with high refractive errors and dark fundus pigmentation are at a slightly lower risk. Patients complain of decreased vision, central scotomata, dyschromatopsia, metamorphopsia, micropsia, and frontal or temporal headache within hours of exposure. Visual acuity is typically reduced to 20/25–20/100 but may be worse depending on exposure. Most patients recover within 3–6 months, with vision returning to the level of 20/20–20/40, but residual metamorphopsia and paracentral scotomata may remain.

The fundus findings are variable and usually bilateral. The characteristic finding in the first few days after exposure is a yellow-white spot in the fovea, which subsequently is replaced after several days by a reddish dot, often surrounded by a pigment halo. Mild cases, however, often have no fundus changes. After approximately 2 weeks, a small, reddish, well-circumscribed, 100–200 μm lamellar hole or depression may evolve. This lesion may lie at or adjacent to the fovea and is usually permanent. Fluorescein angiography, rarely, reveals leakage in early stages and window defects in late stages.

It is theorized that solar retinopathy is caused by a photochemical injury, perhaps thermally enhanced. The extent of the damage depends on the length of the exposure. Histopathologic studies have shown RPE damage. No known beneficial treatment exists, and prevention by education is critically important.

Phototoxicity from Ophthalmic Instrumentation

The potential for photochemical damage from modern ophthalmic instruments has been studied extensively. Injuries have been reported from operating microscopes and from fiberoptic endoilluminating probes used in vitrectomies. The prevalence of photic retinopathy after cataract surgery has been estimated at 3%–7.4%, with the incidence increasing with prolonged operating times. In retinal surgery, photic injury is more likely with prolonged, focal exposure, especially when the light probe is held in close proximity to the retina, as is the case in macular hole or epiretinal membrane procedures. Most patients are asymptomatic; however, some will notice a paracentral scotoma on the first postoperative day. In general, vision returns to normal after a few months. Acutely affected patients may have a deep, irregular, oval-shaped, yellow-white, retinal lesion adjacent to the fovea that resembles the shape of the light source. The lesion typically evolves to become a zone of mottled RPE that transmits hyperfluorescence on fluorescein angiography. Although animal studies generally exaggerate clinical exposures, recent reports of photic macular lesions following cataract surgery emphasize the need for prevention. Minimizing exposure, avoiding intense illumination, using oblique illumination during nonessential parts of the surgery, filtering out short-wavelength blue light and UV light, and using shielding may prove helpful in reducing the risk of photic retinopathy during ocular surgery. BCSC Section 11, *Lens and Cataract,* lists several precautions to minimize retinal light toxicity.

Food and Drug Administration. Retinal photic injuries from operating microscopes during cataract surgery. FDA Public Health Advisory. Rockville, MD: US Dept Health & Human Services; 1995.

Fuller D, Machemer R, Knighton RW. Retinal damage produced by intraocular fiber optic light. *Am J Ophthalmol.* 1978;85:519–537.

Kleinmann G, Hoffman P, Schechtman E, et al. Microscope-induced retinal phototoxicity in cataract surgery of short duration. *Ophthalmology.* 2002;109:334–338.

Pavilack MA, Brod RD. Site of potential operating microscope light-induced phototoxicity on the human retina during temporal approach eye surgery. *Ophthalmology.* 2001;108: 381–385.

Ambient Light

Although there is much speculation that ambient exposure to ultraviolet radiation or visible light is a potential cause of retinal toxicity or degeneration, further study and documentation are required.

West SK, Rosenthal FS, Bressler NM, et al. Exposure to sunlight and other risk factors for age-related macular degeneration. *Arch Ophthalmol.* 1989;107:875–879.

Occupational Light Toxicity

Occupational exposure to bright lights can lead to retinal damage. One of the most common causes of occupational injury is arc welding without the use of protective goggles. The damage from the visible blue light of the arc welder leads to photochemical damage similar to that seen in solar retinopathy. Occupational injury from stray laser exposure is also a serious concern. Photic retinal injury has been reported as well after exposure to laser pointers. Robertson and colleagues noted damage after exposing the retina to light from class 3A laser pointers for durations greater than 15 minutes.

Robertson DM, Lim TH, Salomao DR, et al. Laser pointers and the human eye: a clinico-pathologic study. *Arch Ophthalmol.* 2000;118:1686–1691.

PART III

Selected Therapeutic Topics

CHAPTER 15

Laser Therapy for Posterior Segment Diseases

Basic Principles of Photocoagulation

Photocoagulation is a therapeutic technique employing a strong light source to coagulate tissue. Light energy is absorbed by the target tissue and converted into thermal energy. When tissue temperature rises above 65°C, denaturation of tissue proteins and coagulative necrosis occur.

Most surgeons currently perform photocoagulation with lasers spanning the visible light spectrum of 400–780 nm and venturing into the infrared wavelengths. Current posterior segment laser delivery systems include green, red, yellow, and infrared. Delivery systems may employ a transpupillary approach with slit-lamp delivery, indirect ophthalmoscopic application, endophotocoagulation during vitrectomy surgery, and transscleral application with a contact probe.

The effectiveness of any photocoagulator depends on how well its light penetrates the ocular media and how well that light is absorbed by pigment in the target tissue. Light is principally absorbed in ocular tissues that contain melanin, xanthophyll, or hemoglobin. Figure 15-1 illustrates the absorption spectra of the key pigments found in ocular tissues:

- *Melanin* is an excellent absorber of green, yellow, red, and infrared wavelengths.
- Macular *xanthophyll* readily absorbs blue but minimally absorbs yellow or red wavelengths.
- *Hemoglobin* easily absorbs blue, green, and yellow, with minimal absorption of red wavelengths.

Choice of Laser Wavelength

Depending on the specific goals of treatment, the surgeon considers the absorption properties of the key ocular pigments in choosing the appropriate wavelength of light to selectively deliver focal photocoagulation to target tissues while attempting to spare adjacent normal tissues. However, the *area* of effective coagulation (depth and diameter) is also related directly to the *intensity* and *duration* of the irradiation, and these factors can often supersede the theoretic differences of various wavelengths. For a specific set of laser parameters (spot size, duration, and power), the intensity of the burn obtained depends

313

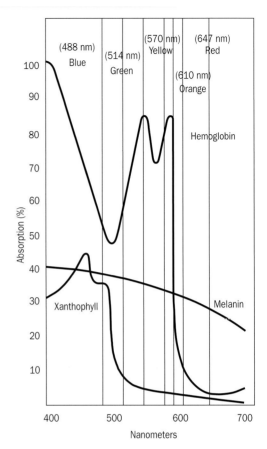

Figure 15-1 Absorption spectra of xantho-phyll, hemoglobin, and melanin. *(Reproduced with permission from Folk JC, Pulido JS. Laser Photo-coagulation of the Retina and Choroid. Ophthalmology Monograph 11. San Francisco: American Academy of Ophthalmology; 1997:9.)*

on the clarity of the ocular media and the degree of pigmentation of the fundus in the individual eye. Table 15-1 specifies the preferred laser wavelengths for treatment of particular retinal and choroidal pathology.

The *green laser* produces light that is absorbed well by melanin and hemoglobin and less completely by xanthophyll. Because of these characteristics and the absence of blue wavelengths, it has replaced the blue-green laser for the treatment of retinal vascular abnormalities and choroidal neovascularization (CNV). The *blue-green laser* emits both blue and green wavelengths. The initial hope that this combination of wavelengths would close elevated neovascular fronds has not been realized. The disadvantages of blue-green laser, principally associated with the blue wavelengths, include increased scatter and absorption by cataractous lenses, uptake by macular xanthophyll, and potential photo-chemical toxicity. It is noted here only for historical comparison because this wavelength is no longer used in clinical practice.

The *red laser* penetrates through nuclear sclerotic cataracts and moderate vitreous hemorrhages better than other wavelengths. In addition, it is minimally absorbed by xanthophyll and thus may be useful in the treatment of CNV adjacent to the fovea. The *infrared laser* has similar characteristics to the red laser, but it offers deeper tissue penetration.

Table 15-1 Preferred Wavelengths for Specific Diseases of Retina and Choroid

Disease	Preferred	Acceptable	Unacceptable	Reason
Proliferative retinopathies (eg, diabetes, vein occlusions)				
Routine	Green (514 nm)	All others	—	Green is safe and proven effective.
With vitreous hemorrhage	Red (647 nm)	Green (514 nm) Infrared (810 nm)	Yellow (577 nm)	Red is absorbed less by blood. Green can often be used if vitreous blood is avoided.
With moderate or severe inner retinal hemorrhage	Red (647 nm)	Infrared (810 nm)	Green (514 nm) Yellow (577 nm)	Green and yellow are absorbed by inner retinal hemorrhage.
With increased vitreoretinal traction	Red (647 nm) Infrared (810 nm)	Green (514 nm)	—	Red and infrared cause "deeper" burns and theoretically decreased chance of increasing traction. Green is usually acceptable unless too many intense burns are given in one session.
Macular edema secondary to diabetes or branch retinal vein occlusion	Green (514 nm) Yellow (577 nm)	All others	—	Green is safe and proven effective. Yellow is better for treating microaneurysms but may not matter.

(Continued)

Table 15-1 Preferred Wavelengths for Specific Diseases of Retina and Choroid (Continued)

Disease	Preferred	Acceptable	Unacceptable	Reason
Choroidal neovascularization				
General	Green (514) nm Red (647 nm)	Yellow (577 nm) Perhaps infrared (810 nm)	—	Green and red are proven effective.
With moderate or severe subretinal blood	Red (647 nm)	Green (514 nm) Infrared (810 nm)	Yellow (577 nm)	Red is absorbed less by blood. Infrared is also less absorbed by blood, but efficacy is unproven. Green can still be used in many cases even with blood present.
In maculopapillary bundle or peripapillary location	Red (647 nm)	Green (514 nm) Infrared (810 nm)	—	Red and infrared cause "deeper" burns with less chance of nerve fiber layer or superficial retinal damage. Red is proven effective; infrared is not.
With preretinal membrane or internal limiting membrane wrinkling	Red (647 nm)	Infrared (810 nm) Green (514 nm) Yellow (577 nm)	—	Red and infrared cause "deeper" burns with less chance of nerve fiber layer or superficial retinal damage. Red is proven effective; infrared is not.
Coats disease and retinal angioma	Yellow (577 nm)	Green (514 nm)	Red (647 nm) Infrared (810 nm)	Need absorption by hemoglobin.
Retinal breaks	Green (514 nm)	All others	—	Green is effective and less painful. Others are acceptable.

(Adapted with permission from Folk JC, Russell SR. Appropriate wavelengths for posterior segment laser photocoagulation. In: *Focal Points: Clinical Modules for Ophthalmologists*. San Francisco: American Academy of Ophthalmology; 1988: vol 6, no 7.)

Yellow laser has, among its advantages, minimal scatter through nuclear sclerotic lenses, low xanthophyll absorption, and little potential for photochemical damage. It appears to be useful for destroying vascular structures with little damage to adjacent pigmented tissue; thus, it may be valuable for treating retinal vascular and choroidal neovascular lesions.

Bressler SB. Does wavelength matter when photocoagulating eyes with macular degeneration or diabetic retinopathy? *Arch Ophthalmol.* 1993;111:177–180.

Practical Aspects of Laser Photocoagulation

Topical, peribulbar, or retrobulbar anesthesia may be needed to facilitate delivery of laser photocoagulation. The choice of which method to use is often guided by the laser wavelength being used, the length of treatment, the type of treatment, and the importance of immobilizing the eye.

Two types of contact lenses are available to assist in slit-lamp delivery of photocoagulation: negative power planoconcave lenses and high-plus-power lenses. The planoconcave lenses provide an upright image with superior resolution of a small retinal area. Most clinicians favor these lenses for macular treatments. Mirrored planoconcave lenses direct photocoagulation to more peripheral regions by employing different angles on the mirror. Where these mirrors are in use, the macula will not be in the surgeon's view; therefore, he or she must be mindful of where the mirror is directing the location of the laser beam in the fundus to avoid accidental treatment of the macula. High-plus-power lenses provide an inverted image with some loss of fine resolution, but they offer a wide field of view, facilitating efficient treatment over a broad area. The macula may be kept in view while the midperiphery of the retina is being treated, making these lenses ideal for panretinal photocoagulation. The type of contact lens selected affects the actual burn size on the retina, as planoconcave lenses generally provide the same retinal spot size as that selected on the slit-lamp setting, whereas the spot size with high-plus-power lenses is magnified over the laser setting size, depending on the lens used (Table 15-2).

Selection of laser setting parameters depends on the intent of the treatment, the clarity of the ocular media, and the fundus pigmentation. As a general rule, smaller spot sizes require less energy than larger spot sizes, and longer-duration exposures require less energy than shorter-duration exposures to achieve the same intensity effects. For further discussion of laser characteristics and techniques, see also BCSC Section 3, *Clinical Optics.*

Folk JC, Pulido JS. *Laser Photocoagulation of the Retina and Choroid.* Ophthalmology Monograph 11. San Francisco: American Academy of Ophthalmology; 1997.

L'Esperance FA Jr. Photocoagulation of ocular disease: application and technique. In: L'Esperance FA Jr, ed. *Ophthalmic Lasers.* 3rd ed. St Louis: Mosby; 1989.

Indications

Indications for retinal photocoagulation include the following:

- panretinal scatter treatment to ablate ischemic tissue in order to eliminate retinal, iris, and disc neovascularization and the stimulus for further proliferation in

Table 15-2 Magnification Factors for Common Laser Lenses

Panretinal photocoagulation lenses

Ocular Mainster PRP 165	0.51× magnification	1.96× laser spot magnification
Ocular Mainster Wide Field PDT	0.68× magnification	1.50× laser spot magnification
Ocular Mainster Ultra Field PRP	0.53× magnification	1.89× laser spot magnification
Rodenstock Panfunduscope	0.7× magnification	1.43× laser spot magnification
Volk SuperQuad 160	0.5× magnification	2.0× laser spot magnification
Volk QuadrAspheric	0.51× magnification	1.97× laser spot magnification
Volk Equator Plus	0.44× magnification	2.27× laser spot magnification

Focal laser lenses

Goldmann 3-mirror (central)	0.93× magnification	1.08× laser spot magnification
Ocular Mainster High Magnification	1.25× magnification	0.80× laser spot magnification
Ocular PDT 1.6×	0.63× magnification	1.6× laser spot magnification
Ocular Reichel-Mainster 1× Retina	0.95× magnification	1.05× laser spot magnification
Ocular Yannuzzi Fundus	0.93× magnification	1.08× laser spot magnification
Volk PDT Lens	0.66× magnification	1.5× laser spot magnification
Volk Area Centralis	1.06× magnification	0.94× laser spot magnification

proliferative diseases such as proliferative diabetic retinopathy and venous occlusive diseases

- to a limited degree, focal ablation of nonelevated neovascularization associated with proliferative diseases such as proliferative diabetic retinopathy
- closure of intraretinal vascular abnormalities such as microaneurysms, telangiectasis, and perivascular leakage
- focal ablation of CNV, such as neovascularization associated with OHS or AMD
- creation of chorioretinal adhesions, as in the area surrounding retinal breaks or limited retinal detachment
- focal treatment of pigment epithelium abnormalities, including leakage associated with central serous chorioretinopathy
- to a limited degree, management of selected ocular tumors

Complications of Photocoagulation

Like any other surgical procedure, photocoagulation may occasionally be associated with complications. The most serious complications are caused by excessive energy or misdirected light. Constant attention to the foveal center during any laser treatment is imperative to avoid hitting this vital structure. Wide-field lenses makes avoiding the fovea easier because it is always in the field of view. Proper selection of wavelength, power, exposure time, and spot size is critical. If appropriate laser settings do not produce the desired tissue effect, the procedure should be stopped. Slowly titrate the laser power and exposure to avoid unnecessary treatment or burns that break through Bruch's membrane, risking bleeding or future CNV.

Patient preparation is also important in minimizing complications. Carefully explaining the laser procedure to the patient preoperatively will help to elicit cooperation, steady fixation, and proper positioning of both patient and surgeon for comfort and safety.

Among the complications that may be associated with photocoagulation are inadvertent corneal burns, which can lead to opacities. Treatment of the iris may cause iritis and zones of atrophy. Pupillary abnormalities may arise from thermal damage to the ciliary nerves in the suprachoroidal space. Absorption by lens pigments may create lenticular burns and resultant opacities. Optic neuritis from treatment directly to or adjacent to the disc may occur, and nerve fiber damage may follow intense absorption in zones of increased pigmentation or retinal thinning. Chorioretinal complications include foveal burns, Bruch's membrane ruptures, creation of retinal or choroidal lesions, choroidal detachment, and exudative retinal detachment.

Accidental foveal burns

Great care should be taken to identify the fovea by means of biomicroscopy; comparison with fluorescein angiography may further facilitate this identification. Frequent reference to the foveal center throughout the session is helpful to avoid losing track of where, in the fundus, treatment is taking place. The patient's ability to fixate steadily is important in avoiding foveal burns. The risk of foveal burns may be reduced in some instances by immobilizing the globe with peribulbar or retrobulbar anesthesia, especially when juxtafoveal treatment is being performed.

Bruch's membrane ruptures

Small spot size, high intensity, and long duration of applications all increase the risk of Bruch's membrane rupture, which may subsequently give rise to hemorrhage from the choriocapillaris and development of CNV. Increasing digital pressure on the contact lens is often sufficient to allow for thrombosis and cessation of acute bleeding.

Retinal lesions

Intense photocoagulation may cause fibrous proliferation that can lead to retinal tears. Similarly, intense treatment may create striae and foveal distortion, with resultant metamorphosia or diplopia. Focal treatment with small-diameter, high-intensity burns may cause vascular occlusion or perforate blood vessels, leading to preretinal or vitreous hemorrhage with resultant visual loss. In addition, extensive panretinal treatment may induce or exacerbate macular edema.

Choroidal lesions

Treatment of CNV may be complicated by subretinal hemorrhage; choroidal ischemia; and additional choroidal neovascularization, chorioretinal neovascularization, or chorioretinal anastomosis. Active subretinal hemorrhage that occurs during treatment should be immediately addressed by increasing digital pressure on the contact lens while continuing with the treatment to the remaining portions of the CNV lesion. Interruption of the treatment may allow the new blood to obscure the landmarks that the surgeon is following to define the area of treatment, and it may hinder absorption of the laser at the level of the RPE and choroid. Progressive retinal pigment epithelial atrophy may develop at the margin of photocoagulation scars, resulting in enlarged or even central scotomata. Finally, rips of the pigment epithelium may be precipitated by photocoagulation.

Exudative retinal detachment

Extensive, intense photocoagulation may result in massive chorioretinal edema, with sensory retinal detachment, choroidal detachment, and shallowing of the anterior chamber angle associated with elevated IOP (Fig 15-2).

Burgess D, Boniuk I. Retinal photocoagulation and cryotherapy. In: Krupin T, Kolker AE, eds. *Atlas of Complications in Ophthalmic Surgery.* New York: Gower; 1993; chap 15:15.2–15.8.

Gass JD, ed. *Stereoscopic Atlas of Macular Disease: Diagnosis and Treatment.* 4th ed. St Louis: Mosby; 1997.

Mainster MA. Laser light, interactions and clinical systems. In: L'Esperance FA Jr, ed. *Ophthalmic Lasers.* 3rd ed. St Louis: Mosby; 1989.

Transpupillary Thermotherapy

Transpupillary thermotherapy (TTT) acts in a subthreshold manner by slightly raising the choroidal temperature, thereby treating the CNV with minimal damage to the overlying retina. TTT is administered with an infrared laser (810 nm) with beam sizes ranging from 0.8 and 3.0 mm, power settings between 250 and 750 mW, and a 1-minute exposure, with the endpoint being no visible change or a slight graying of the retina. A pilot study using TTT in predominantly occult CNV demonstrated that 56% of treated eyes remained stable 1 year after treatment, with only 25% losing 2 lines of visual acuity. The Transpupillary Thermotherapy for Choroidal Neovascularization (TTT4CNV) study is a randomized, double-blind trial evaluating TTT for the management of predominantly occult CNV in AMD. TTT has also been shown to be beneficial in the management of intraocular tumors, including retinoblastoma and choroidal malignant melanoma.

Newsom RS, McAlister JC, Saeed M, et al. Transpupillary thermotherapy (TTT) for the treatment of choroidal neovascularisation. *Br J Ophthalmol.* 2001;85:173–178. Erratum in: *Br J Ophthalmol.* 2001;85:505.

Subramanian ML, Reichel E. Current indications of transpupillary thermotherapy for the treatment of posterior segment diseases. *Curr Opin Ophthalmol.* 2003;14:155–158.

Photodynamic Therapy

A variety of photosensitizing drugs and specific lasers that deliver light at the absorption peak of the individual drugs are presently under development and being tested for ophthalmic use. Photodynamic therapy with verteporfin (PDT) has recently been approved for the treatment of

- subfoveal, predominantly classic CNV in age-related macular degeneration
- subfoveal CNV secondary to ocular histoplasmosis syndrome
- subfoveal CNV secondary to pathologic myopia

In addition, the AAO Ophthalmic Technology Assessment Committee recommends PDT with verteporfin for the treatment of occult with no CNV in AMD. PDT with other photosensitizing drugs, as well as other indications for PDT, including treating ocular

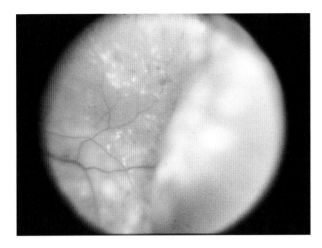

Figure 15-2 Choroidal detachment following panretinal scatter photocoagulation for the management of diabetic retinopathy. *(Photograph courtesy of M. Gilbert Grand, MD.)*

tumors and central serous chorioretinopathy, are currently under investigation. The process of PDT consists of 2 steps:

1. intravenous administration of the photosensitizing drug that localizes to actively proliferating endothelial cells such as those in CNV and tumors
2. local activation of the drug by a specific laser wavelength and a nonthermal laser light

The laser does not heat or photocoagulate tissues; instead, the laser energy produces a photochemical reaction that excites the drug into a higher energy state. The activated drug then releases its energy to surrounding oxygen molecules, leading to the formation of reactive oxygen species and free radicals. This process, in turn, leads to endothelial cell damage, platelet adherence, vascular thrombosis, and capillary closure. The technique and clinical studies of PDT are discussed at length in Chapter 4.

Ophthalmic Technology Assessment Committee. Photodynamic therapy with verteporfin for age-related macular degeneration. San Francisco: American Academy of Ophthalmology; 2000.

Complications of Photodynamic Therapy

The most serious side effect of PDT is photosensitivity reactions that range from mild sunburns to second-degree burns. Photosensitivity reactions occurred in 3.5% of patients in the Treatment of Age-Related Macular Degeneration with Photodynamic Therapy (TAP) Study and in 0.4% in the Verteporfin in Photodynamic Therapy (VIP) Study. This complication is easily avoided with good patient education, including minimizing exposure to sunlight and wearing protective clothing, special glasses, and a hat during the period of total body photosensitivity. For verteporfin, this lasts 48 hours after treatment. Other photodynamic compounds have different precautionary periods. Back, side, and chest pain was reported in 2.2%–2.5% of patients in the studies and is related to the infusion of the drug. The pain resolves after the infusion finishes. No treatment has been shown to prevent this pain. Finally, 0.7%–2.2% of patients experienced a severe loss of vision within 7 days of treatment with PDT. This complication is more common in lesions that are minimally classic or occult with no classic and may lead to permanent acuity loss.

Blinder KJ, Blumenkranz MS, Bressler NM, et al. Verteporfin therapy of subfoveal choroidal neovascularization in pathologic myopia: 2-year results of a randomized clinical trial—VIP report 3. *Ophthalmology*. 2003;110:667–673.

Bressler NM, Treatment of Age-Related Macular Degeneration with Photodynamic Therapy (TAP) Study Group. Photodynamic therapy of subfoveal choroidal neovascularization in age-related macular degeneration with verteporfin: two-year results of two randomized clinical trials—TAP report 2. *Arch Ophthalmol*. 2001;119:198–207.

Saperstein DA, Rosenfeld PJ, Bressler NM, et al. Photodynamic therapy of subfoveal choroidal neovascularization with verteporfin in the ocular histoplasmosis syndrome: one-year results of an uncontrolled, prospective case series. *Ophthalmology*. 2002;109:1499–1505.

Verteporfin in Photodynamic Therapy (VIP) Study Group. Verteporfin therapy of subfoveal choroidal neovascularization in age-related macular degeneration: two-year results of a randomized clinical trial including lesions with occult with no classic choroidal neovascularization—Verteporfin in Photodynamic Therapy report 2. *Am J Ophthalmol*. 2001;131:541–560.

CHAPTER 16

Vitreoretinal Surgery

Pars Plana Vitrectomy

Pars plana vitrectomy is a closed-system technique that typically utilizes 3 ports, placed 3–4 mm posterior to the surgical limbus. One port is used to allow intraocular infusion of a balanced saline solution. Intraocular pressure can be maintained at any level and is controlled by the surgeon. The remaining ports are used to introduce various instruments into the vitreous cavity to illuminate the posterior segment and manipulate intraocular tissues.

Vitrectomy is performed using an operating microscope in conjunction with a contact lens or non–contact lens viewing system. Direct and indirect visualization is possible. The advantages of indirect visualization include a wider viewer angle and better visualization through media opacities, miotic pupils, and gas-filled eyes. The direct viewing systems allow greater magnification and enhanced stereopsis at the expense of a smaller field of view.

A recent advance in vitreous surgery has been the development of minimally invasive transconjunctival vitrectomy systems. Twenty-five-gauge or 23-gauge trocars are placed that allow access into the vitreous cavity. Specially designed vitrectomy instruments are available for use with these systems. Unlike sclerotomies made using standard 19- or 20-gauge instruments, those made using 25- or 23-gauge instruments do not require suture closure (Fig 16-1).

Fujii GY, De Juan E Jr. Humayun MS, et al. Initial experience using the transconjunctival sutureless vitrectomy system for vitreoretinal surgery. *Ophthalmology*. 2002;109:1814–1820.

Vitrectomy for Selected Macular Diseases

Macular Epiretinal Membrane

Macular epiretinal membranes (ERMs) have a variable clinical course but usually reach maximal formation within a few months before stabilizing. Most eyes maintain excellent visual acuity with minimal distortion of central vision, but the small percentage of patients who do develop marked distortion of central vision may be candidates for pars plana vitrectomy. Patients primarily complaining of metamorphopsia may derive the most benefit from this surgery.

Figure 16-1 A, 25-gauge vitrectomy instruments. **B, C,** Placement of a flexible polyamide 25-gauge trocar transconjunctivally. *(Photographs courtesy of Tom S. Chang, MD.)*

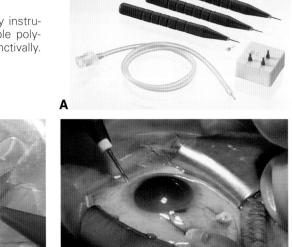

A

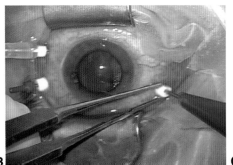

B C

Following surgery, approximately 60%–80% of patients achieve 2 or more lines of visual acuity improvement, often continuing to improve for 6–12 months after surgery. Intraoperative complications of this surgery include retinal tear or retinal detachment in less than 5% of cases. Progressive nuclear sclerosis occurs postoperatively in the majority of patients, and the rate increases over time (Fig 16-2).

McDonald HR, Verre WP, Aaberg TM. Surgical management of idiopathic epiretinal membranes. *Ophthalmology.* 1986;93:978–983.

Vitreomacular Traction Syndrome

Vitreomacular traction syndrome (VMT) is a special subset of macular ERMs with an incomplete posterior vitreous separation at the macula and the optic nerve head. Glial cells are the predominant cell type in the ERM. Vitreomacular traction syndrome may create a shallow retinal detachment in addition to distortion of the macula from the ERM. Optical coherence tomography (OCT) may be useful in helping to differentiate between VMT and idiopathic ERMs. This syndrome is often progressive and is associated with a greater visual loss than that from ERMs alone. Surgery consists of a standard pars plana vitrectomy and peeling of the ERM after removal of the posterior vitreous traction (Fig 16-3).

Hikichi T, Yoshida A, Trempe CL. Course of vitreomacular traction syndrome. *Am J Ophthalmol.* 1995;119:55–61.

McDonald HR, Johnson RN, Schatz H. Surgical results in the vitreomacular traction syndrome. *Ophthalmology.* 1994;101:1397–1403.

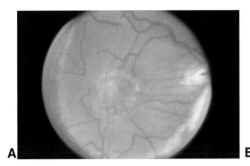 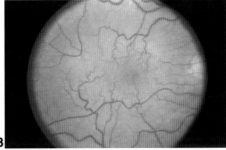

Figure 16-2 Macular epiretinal membrane (ERM). **A,** Patient with macular ERM and complaints of distortion and reduced visual acuity (20/200). **B,** Following pars plana vitrectomy and membrane peeling, distortion is markedly reduced and visual acuity is 20/30. *(Photographs courtesy of Harry W. Flynn Jr, MD.)*

Idiopathic Macular Hole

Vitrectomy surgery is indicated for full-thickness macular holes (stages 2, 3, and 4). Early surgery is considered an important prognostic factor, leading to improved functional and anatomic outcomes. Because stage 1 macular holes have a high rate of spontaneous resolution and reported studies have failed to demonstrate a benefit from vitrectomy, surgery is not generally recommended for this earliest stage. Surgery for full-thickness macular holes (stages 2, 3, or 4) consists of a standard pars plana vitrectomy, removal of the posterior cortical vitreous, a variable degree of preretinal tissue dissection, and use of an intraocular tamponade with face-down positioning. That is, the patient is positioned face down postoperatively for tamponade of the macular hole. Various pharmacologic adjuvants, including transforming growth factor–beta2 (TGF-β2), autologous serum, whole blood, and plasma–thrombin mixture, have been applied intraoperatively in an attempt to increase the rate of successful hole closure. Internal limiting membrane peeling (with or without indocyanine green dye staining) has also been advocated for enhancement of surgical outcomes. To date, however, no definitive evidence has demonstrated improved efficacy for ILM peeling or pharmacologic adjuvants. The use of ILM peeling and/or adjuvants remains controversial.

The first series of patients undergoing vitrectomy for idiopathic macular hole was reported in 1991. In 58% of eyes, the hole was closed, and visual acuity improved by 2 lines or more in 42%. Subsequent series have reported hole closure rates after vitrectomy as high as 92% (Fig 16-4).

Complications of macular hole include cataract, secondary glaucoma, retinal detachment, visual field loss, late reopening of the hole, and other complications related specifically to vitrectomy surgery.

Gass JD. Reappraisal of biomicroscopic classification of stages of development of a macular hole. *Am J Ophthalmol.* 1995;119:752–759.

Kelly NE, Wendel RT. Vitreous surgery for idiopathic macular holes: results of a pilot study. *Arch Ophthalmol.* 1991;109:654–659.

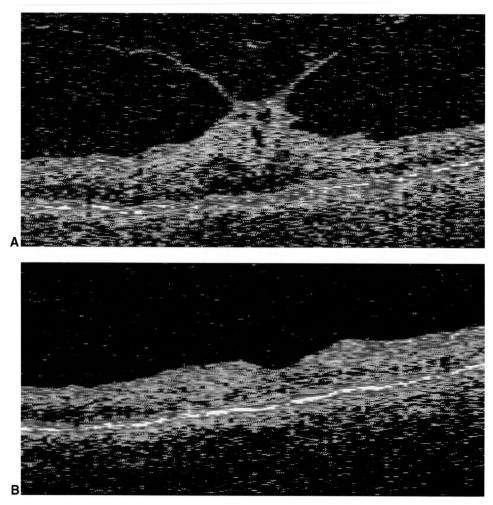

Figure 16-3 Vitreomacular traction syndrome. **A,** Patient with vitreomacular traction, no PVD, and reduced visual acuity (20/200). **B,** After pars plana vitrectomy and removal of macular traction, visual acuity improved to 20/30. *(Photographs courtesy of Mark W. Johnson, MD.)*

Leonard RE 2nd, Smiddy WE, Flynn HW Jr, et al. Long-term visual outcomes in patients with successful macular hole surgery. *Ophthalmology.* 1997;104:1648–1652.

Submacular Hemorrhage

The clinical course of submacular hemorrhages is variable. Many smaller submacular hemorrhages resolve spontaneously, yielding acceptable visual acuity. However, patients with submacular neovascular AMD and larger hemorrhages generally have poor visual outcomes. For removal of thick submacular hemorrhage, pars plana vitrectomy techniques can be considered. An alternative technique involving intravitreal injection of expansile gas (eg, SF_6 or C_3F_8) with or without adjunctive intravitreal or subretinal tissue plasminogen activator (t-PA) has been reported.

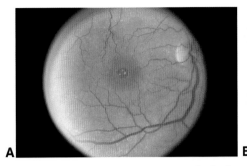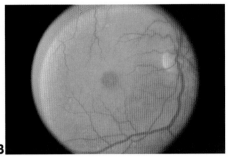

A   B

Figure 16-4 Idiopathic macular hole. **A,** Patient with macular hole and reduced visual acuity (20/100) for 5 months. **B,** Following vitrectomy, membrane peeling, and fluid–gas exchange, the macular hole closed and visual acuity improved to 20/25. *(Photographs courtesy of Harry W. Flynn, Jr, MD.)*

The Submacular Surgery Trial was a randomized, prospective trial evaluating the outcomes of observation versus surgery for eyes with submacular hemorrhage from choroidal neovascularization (CNV) due to AMD (Fig 16-5). The study found that vitrectomy surgery did not improve or stabilize vision in eyes with submacular hemorrhage compared to observation. However, eyes undergoing surgery in the trial were more likely to avoid severe vision loss despite a higher risk of complications.

Bennett SR, Folk JC, Blodi CF, et al. Factors prognostic of visual outcome in patients with subretinal hemorrhage. *Am J Ophthalmol.* 1990;109:33–37.

Berrocal MH, Lewis ML, Flynn HW Jr. Variations in the clinical course of submacular hemorrhage. *Am J Ophthalmol.* 1996;122:486–493.

Bressler NM, Bressler SB, Childs AL, et al. Submacular Surgery Trials (SST) Research Group. Surgery for hemorrhagic choroidal neovascular lesions of age-related macular degeneration: ophthalmic findings. SST report no. 13. *Ophthalmology.* 2004;111:1993–2006.

Hassan AS, Johnson MW, Schneiderman TE, et al. Management of submacular hemorrhage with intravitreal tissue plasminogen activator injection and pneumatic displacement. *Ophthalmology.* 1999;106:1900–1907.

Subfoveal Choroidal Neovascularization

The alternatives for nonsurgical management of patients with subfoveal CNV include laser photocoagulation, photodynamic therapy, and pharmacologic therapy. Surgical management options include pars plana vitrectomy and removal of subfoveal CNV (Fig 16-6) or para plana vitrectomy and macular translocation. The SST showed that vitrectomy surgery was not beneficial for subfoveal CNV due to AMD. However, the surgery was found to be of modest benefit for subfoveal CNV due to OHS and idiopathic causes if the preoperative visual acuity was worse than 20/100.

Hawkins BS, Bressler NM, Bressler SB, et al. Surgical removal vs observation for subfoveal choroidal neovascularization, either associated with the ocular histoplasmosis syndrome or idiopathic. I. Ophthalmic findings from a randomized clinical trial. Submacular Surgery Trials (SST) Group H Trial. SST report no. 9. *Arch Ophthalmol.* 2004;122:1597–1611.

Hawkins BS, Bressler NM, Miskala PH, et al. Surgery for subfoveal choroidal neovascularization in age-related macular degeneration: ophthalmic findings. Submacular Surgery Trials (SST) Research Group. SST report no. 11. *Ophthalmology.* 2004;111:1967–1980.

Melberg NS, Thomas MA, Burgess DB. The surgical removal of subfoveal choroidal neovascularization: ingrowth site as a predictor of visual outcome. *Retina.* 1996;16:190–195.

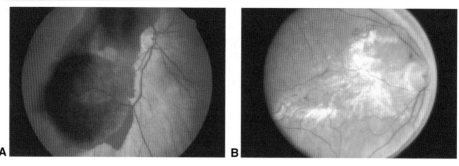

Figure 16-5 Submacular hemorrhage in AMD. **A,** Patient with submacular hemorrhage for 5 days and visual acuity of 3/200. **B,** After pars plana vitrectomy, injection of subretinal t-PA, drainage of subretinal hemorrhage, and fluid–gas exchange, the visual acuity improved to 20/400. RPE atrophic changes in the macula limited visual improvement, however. *(Photographs courtesy of Harry W. Flynn, Jr, MD.)*

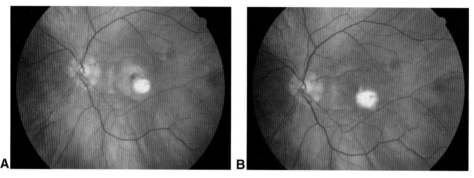

Figure 16-6 A 59-year-old man with recurrent choroidal neovascularization in ocular histoplasmosis. **A,** Preoperatively, subfoveal CNV is adjacent to previous laser scar (VA = 20/300). **B,** One month after pars plana vitrectomy and removal of CNV, visual acuity is 20/25. *(Photographs courtesy of Mark W. Johnson, MD.)*

Vitrectomy for Posterior Segment Complications of Anterior Segment Surgery

Postoperative Endophthalmitis

The clinical features of endophthalmitis following anterior segment surgery include marked intraocular inflammation, often with hypopyon. Conjunctival vascular congestion, corneal edema, and eyelid edema are additional signs associated with intraocular infection. Symptoms often include pain and marked loss of vision. In eyes with endophthalmitis, the loss of vision is usually profound and out of proportion to the typical postoperative visual acuity measured during the first days or weeks after intraocular surgery.

Management of postoperative endophthalmitis includes obtaining intraocular cultures and administering intravitreal antibiotics. An anterior chamber specimen is typically obtained using a 30-gauge needle on a tuberculin syringe. After a povidone-iodide prep, a vitreous specimen can be obtained either by needle tap or by using a vitrectomy instrument. The needle tap of the vitreous generally is accomplished with a 25-gauge 1-inch needle introduced through the pars plana and directed toward the midvitreous cavity. Neither a conjunctival incision nor suture closure is necessary for the needle tap. A small specimen (0.2–0.5 mL) is obtained and directly inoculated on culture media. Vitreous specimens are more likely to yield a positive culture result than simultaneously obtained aqueous specimens.

This classification of postoperative endophthalmitis includes the time of onset and the organisms most frequently isolated:

- acute-onset endophthalmitis (within 6 weeks of intraocular surgery): coagulase-negative *Staphylococcus, S aureus, Streptococcus* spp, gram-negative organisms
- chronic (delayed-onset) endophthalmitis (beyond 6 weeks after surgery): *Propionibacterium acnes,* coagulase-negative *Staphylococcus,* fungi
- bleb-associated endophthalmitis (months or years after surgery): *Streptococcus* spp, *Haemophilus* spp, gram-positive organisms

Acute-onset postoperative endophthalmitis

Vitrectomy for acute postoperative endophthalmitis is guided by the results of the Endophthalmitis Vitrectomy Study (EVS; Clinical Trial 16-1). In the EVS, patients were randomized to undergo either vitrectomy or vitreous tap/biopsy. Both groups received intravitreal and subconjunctival antibiotics (vancomycin and amikacin) injections. The EVS concluded that vitrectomy surgery was indicated in patients who presented with acute-onset (within 6 weeks of cataract extraction) postoperative endophthalmitis with light perception vision (Fig 16-7). Patients with hand motions visual acuity or better had equivalent postoperative outcomes in both treatment groups.

Ceftazidime has largely replaced amikacin in clinical practice, largely because of concerns for potential aminoglycoside toxicity. Intravitreal dexamethasone may reduce post-treatment inflammation, but its role in endophthalmitis management remains controversial.

Han DP. Endophthalmitis. In: Albert DM, ed. *Ophthalmic Surgery: Principles and Techniques.* Malden, MA: Blackwell Science; 1999:650–662.

Results of the Endophthalmitis Vitrectomy Study: a randomized trial of immediate vitrectomy and of intravenous antibiotics for the treatment of postoperative bacterial endophthalmitis. Endophthalmitis Vitrectomy Study Group. *Arch Ophthalmol.* 1995;113:1479–1496.

Chronic (delayed-onset) endophthalmitis

Patients with chronic endophthalmitis present with progressive intraocular inflammation and a chronic indolent course over months or years following cataract surgery. *P acnes* endophthalmitis characteristically induces a peripheral white plaque within the capsular bag and an associated chronic granulomatous inflammation. Treatment by injection of antibiotics into the capsular bag or into the vitreous cavity is usually unsuccessful in eliminating the infection. A preferred approach is pars plana vitrectomy, partial capsulectomy with selected removal of intracapsular white plaque, and injection of intravitreal vancomycin 1 mg adjacent to or inside the capsular bag. If the condition recurs after

Endophthalmitis Vitrectomy Study

Objective: Evaluate the role of pars plana vitrectomy and intravenous antibiotics in management of postoperative bacterial endophthalmitis.

Participants: Patients with clinical signs and symptoms of bacterial endophthalmitis in an eye following cataract surgery or lens implantation within 6 weeks of onset of infection.

Randomization: Patients randomized to receive systemic antibiotics or no systemic antibiotics and evaluated at regular intervals after treatment. Patients were randomized to immediate pars plana vitrectomy or to immediate tap/biopsy.

Outcome Measures: Standardized visual acuity testing and media clarity.

Results:

1. No difference in final visual acuity or media clarity whether or not EVS systemic antibiotics (amikacin/ceftazidime) were employed.
2. No difference in outcomes between the three-port pars plana vitrectomy group compared to the immediate tap/biopsy group for patients with better than light perception visual acuity at the study entry examination.
3. For patients with light perception visual acuity, much better results in the immediate pars plana vitrectomy group:
    a. Three times more likely to achieve ≥20/40 (33% versus 11%)
    b. Two times more likely to achieve ≥20/100 (56% versus 30%)
    c. Less likely to incur <5/200 (20% versus 47%)

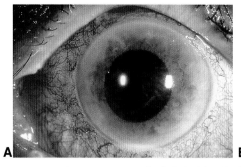 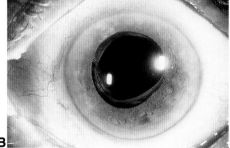

A   **B**

Figure 16-7 Acute-onset endophthalmitis. **A,** Patient with marked intraocular inflammation, hypopyon, and endophthalmitis 5 days after cataract surgery. **B,** After needle tap of vitreous and injection of intravitreal antibiotics, inflammation resolved and visual acuity improved to 20/30. *(Photographs courtesy of Harry W. Flynn, Jr, MD.)*

vitrectomy and subtotal capsulectomy, removal of the entire capsular bag, with removal or exchange of the IOL should be considered (Fig 16-8).

Clark WL, Kaiser PK, Flynn HW Jr, et al. Treatment strategies and visual acuity outcomes in chronic postoperative *Propionibacterium acnes* endophthalmitis. *Ophthalmology.* 1999; 106:1665–1670.

Fox GM, Joondeph BC, Flynn HW Jr, et al. Delayed-onset pseudophakic endophthalmitis. *Am J Ophthalmol.* 1991;111:163–173.

Endophthalmitis associated with conjunctival filtering blebs

Except for the additional sign of a purulent bleb, the clinical features of conjunctival filtering bleb–associated endophthalmitis are similar to acute-onset postoperative endophthalmitis. These features include conjunctival vascular congestion and marked intraocular inflammation, often with hypopyon (occurring months or years after glaucoma filtering surgery or cataract surgery resulting in an unintentional bleb). The initial infection may involve the bleb only *(blebitis)* without anterior chamber or vitreous involvement. Blebitis without endophthalmitis can be treated with frequent applications of topical and subconjunctival antibiotics with close follow-up. However, when blebitis leads to bleb-associated endophthalmitis, these patients are treated by intravitreal antibiotics with or without vitrectomy. The recommended intravitreal antibiotics are similar to those used in acute-onset postoperative endophthalmitis. However, the most common causative organisms in bleb-associated endophthalmitis (eg, *Streptococcus* or *Haemophilus* spp) are more virulent than the most frequent organisms in other postoperative categories. In spite of prompt treatment, the visual outcomes in this category are generally worse than for acute-onset endophthalmitis following cataract surgery (Fig 16-9).

Brown RH, Yang LH, Walker SD, et al. Treatment of bleb infection after glaucoma surgery. *Arch Ophthalmol.* 1994;112:57–61.

Greenfield DS. Dysfunctional glaucoma filtration blebs. *Focal Points: Clinical Modules for Ophthalmologists.* San Francisco: American Academy of Ophthalmology; 2002, module 4.

Kangas TA, Greenfield DS, Flynn HW Jr, et al. Delayed-onset endophthalmitis associated with conjunctival filtering blebs. *Ophthalmology.* 1997;104:746–752.

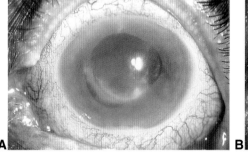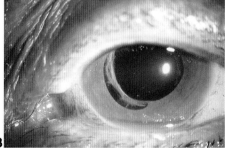

Figure 16-8 Chronic (delayed-onset) postoperative endophthalmitis. **A,** Endophthalmitis patient with progressive intraocular inflammation 3 months after cataract surgery. **B,** Same patient after pars plana vitrectomy, capsulectomy, and injection of intravitreal antibiotics. Culture confirmed diagnosis of *P acnes* endophthalmitis. *(Photographs courtesy of Harry W. Flynn, Jr, MD.)*

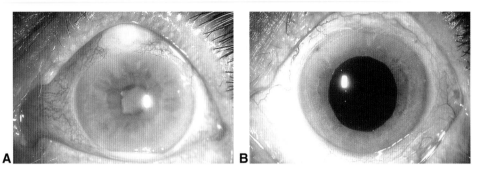

Figure 16-9 Bleb-associated endophthalmitis. **A,** Patient with endophthalmitis with sudden onset of decreased vision, redness, and pain 2 years after glaucoma filtering surgery. **B,** Same patient after treatment with pars plana vitrectomy and injection of intravitreal antibiotics. *(Photographs courtesy of Harry W. Flynn, Jr, MD.)*

Cystoid Macular Edema

Cystoid macular edema (CME) following anterior segment surgery usually resolves spontaneously. Treatment with topical medications is the first-line approach for patients with persistent CME. Periocular and intraocular corticosteroids may be used in recalcitrant cases. When visual loss is unresponsive to medical therapy and vitreous adhesions to anterior segment structures are present, pars plana vitrectomy with removal of these adhesions may promote resolution of CME and improve visual acuity (Fig 16-10). Optical coherence tomography may be helpful in identifying vitreous traction that can be relieved with vitrectomy surgery.

Harbour JW, Smiddy WE, Rubsamen PE, et al. Pars plana vitrectomy for chronic pseudophakic cystoid macular edema. *Am J Ophthalmol.* 1995;120:302–307.

Heier JS, Topping TM, Baumann W, et al. Keteroloc versus prednisolone versus combination therapy in the treatment of acute pseudophakic cystoid macular edema. *Ophthalmology.* 2000;107:2034–2039.

Pendergast SD, Margherio RR, Williams GA, et al. Vitrectomy for chronic pseudophakic cystoid macular edema. *Am J Ophthalmol.* 1999;128:317–323.

Suprachoroidal Hemorrhage

Suprachoroidal hemorrhage may occur during or after any form of intraocular surgery, particularly glaucoma surgery. It may be limited to 1 or 2 quadrants, or it can be massive, resulting in extrusion of intraocular contents or forcing the retinal surfaces into apposition. Reported risk factors for suprachoroidal hemorrhage include

- advanced age
- glaucoma
- myopia
- aphakia
- arteriosclerotic cardiovascular disease
- hypertension
- Sturge-Weber-associated choroidal hemangiomas
- intraoperative tachycardia

Transient hypotony is a common feature during or after all intraocular surgery, and this may be associated with suprachoroidal hemorrhage from rupture of the long or short posterior ciliary arteries in a small percentage of patients.

Surgical management strategies are controversial. Most authors recommend immediate closure of ocular surgical incisions and removal of vitreous prolapse into the wound, if possible. Intraoperative suprachoroidal hemorrhage drainage is almost never successful (Fig 16-11). Most surgeons recommend observation for 7–14 days in order to allow some degree of liquefaction of the suprachoroidal hemorrhage. B-scan ultrasound, specifically in looking for echographic features of liquefaction of the clot, is helpful in determining the timing of secondary surgical intervention. Indications for surgical drainage of suprachoroidal hemorrhage include recalcitrant pain, increased intraocular pressure, retinal detachment, or appositional choroidal detachments (ie, "kissing" choroidals).

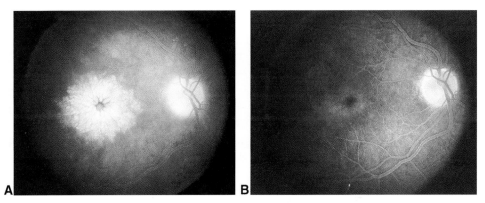

Figure 16-10 Pseudophakic cystoid macular edema (CME). **A,** Patient with nonresolving CME, vitreous strands to cataract wound, and dislocated IOL. **B,** Same patient after pars plana vitrectomy, removal of vitreous strands, repositioning of IOL, and periocular administration of corticosteroids. CME has markedly improved. *(Photographs courtesy of Harry W. Flynn, Jr, MD.)*

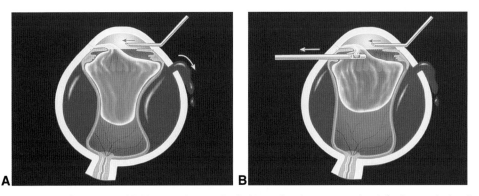

Figure 16-11 Suprachoroidal hemorrhage. **A,** Schematic shows anterior infusion and simultaneous drainage of suprachoroidal hemorrhage through pars plana sclerotomy. **B,** Schematic shows pars plana vitrectomy to remove vitreous prolapse as drainage of suprachoroidal hemorrhage continues. *(Images courtesy of Harry W. Flynn, Jr, MD.)*

Surgical management of suprachoroidal hemorrhage involves placing an anterior chamber infusion line to maintain intraocular pressure. A full-thickness sclerotomy is then placed subjacent to the site of maximum accumulation of blood. After drainage of suprachoroidal blood, pars plana vitrectomy may be performed. Appositional suprachoroidal hemorrhage generally has a poor visual prognosis.

Scott IU, Flynn HW Jr, Schiffman J, et al. Visual acuity outcomes among patients with appositional suprachoroidal hemorrhage. *Ophthalmology.* 1997;104:2039–2046.

Pollack AL, McDonald HR, Ai E, et al. Massive suprachoroidal hemorrhage during pars plana vitrectomy associated with Valsalva maneuver. *Am J Ophthalmol.* 2001;132:383–387.

Retinal Detachment

The incidence of retinal detachment following cataract surgery is approximately 1% (Fig 16-12). However, when cataract surgery is accompanied by vitreous loss, the incidence of retinal detachment increases to 5% or more. Another risk factor for pseudophakic retinal detachment is Nd:YAG laser capsulotomy. In one reported study, the performance of Nd:YAG laser capsulotomy doubled the incidence of retinal detachment.

Management options include laser demarcation, pneumatic retinopexy, scleral buckling surgery, and vitrectomy with or without a scleral buckle. Observation can be considered in selected patients with localized retinal detachment and no associated symptoms.

Selection of treatment options for retinal detachment depends on the surgeon and remains a topic of debate within the retina community. Understanding the principles and limitations of these treatment modalities is essential in optimizing visual outcomes.

Brod RD, Flynn HW Jr, Lightman DA. Asymptomatic rhegmatogenous retinal detachments. *Arch Ophthalmol.* 1995;113:1030–1032.

Campo RV, Sipperley JO, Sneed SR, et al. Pars plana vitrectomy without scleral buckle for pseudophakic retinal detachments. *Ophthalmology.* 1999;106:1811–1816.

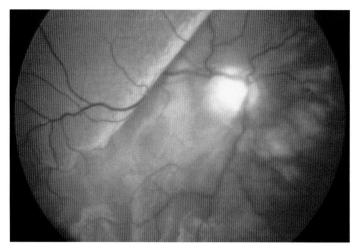

Figure 16-12 Retinal detachment: patient with symptomatic retinal detachment following cataract surgery. *(Photograph courtesy of Harry W. Flynn, Jr, MD.)*

Hilton GF, McLean EB, Brinton DA. *Retinal Detachment: Principles and Practice.* 2nd ed. Ophthalmology Monograph 1. San Francisco: American Academy of Ophthalmology; 1995.

Wilkinson CP, Rice TA. *Michel's Retinal Detachment.* 2nd ed. St Louis: Mosby; 1997:641–729.

Surgical repair of retinal detachments

Three surgical techniques have been described for patients who develop a primary un-complicated rhegmatogenous retinal detachment: pneumatic retinopexy, scleral buckle, and primary vitrectomy.

Pneumatic retinopexy The principle behind pneumatic retinopexy involves creating an intraocular tamponade of the retinal breaks to allow sufficient time for subretinal fluid to be resorbed and a chorioretinal adhesion to form around the break. The classic in-dications for pneumatic retinopexy include: retinal breaks confined to the superior 8 clock-hours, retinal break or breaks with 1–2 clock-hours, absence of proliferative vi-treoretinopathy (PVR) grade C or D, the ability to maintain head position, and clear media. With direct pneumatic tamponade of the causative retinal breaks, complete sub-retinal fluid resorption often takes place within 6–8 hours in acute detachments. Pneu-matic retinopexy may even be possible with inferior retinal detachments in particularly flexible patients who can maintain head position for 6–8 hours.

The procedure can be performed with topical, subconjunctival or retrobulbar an-esthesia. Using a lid speculum, an application of 5% povidine-iodine is instilled into the conjunctival cul-de-sac and lid margin. Transconjunctival cryopexy of the causative reti-nal breaks can be applied. Alternatively, laser retinopexy may be performed following retinal apposition. Gas is then injected transconjunctivally through the pars plana. A variety of intraocular gases has been used (air, SF_6 and C_3F_8). Frequently, an anterior chamber paracentesis is required to lower the intraocular pressure that results from the gas application. To tamponade all causative retinal breaks, the patient must maintain the demonstrated head position.

A prospective, multicenter, randomized clinical trial comparing pneumatic retino-pexy to scleral buckle demonstrated successful retinal reattachment in 73% of patients who underwent pneumatic retinopexy and 82% success in those who were randomized to scleral buckles. This was not a statistically significant difference. For patients who required more than one procedure, 99% of patients originally randomized to pneumatic retinopexy and 98% of patient in the scleral buckle group achieved anatomic success.

The functional outcome was equivalent between the 2 groups for macula-on retinal detachments. For patients with macula-off retinal detachments of recent duration (<14 days), pneumatic retinopexy was superior to scleral buckling in regard to visual outcome.

Complications from pneumatic retinopexy include subretinal gas migration, anterior chamber gas migration, endophthalmitis, cataract, and new retinal break formation.

Chang TS, Pelzek CD, Nguyen RL, et al. Inverted pneumatic retionpexy: a method of treating retinal detachments associated with inferior retinal breaks. *Ophthalmology.* 2003;110: 589–594.

Tornambe PE, Hilton GF. Pneumatic retinopexy: a multicenter randomized controlled clinical trial comparing pneumatic retinopexy with scleral buckling. The Retinal Detachment Study Group. *Ophthalmology.* 1989;96:772–784.

Scleral buckle The principle behind scleral buckling is to relieve vitreous traction on retinal breaks, alter intraocular fluid currents, and reappose retinal/RPE anatomy. Scleral buckling in conjunction with retinal cryopexy is used to create a permanent adhesion at the sites of retinal breaks.

Choosing a scleral buckling technique (eg, encircling vs segmental vs radial sponge) is a multifactorial decision that takes into account the number and position of retinal breaks, the size of the eye, surgeon preference, associated vitreoretinal findings (ie, lattice, vitreoretinal traction, aphakia).

External drainage of subretinal fluid and/or intraocular gas tamponade may be indicated if intraocular pressure increases due to displaced volume from the buckling effect, chronic viscous subretinal fluid, fish-mouthing of large retinal breaks, and bullous retinal detachments.

Complications of scleral buckles include induced myopia, ocular ischemia, diplopia, ptosis, orbital cellulitis, subretinal hemorrhage from drainage, and retinal incarceration at drainage site.

Primary vitrectomy The principles behind primary vitrectomy involve release of vitreous traction, internal drainage of subretinal fluid, intraocular tamponade (air, gas, silicone oil, perfluorocarbon liquids), and creation of chorioretinal adhesions with endolaser photocoagulation or cryopexy.

Needle Penetration of the Globe

Factors predisposing to needle penetration of the globe include

- axial high myopia
- posterior staphyloma
- previous scleral buckling surgery
- poor patient cooperation at the time of the injection

Another risk factor may be injection by those who may have limited experience in providing ocular anesthesia.

Management options vary with the severity of the intraocular damage. Often, blood obscures and surrounds the retinal penetration site, making laser treatment difficult. Observation or transscleral cryotherapy may be considered in such cases. When associated retinal detachment is present, early vitrectomy combined with scleral buckling is often recommended. Eyes without retinal detachment have a much better visual prognosis than eyes with retinal detachment. Posterior pole damage from needle extension into the macula or optic nerve is associated with a very poor visual prognosis (Fig 16-13).

Duker JS, Belmont JB, Benson WE, et al. Inadvertent globe perforation during retrobulbar and peribulbar anesthesia: patient characteristics, surgical management, and visual outcome. *Ophthalmology.* 1991;98:519–526.

Hay A, Flynn HW Jr, Hoffman JI, et al. Needle penetration of the globe during retrobulbar and peribulbar injections. *Ophthalmology.* 1991;98:1017–1024.

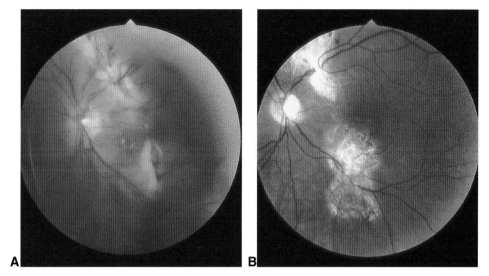

Figure 16-13 Needle penetration of the globe. **A,** Needle penetration of the globe has caused multiple retinal breaks, including damage to the macula. **B,** After retinal detachment occurred, treatment consisted of vitrectomy, fluid–gas exchange, and endolaser photocoagulation of retinal breaks. Retinal reattachment was achieved, but the visual acuity remained very poor. *(Photographs courtesy of Harry W. Flynn, Jr, MD.)*

Retained Lens Fragments After Phacoemulsification

The incidence of posteriorly displaced lens fragments ranges between 0.3% and 1.1% in reported series. Retained lens fragments may cause severe intraocular inflammation and secondary glaucoma. The postoperative intraocular inflammation is generally associated with the amount of retained lens material and the induced surgical trauma. Nuclear fragments usually continue to cause chronic intraocular inflammation, whereas cortical remnants may be reabsorbed. Eyes with posteriorly retained lens fragments may have undergone significant trauma during the initial cataract surgery and therefore often have associated corneal edema, retinal detachment, and CME. The postoperative inflammation may be exacerbated by the patient's individual inflammatory response to retained lens material.

Use of phacoemulsification in the setting of vitreous prolapse into the anterior segment can create excessive vitreoretinal traction that can lead to retinal detachment. Vitreous and/or remaining lens fragments should be removed from the anterior segment using a cutting instrument. At the time of the initial cataract surgery, attempts at retrieving lens fragments can lead to increased vitreoretinal complications and should be avoided by anterior segment surgeons.

Small chips of nucleus in the posterior segment may sometimes be tolerated without the need for surgical intervention. However, larger pieces (>2 mm in diameter) nearly always require removal (Table 16-1).

Indications for vitrectomy to remove posteriorly retained lens fragments include secondary glaucoma, lens-induced uveitis, and large nuclear fragments. In the 4 largest reported series, 52% of patients with retained lens fragments had an IOP ≥30 mm Hg

Table 16-1 General Recommendations for Management of Retained Lens Fragments

For the anterior segment surgeon

Attempt retrieval of displaced lens fragments if fragments are readily accessible.

Perform anterior vitrectomy as necessary to avoid vitreous prolapse into the wound.

Insert an intraocular lens if possible.

Close the cataract wound with interrupted sutures.

Prescribe topical medications as needed.

Refer the patient to a vitreoretinal consultant.

For the vitreoretinal surgeon

Observe eyes with minimal inflammation and/or a small lens fragment.

Continue topical medications as needed.

Schedule vitrectomy:

if inflammation or IOP is not controlled

if fragment is >2 mm in size

Delay vitrectomy if necessary to allow clearing of corneal edema.

Perform adequate core vitrectomy before phacoemulsification.

Start with low fragmentation power (5%–10%) for more efficient removal of the nucleus.

Prepare for secondary IOL insertion if necessary.

Examine the retinal periphery for retinal tears or retinal detachment.

(Modified from Flynn HW Jr, Smiddy WE, Vilar NF. Management of retained lens fragments after cataract surgery. In: Saer JB, ed. *Vitreo-Retinal and Uveitis Update*. The Hague, Netherlands: Kugler; 1998:149, 150.)

prior to vitrectomy. Vitrectomy and removal of retained lens fragments reduced this incidence by 50% or more in these reported series.

Vilar NF, Flynn HW Jr, Smiddy WE, et al. Removal of retained lens fragments after phacoemulsification reverses secondary glaucoma and restores visual acuity. *Ophthalmology*. 1997;104:787–791.

The preferred approach for removal includes pars plana vitrectomy with or without ultrasonic emulsification (with the fragmatome—posterior segment ultrasonic fragmenter) to remove harder pieces of lens nucleus (Fig 16-14). In the setting of concurrent retinal detachment, the perfluorocarbon liquids may be useful in floating the lens material anteriorly while stabilizing the retinal detachment. After the vitreous is removed, the fragmatome can be used at a low power setting to maintain contact between the fragmentation probe and the nuclear fragment. The retinal periphery should be examined for the presence of retinal tears or retinal detachment in these patients.

Borne MJ, Tasman W, Regillo C, et al. Outcomes of vitrectomy for retained lens fragments. *Ophthalmology*. 1996;103:971–976.

Gilliland GD, Hutton WL, Fuller DG. Retained intravitreal lens fragments after cataract surgery. *Ophthalmology*. 1992;99:1263–1269.

Lewis H, Blumenkranz MS, Chang S. Treatment of dislocated crystalline lens and retinal detachment with perfluorocarbon liquids. *Retina*. 1992;12:299–304.

Reported series with long-term follow-up have found that retinal detachment occurs in about 15% of eyes with retained lens fragments. If the lens fragments are in the posterior vitreous, aggressive attempts to retrieve them from a limbal approach are some-

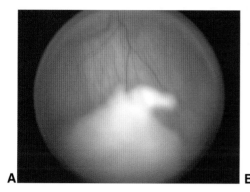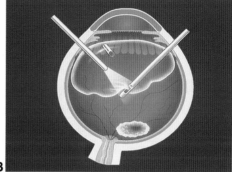

Figure 16-14 Retained lens fragments after phacoemulsification. **A,** Clinical photograph of large lens fragment on the retina. **B,** Schematic shows pars plana vitrectomy for removal of formed vitreous before approaching the lens fragment. *(Reproduced with permission from Smiddy WE, Flynn HW Jr. Managing retained lens fragments and dislocated posterior chamber IOLs after cataract surgery. Focal Points: Clinical Modules for Ophthalmologists. San Francisco: American Academy of Ophthalmology; 1996, module 7.)*

times complicated by retinal detachment with giant retinal tear. Giant retinal tear is more common in the inferior quadrants when a superior limbal approach was used for cataract surgery.

Aaberg TM Jr, Rubsamen PE, Flynn HW Jr, et al. Giant retinal tear as a complication of attempted removal of intravitreal lens fragments during cataract surgery. *Am J Ophthalmol.* 1997;124:222–226.

The outcomes reported in the literature do not exclude patients with preexisting macular disease, glaucoma, or diabetic retinopathy. Therefore, some unfavorable visual acuity outcomes may reflect adverse events not directly caused by retained lens fragments. Overall, around 60% of these patients will achieve reading vision ($\geq$20/40).

Smiddy WE, Flynn HW Jr. Managing retained lens fragments and dislocated posterior chamber IOLs after cataract surgery. *Focal Points: Clinical Modules for Ophthalmologists.* San Francisco: American Academy of Ophthalmology; 1996, module 7.

Posteriorly Dislocated Intraocular Lenses

Dislocated posterior chamber intraocular lenses (PC IOLs) may not be recognized by the surgeon until the first postoperative day. Even though the capsular support may have seemed satisfactory at the time of the initial cataract surgery, the lens may be seen to be dislocated posteriorly on the first day following surgery. Factors that should be considered when placing a sulcus IOL include the presence of zonular dehiscence, total amount of anterior capsular support (eg, >180°), size of the eye, and haptic-to-haptic length of the IOL. Foldable IOLs have a 12.5- to 13.0-mm haptic-to-haptic length. This is frequently smaller than the sulcus-to-sulcus diameter in which these lenses are placed and may contribute to subluxation or dislocation of the IOL in the postoperative period. Dislocation of a flexible IOL may also follow Nd:YAG laser capsulotomy when performed soon after cataract surgery. Late dislocation of the IOL (several days or weeks after surgery) is less common but may occur as a result of trauma or spontaneous loss of zonular support in eyes with pseudoexfoliation syndrome. The options for treatment include observation only, surgical repositioning, IOL exchange, or IOL removal.

Vitrectomy for posteriorly dislocated IOLs involves removal of all vitreous adhesions to the IOL in order to minimize vitreous traction to the retina when the lens is manipulated back into the anterior chamber. The intraocular lens may be placed into the ciliary sulcus, providing there is adequate support. If there is inadequate capsular support, then one may suture-fixate the IOL to either the iris or the sclera.

Schneiderman TE, Johnson MW, Smiddy WE, et al. Surgical management of posteriorly dislocated silicone plate haptic intraocular lenses. *Am J Ophthalmol.* 1997;123:629–635.

Smiddy WE, Flynn HW Jr. Managing retained lens fragments and dislocated posterior chamber IOLs after cataract surgery. *Focal Points: Clinical Modules for Ophthalmologists.* San Francisco: American Academy of Ophthalmology; 1996, module 7.

Vitrectomy for Complex Retinal Detachment

Complex retinal detachment includes giant retinal tears (retinal breaks that exceed 3 contiguous clock-hours), recurrent retinal detachments, vitreous hemorrhage, and PVR. Pars plana vitrectomy is necessary to remove proliferating tissue, unfold retinal structures, and remove media opacities—features that are commonly seen in patients with complex retinal detachment (see also Chapter 11). Controversy has surrounded the use of long-acting gas versus silicone oil in retinal tamponade for eyes with advanced grades of PVR, an issue addressed in the Silicone Study (Clinical Trial 16-2). This randomized, prospective, multicentered study concluded that tamponade with SF_6 was inferior to both C_3F_8 and silicone oil. For most cases of complex retinal detachment repair, outcomes from the use of C_3F_8 and silicone oil were equivalent. A lower rate of hypotony was noted in patients with silicone oil when compared to those treated with C_3F_8.

Abrams GW, Azen SP, McCuen BW 2nd, et al. Vitrectomy with silicone oil or long-acting gas in eyes with severe proliferative vitreoretinopathy: results of additional and long-term follow-up. Silicone Study report 11. *Arch Ophthalmol.* 1997;115:335–344.

Azen SP, Scott IU, Flynn HW Jr, et al. Silicone oil in the repair of complex retinal detachments: a prospective observational multicenter study. *Ophthalmology.* 1998;105:1587–1597.

Scott IU, Flynn HW Jr, Azen SP, et al. Silicone oil in the repair of pediatric complex retinal detachments: a prospective, observational, multicenter study. *Ophthalmology.* 1999;106:1399–1407.

Vitrectomy with silicone oil or perfluoropropane gas in eyes with severe proliferative vitreoretinopathy: results of a randomized clinical trial. Silicone Study report 2. *Arch Ophthalmol.* 1992;110:780–792.

Vitrectomy with silicone oil or sulfur hexafluoride gas in eyes with severe proliferative vitreoretinopathy: results of a randomized clinical trial. Silicone Study report 1. *Arch Ophthalmol.* 1992;110:770–779.

Silicone Study

Objective: Evaluate the use of various methods of retinal tamponade together with pars plana vitrectomy techniques on eyes with complex retinal detachment and advanced proliferative vitreoretinopathy.

Participants: Randomized, prospective study included patients 18 years of age and older with grade C3 or greater PVR. Subgroups in the study included the following:

> Group 1 eyes: no previous vitrectomy surgery
> Group 2 eyes: one or more previous vitrectomy operations using gas

Randomization: The study eye was randomized to receive either perfluoropropane (C_3F_8) gas or silicone oil after effecting retinal reattachment by way of fluid–gas exchange.

Outcome Measures: Visual acuity of 5/200 or better and macular reattachment for 6 months following the surgical procedure.

Outcomes: The results of the study showed no significant differences between C_3F_8 and silicone oil in achieving visual acuity of 5/200 or better (43% versus 45% for Group 1, 38% versus 33% for Group 2). Overall, silicone oil slightly exceeded C_3F_8 in macular and complete retinal reattachment rates and in final visual acuity outcomes. Keratopathy was more common in C_3F_8 treated eyes and in Group 2 eyes.

Vitrectomy for Diabetic Tractional Retinal Detachments

Vitrectomy is indicated when progression of a tractional retinal detachment threatens the macula. Whenever possible, attempts should be made to add or complete panretinal photocoagulation prior to surgery. The goal of vitrectomy surgery is to relieve vitreoretinal traction to facilitate retinal reattachment. Three categories of tractional forces can be considered. Anteroposterior traction is typically directed along a vector connecting the posterior aspect of the vitreous base to sites of posterior vitreoretinal adhesion (typically along the temporal vascular arcades). Circumferential and centripedal forces are then addressed with a combination of scissors, picks, and forceps, using either unimanual or bimanual techniques. Various approaches to managing fibrovascular tissue removal have been described; these include segmentation, delamination, and en bloc and modified en bloc excision.

Following removal of all tractional membranes, diathermy is applied to all fibrovascular tufts, and supplemental laser is applied. At the completion of the surgery, it is essential that the retinal periphery be carefully examined for retinal breaks.

Ryan SJ, ed. *Retina.* 3rd ed. St Louis: Mosby; 2001:pp 2436–2476.

Complications of Pars Plana Vitrectomy

Pars plana vitrectomy can be associated with cataract, secondary glaucoma, retinal tears and detachment, subretinal perfluorocarbon, retinal and/or vitreous incarcerations, endophthalmitis, and recurrent vitreous hemorrhage. Endophthalmitis after vitrectomy is rare, but it is more common in patients with diabetes and in eyes with retained intraocular foreign bodies. Table 16-2 lists the most common complications of pars plana vitrectomy.

Banker AS, Freeman WR, Kim JW, et al. Vision-threatening complications of surgery for full-thickness macular holes. Vitrectomy for Macular Hole Study Group. *Ophthalmology.* 1997;104:1442–1453.

Cohen SM, Flynn HW Jr, Murray TG, et al. Endophthalmitis after pars plana vitrectomy. The Postvitrectomy Endophthalmitis Study Group. *Ophthalmology.* 1995;102:705–712.

Gass JD. Sympathetic ophthalmia following vitrectomy. *Am J Ophthalmol.* 1982;93:552–558.

Table 16-2 Complications of Pars Plana Vitrectomy

Complications more commonly associated with pars plana vitrectomy
Intraoperative or postoperative retinal break
Intraoperative or postoperative retinal detachment
Intraoperative or postoperative cataract
Postoperative vitreous hemorrhage
Postoperative massive fibrin accumulation
Postoperative anterior segment neovascularization

Complications associated with silicone oil
Glaucoma
Band keratopathy

Complications of intraocular surgery in general
Endophthalmitis
Sympathetic ophthalmia
Recurrent corneal erosion

The authors wish to acknowledge the contributions of Robert Equi, MD, to this chapter.

Basic Texts

Retina and Vitreous

Albert DM, ed. *Ophthalmic Surgery: Principles and Techniques.* Malden, MA: Blackwell Science; 1999.

Albert DM, Jakobiec FA, eds. *Principles and Practice of Ophthalmology.* 2nd ed. Philadelphia: Saunders; 2000.

Alfaro DV III, Liggett PE, eds. *Vitreorenial Surgery of the Injured Eye.* Philadelphia: Lippincott; 1999.

Dibernardo CW, Schachat AP, Fekrat S. *Ophthalmic Ultrasound: A Diagnostic Atlas.* New York: Thieme; 1998.

Gass JD. *Stereoscopic Atlas of Macular Diseases: Diagnosis and Treatment.* 4th ed. St Louis: Mosby; 1997.

Guyer DR, Yannuzzi LA, Chang S, et al, eds. *Retina–Vitreous–Macula.* Philadelphia: Saunders; 1999.

Heckenlively JR, Arden GB, Adachi-Usami E, et al, eds. *Principles and Practice of Clinical Electrophysiology of Vision.* St Louis: Mosby; 1991.

Kertes PJ, Conway MD, eds. *Clinical Trials in Ophthalmology: A Summary and Practice Guide.* Baltimore: Williams & Wilkins; 1998.

Meredith T. *Atlas of Retinal and Vitreous Surgery.* St Louis: Mosby; 1999.

Parrish RK II, ed. *The University of Miami Bascom Palmer Eye Institute Atlas of Ophthalmology.* Philadelphia: Current Medicine; 2000.

Peyman GA, Meffert SA, Chou F, et al, eds. *Vitreoretinal Surgery Techniques.* London: Martin Dunitz; 2000.

Regillo CD, Benson WE. *Retinal Detachment: Diagnosis and Management.* 3rd ed. Philadelphia: Lippincott; 1998.

Regillo CD, Brown GC, Flynn HW Jr, eds. *Vitreoretinal Disease: The Essentials.* New York: Thieme; 1999.

Ryan SJ, ed. *Retina.* 3rd ed. St Louis: Mosby; 2001.

Tasman WS, Jaeger EA, eds. *Duane's Clinical Ophthalmology.* Philadelphia: Lippincott; 2001.

Wilkinson CP, Rice TA. *Michel's Retinal Detachment.* 2nd ed. St Louis: Mosby; 1997.

Yannuzzi LA, Flower RW, Slakter JS, eds. *Indocyanine Green Angiography.* St Louis: Mosby; 1997.

Yannuzzi LA, Guyer DR, Green RW, Green WR. *The Retina Atlas.* St Louis; Mosby; 1996.

Websites

Diabetes 2000. http://www.eyenet.org/member/clinical/eyecon
National Eye Institute. http://www.nei.nih.gov
RetNet, the Retinal Information Network. http://www.sph.uth.tmc.edu/retnet

Related Academy Materials

Focal Points: Clinical Modules for Ophthalmologists

Bressler SB. Age-related macular degeneration (Module 2, 1995).

Brown GC. Retinal arterial obstruction (Module 1, 1994).

Capone A Jr. Macular surface disorders (Module 4, 1996).

Colucciello M. Evaluation and management of macular holes (Module 1, 2003).

Doft BH. Managing infectious endophthalmitis: results of the EVS (Module 3, 1997).

Eller AW. Diagnosis and management of vitreous hemorrhage (Module 10, 2000).

Finkelstein D, Clarkson JG, Hillis A. Branch and central vein occlusions (Module 9, 1997).

Fishkind WJ. The torn posterior capsule: prevention, recognition, and management (Module 4, 1999).

Fong DS, Ferris FL III. Practical management of diabetic retinopathy (Module 3, 2003).

Haller JA. Retinal detachment (Module 5, 1998).

Ip MS, Duker JS. Advances in posterior segment imaging techniques (Module 7, 1999).

Lee BL, van Heuven WAJ. Peripheral lesions of the fundus (Module 8, 2000).

Mieler WF. Syutemic therapeutic agents and retinal toxicity (Module 12, 1997).

Rosenfeld PJ, Weissgold DJ. Ocular photodynamic therapy with verteporfin: clinical trial results and current indications for treatment (Module 12, 2002).

Smiddy WE, Flynn HW Jr. Managing retained lens fragments and dislocated posterior chamber IOLs after cataract surgery (Module 7, 1996).

Tiedeman JS. Retinal breaks, holes, and tears (Module 3, 1996).

Vinger PF. Athletic eye injuries and appropriate protection (Module 8, 1997).

Weissgold DJ, Fardin B. Advances in the treatment of exudative age-related macular degeneration (Module 6, 2003).

Weissgold DJ, Fardin B. Advances in the treatment of nonexudative age-related macular degeneration (Module 5, 2003).

Publications

Berkow JW, Flower RW, Orth DH, et al. *Fluorescein and Indocyanine Green Angiography: Technique and Interpretation.* 2nd ed. (Ophthalmology Monograph 5, 1997).

Fishman GA, Birch DG, Holder GE, et al. *Electrophysiologic Testing in Disorders of the Retina, Optic Nerve, and Visual Pathway.* 2nd ed. (Ophthalmology Monograph 2, 2001).

Flynn HW Jr, Smiddy WE, eds. *Diabetes and Ocular Disease: Past, Present, and Future Therapies* (Ophthalmology Monograph 14, 2000).

Folk JC, Pulido JS. *Laser Photocoagulation of the Retina and Choroid* (Ophthalmology Monograph 11, 1997).

Lane SS, Skuta GL. *ProVision: Preferred Responses in Ophthalmology,* Series 3 (Self-Assessment Program, 1999).

Skuta GL, ed. *ProVision: Preferred Responses in Ophthalmology,* Series 2 (Self-Assessment
    Program, 1996).

Continuing Ophthalmic Video Education

Al-Torbak AA. *Capsulorrhexis in Mature Cataract;* Dewey SH, Werner L, Apple DJ, et al.
    Cortical Removal by J-Cannula Irrigation to Reduce Posterior Capsule Opacification;
    Assi AC, Lacey A, Aylward B. *Basic Properties of Intraocular Gases;* Busin M, Arffa
    RC. *Deep Suturing Techniques for Penetrating Keratoplasty;* Teichmann KD, Al-Rajhi
    AA. *Maximum Depth Lamellar Keratoplasty for Keratoconus With Anwar's Big Bubble*
    (2001).
DRS Research Group, ETDRS Research Group, DRVS Research Group. *Evaluation and
    Treatment of Diabetic Retinopathy* (1999).
DRS Research Group, ETDRS Research Group. *Management of Diabetic Retinopathy for
    the Primary Care Physician* (1999).
Kelly MP. *Basic Techniques of Fluorescein Angiography* (1994).
Wallace P, Evans M. *Fundus Photography* (1989).

Multimedia

Lambert HM, Barr CC, Baumann WC, et al. *LEO Clinical Update Course: Retina* (CD-
    ROM, 2002).

Preferred Practice Patterns

Preferred Practice Patterns Committee, Retina Panel. *Age-Related Macular Degeneration*
    (2003).
Preferred Practice Patterns Committee, Retina Panel. *Diabetic Retinopathy* (2003).
Preferred Practice Patterns Committee, Retina Panel. *Idiopathic Macular Hole* (2003).
Preferred Practice Patterns Committee, Retina Panel. *Management of Posterior Vitreous
    Detachment, Retinal Breaks, and Lattice Degeneration* (1998).

Ophthalmic Technology Assessments

Ophthalmic Technology Assessment Committee. *Indocyanine Green Angiography* (1998).
Ophthalmic Technology Assessment Committee. *Macular Translocation* (2000).
Ophthalmic Technology Assessment Committee. *Photodynamic Therapy With Verteporfin
    for Age-Related Macular Degeneration* (2000).
Ophthalmic Technology Assessment Committee. *The Repair of Rhegmatogenous Retinal
    Detachments* (1996).
Ophthalmic Technology Assessment Committee. *Surgical Management of Macular Holes*
    (2001).

Complementary Therapy Assessments

Complementary Therapy Task Force. *Antioxidant Supplements and Age-Related Macular Degeneration* (2002).

Complementary Therapy Task Force. *Apheresis for Age-Related Macular Degeneration* (2003).

Complementary Therapy Task Force. *Microcurrent Stimulation for Macular Degeneration* (2000).

To order any of these materials, please call the Academy's Customer Service number at (415) 561-8540, or order online at www.aao.org.

Credit Reporting Form

Basic and Clinical Science Course, 2007–2008
Section 12

The American Academy of Ophthalmology is accredited by the Accreditation Council for Continuing Medical Education to provide continuing medical education for physicians.

The American Academy of Ophthalmology designates this educational activity for a maximum of 40 *AMA PRA Category 1 Credits*™. Physicians should only claim credit commensurate with the extent of their participation in the activity.

If you wish to claim continuing medical education credit for your study of this section, you may claim your credit online or fill in the required forms and mail or fax them to the Academy.

To use the forms:

1. Complete the study questions and mark your answers on the Section Completion Form.
2. Complete the Section Evaluation.
3. Fill in and sign the statement below.
4. Return this page and the required forms by mail or fax to the CME Registrar (see below).

To claim credit online:

1. Log on to the Academy website (www.aao.org/cme).
2. Select Review/Claim CME.
3. Follow the instructions.

Important: These completed forms or the online claim must be received at the Academy within 3 years of purchase.

I hereby certify that I have spent _____ (up to 40) hours of study on the curriculum of this section and that I have completed the Study Questions.

Signature: _____

Date

Name: _____

Address: _____

City and State: _____ Zip: _____

Telephone: (_____) _____ Academy Member ID# _____
area code

Please return completed forms to: **Or you may fax them to:** 415-561-8575
American Academy of Ophthalmology
P.O. Box 7424
San Francisco, CA 94120-7424
Attn: CME Registrar, Customer Service

2007–2008
Section Completion Form

Basic and Clinical Science Course

Answer Sheet for Section 12

Question	Answer	Question	Answer
1	a b c d	22	a b c d e
2	a b c d	23	a b c d e
3	a b c d	24	a b c d e
4	a b c d	25	a b c d e
5	a b c d	26	a b c d
6	a b c d	27	a b c d e
7	a b c d	28	a b c d
8	a b c d	29	a b c d
9	a b c d e	30	a b c d e
10	a b c d e	31	a b c d
11	a b c d e	32	a b c d
12	a b c d e	33	a b c d e
13	a b c d e	34	a b c d e
14	a b c d e	35	a b c d e
15	a b c d e	36	a b c d e
16	a b c d e	37	a b c d e f
17	a b c d e	38	a b c d
18	a b c d	39	a b c d
19	a b c d e	40	a b c d e
20	a b c d	41	a b c d e
21	a b c d		

Section 12 Evaluation

Please complete this CME questionnaire.

1. To what degree will you use knowledge from BCSC Section 12 in your practice?
   - ☐ Regularly
   - ☐ Sometimes
   - ☐ Rarely

2. Please review the stated objectives for BCSC Section 12. How effective was the material at meeting those objectives?
   - ☐ All objectives were met.
   - ☐ Most objectives were met.
   - ☐ Some objectives were met.
   - ☐ Few or no objectives were met.

3. To what degree is BCSC Section 12 likely to have a positive impact on health outcomes of your patients?
   - ☐ Extremely likely
   - ☐ Highly likely
   - ☐ Somewhat likely
   - ☐ Not at all likely

4. After you review the stated objectives for BCSC Section 12, please let us know of any additional knowledge, skills, or information useful to your practice that were acquired but were not included in the objectives. [Optional]

5. Was BCSC Section 12 free of commercial bias?
   - ☐ Yes
   - ☐ No

6. If you selected "No" in the previous question, please comment. [Optional]

7. Please tell us what might improve the applicability of BCSC to your practice. [Optional]

Study Questions

Although a concerted effort has been made to avoid ambiguity and redundancy in these questions, the authors recognize that differences of opinion may occur regarding the "best" answer. The discussions are provided to demonstrate the rationale used to derive the answer. They may also be helpful in confirming that your approach to the problem was correct or, if necessary, in fixing the principle in your memory. Where relevant, additional references are given.

1. A 32-year-old woman presents for a routine eye examination with no complaints but an elevated choroidal lesion. Ultrasonography reveals an 8-mm-thick lesion with 6 × 10-mm basal dimensions and low internal reflectivity on A-scan. Which of the following statements is *most* correct?

   a. Complete dermatologic evaluation should be scheduled to look for other areas of metastatic malignant melanoma.

   b. Chest radiographs and liver function tests should be ordered to evaluate for metastasis.

   c. The ultrasound findings are most consistent with a choroidal hemangioma.

   d. Immediate enucleation should be considered.

2. A 75-year-old woman presents with sudden visual loss with intraretinal hemorrhages in all 4 quadrants, macular edema, and dilated, tortuous retinal veins. Which of the following statements is *most* correct?

   a. If the patient develops iris neovascularization, panretinal photocoagulation should be performed immediately.

   b. Grid photocoagulation would significantly reduce the macular edema and improve her vision.

   c. Panretinal photocoagulation should be performed immediately to prevent neovascularization.

   d. Younger patients with this diagnosis should receive grid photocoagulation.

3. A 92-year-old man presents with a 6-MPS disc area, 100% classic, well-defined, choroidal neovascular membrane (CNV) that crosses the center of the fovea on fluorescein angiography. What would be the *best* treatment option?

   a. ocular photodynamic therapy

   b. injection of an anti-VEGF inhibitor every month for 1 year

   c. laser photocoagulation with krypton red laser to cover the entire CNV and the 100-μm area surrounding it

   d. laser photocoagulation with krypton red laser to cover the entire CNV but no surrounding area

4. A 64-year-old man presents 3 days after cataract surgery with severe eye pain, decreased vision, and photophobia that started 5 hours previously. On examination, the vision is hand motions at 6 in., and the intraocular pressure is 27. There is 3+ conjunctival injection, 4+ anterior chamber cell, a 3-mm layered hypopyon, a well-centered PC-IOL, and a small section of retained cortex in the inferior trabecular meshwork. Which of the following statements is *most* correct?

   a. The retained lens fragments have induced phacoanaphylactic glaucoma.

   b. The cause of the hypopyon is aggressive postoperative inflammation.

   c. A culture of the capsule in this patient would reveal *Propionibacterium acnes* organisms.

   d. The most likely organism involved is coagulase-negative staphylococci.

5. For the patient in question 4, what would be the *best* treatment option?

   a. aggressive topical steroids to decrease the intraocular inflammation

   b. immediate vitrectomy to remove the retained lens fragments

   c. tap of the anterior chamber and injection of intravitreal antibiotics

   d. immediate vitrectomy and injection of intravitreal antibiotics

6. A 24-year-old man with acquired immunodeficiency syndrome (AIDS) presents with cyto-megalovirus retinitis. According to the findings of the Studies of Ocular Complications of AIDS (SOCA) trials, which statement is *least* correct?

   a. The best initial treatment is intravenous foscarnet.

   b. Color photographs are the best way to follow treatment response.

   c. Combination therapy is no better than monotherapy to prevent progression.

   d. Patients treated with ganciclovir had a higher mortality.

7. A 42-year-old female was recently diagnosed with non–insulin-dependent diabetes. Which statement is *most* correct?

   a. Immediate focal laser photocoagulation should be performed if she has clinically significant macular edema and her vision is 20/20.

   b. According to the Diabetes Control and Complications Trial (DCCT), tight control of the patient's blood sugar would decrease her risk of developing diabetic retinopathy.

   c. Immediate scatter photocoagulation should be applied if neovascularization of the disc and vitreous hemorrhage is present.

   d. Focal laser photocoagulation should be performed if fluorescein leakage is present in the center of the fovea, even if the clinical examination does not show retinal thickening.

8. A 52-year-old man presents with a small visual field defect in his left eye. On examination, his vision is 20/40, and he has a segmental, triangular-shaped distribution of intraretinal hemorrhages extending from an arteriovenous crossing along the superotemporal vascular arcade. Given the patient's clinical presentation, which statement is *most* correct?

   a. If macular edema is present for more than 3 months and no retinal hemorrhages would prevent laser treatment, grid photocoagulation should be applied.

   b. If he has more than 5 disc diameters of capillary nonperfusion on fluorescein angiography, he should receive immediate photocoagulation.

   c. If macular nonperfusion causes visual loss, then no treatment is indicated.

   d. A complete embolic workup should be performed, especially evaluation of the carotid arteries.

9. Fundus albipunctatus is characterized by all of the following *except:*

    a. nyctalopia

    b. reduced scotopic ERG that normalizes after several hours of dark adaptation

    c. normal visual acuity

    d. progressive visual field loss

    e. yellow-white dots in the posterior pole

10. A reduced and delayed cone b-wave is consistent with all of the following diagnoses *except:*

    a. retinitis pigmentosa

    b. central retinal vein occlusion

    c. cone dystrophy

    d. syphilitic chorioretinitis

    e. sectorial retinitis pigmentosa

11. An individual born without red-sensitive cone pigment function (protanopia) is likely to

    a. have poor visual acuity

    b. confuse blue and yellow

    c. perceive the long-wavelength portion of the spectrum as being darker than normal

    d. manifest photophobia

    e. be hypersensitive to green

12. A subnormal EOG in the setting of a normal ERG can be seen in the following condition(s):

    a. retinitis pigmentosa

    b. Best disease

    c. rubella retinopathy

    d. pattern dystrophies

    e. b and d

13. Progressive cone dystrophies are characterized by all of the following *except:*

    a. progressive loss of visual acuity

    b. photoaversion (light intolerance)

    c. better visual function during the day than at dusk

    d. loss of color discrimination

    e. bull's-eye pattern of macular atrophy

14. Which of following macular dystrophies is typically inherited as an autosomal recessive trait?

    a. Best vitelliform dystrophy

    b. Stargardt disease

    c. familial drusen

    d. pattern macular dystrophies

    e. Sorsby macular dystrophy

15. A constant diagnostic feature of congenital X-linked retinoschisis is

    a. peripheral retinoschisis

    b. reduced ERG a-wave amplitudes

    c. macular fluorescein leakage

    d. peripheral pigmentary changes

    e. foveal schisis

16. Each of the following statements is true about monitoring for hydroxychloroquine retinopathy *except:*

    a. The earliest signs of toxicity include relative paracentral scotomata and subtle paracentral macular pigment granularity.

    b. Retinal toxicity is quite common in the United States.

    c. The "safe" daily dose is considered to be less than 6.5 mg/kg/day (based on lean body weight).

    d. Baseline evaluation should include complete ophthalmologic examination, fundus photographs, and evaluation of the central visual field with a red test object.

    e. In addition to higher daily and cumulative doses, other risk factors for retinal toxicity include obesity, kidney or liver disease, older age, and possibly concomitant retinal disease.

17. The most critical and constant finding in retinitis pigmentosa is

    a. dense bone spicule pigmentation in the retinal periphery

    b. an abnormality in the rhodopsin gene

    c. acquired red-green color deficiency

    d. a significantly reduced electroretinogram (ERG)

    e. small tubular visual fields

18. Which of the following statements is *false* in relation to X-linked ocular albinism?

    a. The iris is translucent.

    b. Carrier females cannot be detected.

    c. Macromelanosomes are found in the retinal pigment epithelium.

    d. Nystagmus and reduced vision are features of the disorder.

19. A normal electroretinogram is usually found in all of the following diseases affecting the retina *except:*

    a. vitelliform dystrophy

    b. dominant drusen

    c. juvenile retinoschisis

    d. X-linked ocular albinism

    e. pattern dystrophy

20. Fifty percent of rhegmatogenous retinal detachments associated with blunt trauma in young eyes are found

    a. immediately

    b. within 1 month

    c. within 8 months

    d. within 24 months

21. The Joint Statement of the American Academy of Pediatrics, Section on Ophthalmology; the American Association for Pediatric Ophthalmology and Strabismus; and the American Academy of Ophthalmology recommends at least 2 dilated funduscopic examinations using binocular indirect ophthalmoscopy for all infants with

    a. a birth weight less than 1500 grams

    b. a gestational age of 28 weeks or less

    c. a birth weight between 1500 and 2000 grams and an unstable clinical course

    d. all of the above

22. Which of the following statements about cataract surgery in patients with diabetes is correct?

    a. Patients with diabetes enrolled in the ETDRS who underwent cataract surgery did not show an immediate improvement in visual acuity.

    b. Patients with diabetes with CSME should have cataract surgery performed prior to focal laser.

    c. Patients with diabetes and high-risk proliferative changes visible through their cataract should ideally have scatter laser immediately before cataract extraction.

    d. Patients with diabetes and high-risk proliferative changes visible through their cataract should have scatter laser 1 to 2 months prior to cataract extraction.

    e. Preoperative phenylephrine drops for dilation are contraindicated in patients with diabetes undergoing cataract surgery.

23. Which of the following statements about punctate inner choroidopathy (PIC) is correct?

    a. The condition affects males and females with equal frequency.

    b. Punctate inner choroidopathy is more commonly seen in patients with the ocular histoplasmosis syndrome.

    c. Disease involvement is associated with HLA-DR2 antigen.

    d. The condition is differentiated from MEWDS in that choroidal neovascularization is rarely seen in PIC.

    e. The condition is usually bilateral.

24. The following statement about diffuse unilateral subacute neuroretinitis (DUSN) is correct:

    a. The disease never occurs bilaterally.

    b. DUSN is a common cause of incorrectly diagnosed "unilateral retinitis pigmentosa."

    c. Eradication of the subretinal nematode often results in an intense inflammatory reaction.

    d. Visual loss typically continues after successful eradication of the subretinal nematode.

    e. The condition is seen only in individuals with a history of travel to endemic areas.

25. The following statement is correct about pneumatic retinopexy:

    a. Pneumatic retinopexy works by mechanically reattaching the detached retina.

    b. Pneumatic retinopexy is contraindicated in patients with total retinal detachments.

    c. Pseudophakia is an absolute contraindication to pneumatic retinopexy.

    d. Chronic detachments are a relative contraindication for pneumatic retinopexy.

    e. Pneumatic retinopexy is contraindicated in failed scleral buckles.

26. Features that may help distinguish CRVO from carotid artery occlusive disease include all of the following *except:*

    a. dilated retinal veins

    b. tortuosity of retinal veins

    c. ophthalmodynamometry

    d. retinal artery pressure

27. Multiple evanescent white dot syndrome (MEWDS) is characterized by each of the following clinical features *except:*

    a. enlargement of the physiologic blind spot on visual field testing

    b. individual hyperfluorescent spots on fluorescein angiography arranged in a wreathlike pattern around the fovea

    c. typically presents with unilateral photopsias and loss of vision in young females with myopia

    d. absence of cell in the anterior chamber

    e. granular appearance of the fovea

28. In a randomized, controlled clinical trial, pneumatic retinopexy

    a. was superior to scleral buckle in the anatomic success rate of repairing macula-sparing rhegmatogenous retinal detachments in pseudophakic patients

    b. provided slightly better visual outcome than scleral buckle in patients with macula-involving rhegmatogenous retinal detachments of less than 14-day duration

    c. included patients with causative breaks in the inferior 90° of the retina

    d. led to a worse outcome in patients who required an additional scleral buckle procedure for persistent or recurrent retinal detachment than if a scleral buckle procedure had been performed primarily

29. Patients with acute posterior multifocal placoid pigment epitheliopathy (APMPPE) may have all of the following clinical features *except:*

    a. unilateral or asymmetric fundus involvement

    b. recurrent or relentless progression of fundus lesions leading to permanent loss of central vision

    c. associated cerebral vasculitis

    d. prompt response to oral steroids

30. All of these diagnostic tests are useful in evaluating a patient with a retained magnetic intra-ocular foreign body *except:*

    a. indirect ophthalmoscopy

    b. computed tomography

    c. electrophysiology

    d. magnetic resonance imaging (MRI)

    e. echography

31. In phakic asymptomatic patients, which of the following types of retinal break is almost always treated, whereas the others are rarely treated?

    a. operculated tears

    b. lattice degeneration with or without hole

    c. retinal dialysis

    d. atrophic holes

32. Which of the following statements describing eyes with retained lens fragments after phacoe-mulsificaton is *false?*

    a. Marked intraocular inflammation is common.

    b. Secondary glaucoma is caused by lens particles and proteins obstructing the trabecular meshwork.

    c. The cumulative rate of retinal detachment is approximately 15% in these eyes during fol-low-up.

    d. The visual prognosis is generally poor in spite of treatment.

33. Which of the following is *least* likely to be present in an eye with a purely tractional retinal detachment?

    a. concave surface

    b. sickle cell retinopathy

    c. smooth retinal surface

    d. extension of detachment of the midperiphery

    e. tobacco dust

34. Which of the following is most characteristic of exudative retinal detachment?

    a. shifting fluid

    b. tobacco dust

    c. fixed folds

    d. equatorial traction folds

    e. demarcation lines

35. Based on ETDRS reports, which of the following statements regarding the use of aspirin is *false?*

    a. It has no effect on visual acuity.

    b. It has no effect on progression of retinopathy.

    c. It has no effect on rates of vitreous hemorrhage.

    d. It has no effect on rates of progression to high-risk PDR.

    e. It significantly increases the rate of vitrectomy for nonclearing vitreous hemorrhage

36. In treating CNV associated with ocular histoplasmosis, the ophthalmologist can decrease the risk of recurrent CNV by

    a. using a red laser rather than a green laser

    b. using durations of 0.5 second

    c. covering the entire lesion with laser treatment

    d. attaining a uniform white intensity of the area of photocoagulation at least as great as the minimal intensity standard published by the Macular Photocoagulation Study (MPS)

    e. c and d

37. Laser photocoagulation of subfoveal choroidal neovascularization in age-related macular degeneration has been shown to be successful in certain cases that meet which of the following criteria?

    a. evidence of classic CNV

    b. no evidence of occult CNV

    c. no evidence of blood

    d. well-demarcated boundaries

    e. a and d only

    f. a, b, and d only

38. All of the following are signs of shaken baby syndrome *except:*

    a. intraretinal hemorrhages

    b. retinoschisis cavities

    c. lethargy, irritability, seizures, and hypotonia

    d. optic nerve hypoplasia

39. Sympathetic ophthalmia

    a. occurs in approximately 1 in 1500 penetrating injuries

    b. never causes permanent loss of sight

    c. may be avoided by early enucleation of unsalvageable eyes

    d. does not cause exudative detachment

40. Diffuse and circumscribed choroidal hemangiomas

    a. are really the same thing

    b. may both cause serous detachments

    c. are both commonly associated with glaucoma

    d. are not associated with visual problems

    e. are not associated with systemic disease

41. An area of neovascularization in a patient with age-related macular degeneration shows leakage during fluorescein angiography. What additional fluorescein characteristic is needed to help define the neovascularization as "classic"?

    a. The vessels are well defined.

    b. Soft drusen are present.

    c. The neovascularization is greater than 50% of the lesion.

    d. Fluorescein leakage occurs beyond the boundaries of the neovascularization.

    e. The vessels are seen early in the angiogram.

Answers

1. **b.** Choroidal malignant melanoma is unrelated to dermatologic metastatic melanoma, so no dermatology exam is required. Choroidal hemangioma has high internal reflectivity. The most common sites of metastasis for choroidal malignant melanoma are the liver and lung. Although enucleation could be considered, the preferred treatment would be plaque radiotherapy.

2. **a.** The patient suffered a central retinal vein occlusion. The Central Vein Occlusion Study (CVOS) showed a benefit from panretinal photocoagulation when neovascularization occurred (not immediately) but no benefit from grid photocoagulation for macular edema in older patients. In younger patients, there was a trend toward benefit from grid photocoagulation, but this was not statistically significant.

3. **a.** Although laser photocoagulation could be performed, it would cause immediate and permanent loss of vision. Transpupillary thermotherapy is an investigational treatment of occult-only CNV. Ocular photodynamic therapy is the treatment of choice for this lesion.

4. **d.** This patient has acute postoperative endophthalmitis, most likely caused by coagulase negative staphylococci, as shown in the Endophthalmitis Vitrectomy Study. *P acnes* endophthalmitis is typically delayed, not acute. Inflammatory hypopyon after cataract surgery is rare and does not present so fulminantly.

5. **c.** The Endophthalmitis Vitrectomy Study reported that a tap and inject should be performed when the visual acuity is hand motions or better in patients with acute postoperative endophthalmitis. A vitrectomy would be better if vision is worse.

6. **c.** The Studies of Ocular Complications of AIDS (SOCA) trials reported that patients treated with ganciclovir had a 79% higher mortality than those assigned to foscarnet, with both drugs equal in controlling CMV retinitis and with tolerable side effects. Retinitis progression was best controlled with combination treatment. Color photographs are the gold standard to follow for disease progression.

7. **c.** Although the Early Treatment Diabetic Retinopathy Study (ETDRS) reported that focal laser photocoagulation should be applied in patients with clinically significant macular edema even if the vision is 20/20, this was not mandated, and patients can be observed closely, especially if most of the edema is in the foveal avascular zone. Macular edema in the ETDRS was defined by clinical examination, not imaging methods like fluorescein angiography and optical coherence tomography (OCT). The DCCT findings, although correct, apply only to patients with type 1 diabetes. The Diabetic Retinopathy Study (DRS) reported that immediate panretinal photocoagulation should be applied with high-risk proliferative diabetic retinopathy.

8. **a.** The patient suffered a branch vein occlusion. The Branch Vein Occlusion Study (BVOS) reported that grid photocoagulation should be applied if macular edema is present for more than 3 months and no retinal hemorrhages would prevent laser treatment. PRP should be applied when neovascularization occurs—not if ischemia (>5 disc diameters of capillary nonperfusion) is present. Because patients with macular nonperfusion were excluded from the BVOS, the study findings do not apply. Embolic workups are not required in branch vein occlusion.

9. **d.** Fundus albipunctatus is a form of congenital stationary night blindness characterized by striking yellow-white dots in the posterior pole. Patients have normal visual acuity and color vision. The rod ERG is minimal but normalizes after patients spend several hours in a dark environment. It is nonprogressive and should be differentiated from retinitis punctata albescens, which is a variant of retinitis pigmentosa.

10. **e.** Reduction and delay of cone (or rod) b-waves signifies damage to cells diffusely throughout the retina. This can occur in dystrophic disease, such as retinitis pigmentosa, in widespread ischemic disorders such as central vein occlusion, and in diffuse infections or inflammations such as syphilis. Diffuse cone dysfunction is diagnostic of cone dystrophy. Diseases such as sector retinitis pigmentosa, which destroys only focal regions of retina, may reduce b-wave amplitude, but the shape and timing of the waveforms (being generated by the remaining healthy areas of retina) is usually normal.

11. **c.** A loss of red-sensitive pigment results in a red-green color confusion defect and also makes the longer wavelength portion of the spectrum appear darker than normal. Because cone photoreceptors are not actually missing, acuity and photosensitivity are normal.

12. **e.** A subnormal EOG in the setting of a normal ERG is a consistent, classic finding in Best disease. It can also be seen occasionally with the various forms of adult-onset pattern dystrophies. In retinitis pigmentosa, both the ERG and EOG are subnormal. In rubella retinopathy, the RPE is diffusely affected but the EOG is normal.

13. **c.** Most patients with progressive cone dystrophy develop hemeralopia, or day-blindness. They often describe difficulty seeing on a sunny day and report better vision at dusk or even at night.

14. **b.** The vast majority of cases of Stargardt disease are autosomal recessive. The other dystrophies listed are typically inherited in autosomal dominant fashion.

15. **e.** There is 100% penetrance for foveal schisis in this disorder, even in young children. The a-wave is typically normal whereas the b-wave is reduced, reflecting the Müller cell dysfunction thought to play a role in pathogenesis. Fluorescein leakage is absent in foveal schisis. Peripheral retinoschisis and pigmentary changes are each present in approximately half of affected patients.

16. **b.** Although the incidence of retinal toxicity from hydroxychloroquine is very low in the United States, it is of serious concern because associated visual loss rarely recovers and may even progress after the drug is discontinued. Annual screening examinations are recommended for everyone in higher risk categories (including all patients with more than 5 years of usage).

17. **d.** Pigmentation in retinitis pigmentosa (RP) is variable, and many patients have few or no bone spicules. Rhodopsin gene abnormalities account for only about 30% of dominant RP, and most recessive RP has not been genetically defined. From a clinical standpoint, the ERG is the most critical measure because it documents the diffuse photoreceptor damage that defines the group of hereditary dystrophies that we call RP. Most RP patients have mild tritan (blue-yellow) color deficiency. Small tubular fields are a characteristic late finding in RP, but they are not pathognomic, and many younger patients still have large areas of peripheral vision.

18. **b.** Carrier females can be detected by identification of macromelanosomes of skin biopsy, and the ocular fundus often shows pigmentary mosaicism in the periphery.

19. **c.** Histopathologic study of juvenile retinoschisis reveals significant disruption of the inner nerve fiber layer and inner portions of Müller's cells, and this change most probably accounts for a selective decrease in both photopic and scotopic b-wave amplitudes. Although vitelliform dystrophy, dominant drusen, and butterfly-shaped dystrophy affect the retinal pigment epithelium and sensory retina within the macula, the involvement is generally not sufficient to alter the electroretinographic mass response. In ocular albinism, in spite of foveal hypoplasia, photopic and scotopic b-waves are normal (or sometimes supernormal).

20. **c.** Young eyes rarely develop an acute rhegmatogenous retinal detachment following blunt trauma because their vitreous has not yet undergone syneresis. Therefore, the vitreous provides an internal tamponade. Over several months, however, the vitreous over a tear may liquefy, permitting fluid to pass through the break to detach the retina.

21. **d.** The Joint Statement recommends that infants meeting any of these criteria undergo at least 2 screening examinations for retinopathy of prematurity.

22. **d.** Scatter laser treatment is indicated in patients with high-risk PDR. If a cataract is present, the ideal timing for laser application is 1–2 months pre–cataract extraction to allow the proliferative changes time to respond.

23. **e.** PIC is a bilateral condition that typically affects young, otherwise healthy, women who have a mild to moderate degree of myopia. Choroidal neovascularization remains a major cause of visual loss in affected individuals.

24. **b.** DUSN, although rare, is an important disease to consider, as it is a treatable cause of severe visual loss that often affects children. If left untreated, it will lead to widespread RPE disruption and is frequently mistaken for "unilateral retinitis pigmentosa." The condition has been described in almost every region of the world and is not associated with any specific travel history.

25. **d.** Pneumatic retinopexy works by tamponade of causative breaks and not on buoyant forces on the retina itself. Chronic subretinal fluid typically has delayed resorption, and pneumatic procedures have a poorer success rate in this setting.

26. **a.** Typically, retinal veins are dilated with both CRVO and carotid artery occlusive disease, but often they are tortuous only in CRVO. Ophthalmodynamometry measures the retinal artery pressure, which is normal in CRVO and low in carotid artery occlusive disease.

27. **b.** The hyperfluorescent spots in MEWDS are actually wreathlike clusters of smaller hyperfluorescent dots and not individual spots arranged in a wreathlike configuration around the fovea.

28. **b.** Visual acuity outcome was slightly superior in patients with macula-involving rhegmatogenous retinal detachments of less than 14-day duration who underwent pneumatic retinopexy than in those patients who underwent scleral buckling primarily. Only patients with a causative break(s) in the superior two thirds of the retina were included in the study. Anatomic success rates were slightly greater in patients undergoing primary scleral buckle, but visual outcome was not affected in patients who underwent unsuccessful pneumatic retinopexy and subsequently underwent scleral buckle procedure.

29. **d.** No evidence exists that APMPPE responds to systemic steroid therapy. APMPPE, although typically bilateral, may occur in one eye or be highly asymmetric. Typically a monophasic disease, a recurrent or relentless course may occur and has sometimes been termed "ampiginous choroidopathy."

30. **d.** Magnetic resonance imaging is contraindicated if there is a possible metallic foreign body in the globe or orbit or intracranially. (Weber AL. Radiologic evaluation of the globe. In: Albert DM, Jakobiec FA, eds. *Principles and Practice of Ophthalmology*. Philadelphia: Saunders; 1994:3511–3520.)

31. **c.** Retinal dialysis is usually treated in phakic patients even when asymptomatic. Atrophic holes and operculated tears are treated only in special circumstances.

32. **d.** The visual prognosis is generally good after treatment with pars plana vitrectomy and removal of the retained lens fragments. In eyes with medium to large amounts of retained lens fragments, marked intraocular inflammation is common; secondary glaucoma is also relatively common. Retinal detachment is less common but has been reported in approximately 15% of these eyes in large published series.

33. **e.** Tobacco dust, also known as Shafer's sign, is manifested by small clumps of pigmented cells in the vitreous and is practically diagnostic of rhegmatogenous retinal detachment. Tractional retinal detachments nearly always have a concave surface that is smooth, rather than corrugated; they almost never extend to the ora serrata. Sickle cell retinopathy is a well-known cause of tractional retinal detachment.

34. **a.** Shifting fluid is a hallmark of exudative retinal detachment, although it may occasionally be seen in patients with rhegmatogenous retinal detachment. All of the other findings are characteristic of rhegmatogenous retinal detachment.

35. **e.** In the ETDRS, the use of aspirin was compared with the use of a placebo in 3711 patients with diabetes who had less than high-risk PDR at the baseline examination. Within the follow-up period of at least 3 years, aspirin had no effect on visual acuity, progression of retinopathy, risk of vitreous hemorrhage, or rates of progression to high-risk PDR. Furthermore, there was no statistically significant increase in the incidence of vitrectomy in the aspirin groups of ETDRS patients.

36. **e.** Only one prospective trial compared one laser wavelength to another when treating CNV: the MPS subfoveal trials of CNV associated with AMD. In these trials, wavelength was not shown to affect the incidence of recurrence. Although the duration of treatment should be relatively long to create an intense lesion without suddenly breaking through Bruch's membrane, duration has not been shown to affect the rate of recurrence. However, failure to cover the entire lesion or to achieve a white intensity at least as great as the minimal intensity standards published by the MPS are each factors that independently increased the likelihood of developing persistent CNV.

37. **e.** Laser treatment of subfoveal lesions should be undertaken only in the presence of some classic CNV. However, occult CNV can also be present as long as there is evidence of classic CNV. Because the laser treatment should cover the entire lesion, the boundary of the entire lesion should be well demarcated so that the treating ophthalmologist can clearly recognize the extent of the CNV. Blood can be present as a lesion component provided that the area of CNV is greater than any areas of blood or blocked fluorescence (not from blood) or serous detachment of the RPE.

38. **d.** Optic nerve hypoplasia is more often a congenital abnormality.

39. **c.** Early enucleation of the unsalvageable eyes is thought to dramatically reduce the risk of sympathetic ophthalmia.

40. **b.** Diffuse hemangiomas are associated with Sturge-Weber syndrome, whereas circumscribed ones are not. Both types are associated with serous detachments of the retina.

41. **e.** The additional piece of information needed is the ability to see the vessels early in the fluorescein angiogram. Being "well defined" is not a necessary characteristic. Soft drusen occur in age-related macular degeneration but are not a requisite finding for the designation "classic."

Index

(*i* = image; *t* = table)